Medical Image Registration

Biomedical Engineering Series

Edited by Michael R. Neuman

Published Titles

Electromagnetic Analysis and Design in Magnetic Resonance Imaging, Jianming Jin

Endogenous and Exogenous Regulation and Control of Physiological Systems, Robert B. Northrop

Artificial Neural Networks in Cancer Diagnosis, Prognosis, and Treatment, Raouf N.G. Naguib and Gajanan V. Sherbet

Medical Image Registration, Joseph V. Hajnal, Derek Hill, and David J. Hawkes

Introduction to Dynamic Modeling of Neuro-Sensory Systems, Robert B. Northrop

Forthcoming Titles

Noninvasive Instrumentation and Measurement in Medical Diagnosis, Robert B. Northrop

Handbook of Neuroprosthetic Methods, Warren E. Finn and Peter G. LoPresti

The BIOMEDICAL ENGINEERING Series
Series Editor Michael Neuman

Medical Image Registration

Edited by
Joseph V. Hajnal
Derek L.G. Hill
David J. Hawkes

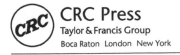

CRC Press
Taylor & Francis Group
Boca Raton London New York

CRC Press is an imprint of the
Taylor & Francis Group, an **informa** business

CRC Press
Taylor & Francis Group
6000 Broken Sound Parkway NW, Suite 300
Boca Raton, FL 33487-2742

First issued in paperback 2019

ISBN-13: 978-0-8493-0064-6 (hbk)
ISBN-13: 978-0-367-39720-3 (pbk)

Library of Congress Cataloging-in-Publication Data

Medical image registration / edited by Joseph Hajnal, David Hawkes, and Derek Hill.
    p. cm.— (Biomedical engineering series)
  Includes bibliographical references and index.
  ISBN 0-8493-0064-9
    1. Diagnostic imaging. I. Hajnal, Joseph. II. Hawkes, D.J. (David J.) III. Hill, Derek (Derek L.G.) IV. Series.

  RC78.7.D53 M436 2001
  616.07′54—dc21   2001028031
                                                                                     CIP

Library of Congress Card Number 2001028031

Visit the Taylor & Francis Web site at
http://www.taylorandfrancis.com

and the CRC Press Web site at
http://www.crcpress.com

Editors

Joseph Hajnal is head of physics and engineering at the Robert Steiner Magnetic Resonance Unit, Hammersmith Hospital, Imperial College School of Medicine and Medical Research Council Clinical Sciences Centre, as well as leader of a research team funded by Marconi Medical Systems. He trained as a physicist at Bristol University, England, and earned a Ph.D. in the physics of electromagnetic waves before working in Australia at Melbourne University and the Australian National University on interactions between atomic beams and laser light. In 1990 Dr. Hajnal began research in medical imaging with a special interest in magnetic resonance imaging. His current research interests include magnetic resonance data acquisition and processing, image registration, and data fusion, as well as novel scanner technology. He has published more than 80 papers in peer-review journals and currently holds six grants from a variety of funding organizations.

Derek Hill earned a B.Sc. in physics from Imperial College, London in 1987, a M.Sc. in medical physics in 1989 and a Ph.D. in medical image registration from the University of London in 1994. He is currently a senior lecturer in the department of radiological sciences in the medical school of King's College, London. Dr. Hill's research interests include rigid and nonrigid registration, intraoperative brain deformation, interventional magnetic resonance imaging, MR imaging, and the study of brain shape and connectivity. He has more than 100 publications in these areas, of which over 30 are peer-review journal articles. During the last five years, Dr. Hill has held five project grants as principle investigator. He has worked extensively with industrial partners on collaborative research to develop imaging technology.

David Hawkes has 25 years experience in medical imaging in hospital and academic environments. He founded the Computational Imaging Science Group in 1989 at Guy's Hospital and recently formed the Medical Imaging Science Interdisciplinary Research Group at the newly merged Guy's, King's, and St. Thomas' School of Medicine, King's College, London. Dr. Hawkes trained as a physicist at Oxford. He earned a master's degree in radiobiology at Birmingham and a Ph.D. on parametrization of the x-ray attenuation coefficient for dual energy computed tomography at Surrey. His current research interests include image matching, data fusion, visualization, shape representation, surface geometry, and modeling tissue deformation, with applications in image-guided interventions, augmented reality in surgery, 3D ultrasound, and interventional magnetic resonance imaging. He has been on the scientific committees of 30 international meetings and is on the editorial boards of five journals. Dr. Hawkes is currently principal investigator of five U.K. Engineering and Physical Sciences Research Council (EPSRC) project grants and manager of three industrially sponsored projects. He has more than 150 publications in the area of medical imaging.

Contributors

Dale L. Bailey Department of Nuclear Medicine, Guy's, King's, and St. Thomas' School of Medicine, Guy's Hospital, London, U.K.

Phillipe Batchelor Department of Radiological Sciences, Guy's, King's, and St. Thomas' School of Medicine, Guy's Hospital, London, U.K.

David Bell Physics Department, Royal Marsden NHS Trust, Sutton, Surrey, U.K.

Graeme M. Bydder Robert Steiner MR Unit, MRC Clinical Sciences Centre, Imperial College School of Medicine, Hammersmith Hospital, London, U.K.

Matthew J. Clarkson Department of Radiological Sciences, Guy's, King's, and St. Thomas' School of Medicine, Guy's Hospital, London, U.K.

D. Louis Collins McConnell Brain Imaging Center, Montreal Neurological Institute, Montreal, Quebec, Canada

Philip J. Edwards Department of Radiological Sciences, Guy's, King's, and St. Thomas' School of Medicine, Guy's Hospital, London, U.K.

Alan C. Evans McConnell Brain Imaging Center, Montreal Neurological Institute, Montreal, Quebec, Canada

J. Michael Fitzpatrick Department of Electrical Engineering and Computer Science, Vanderbilt University, Nashville, Tennessee, U.S.A.

Joseph V. Hajnal Robert Steiner MR Unit, MRC Clinical Sciences Centre, Imperial College School of Medicine, Hammersmith Hospital, London, U.K.

David J. Hawkes Department of Radiological Sciences, Guy's, King's, and St. Thomas' School of Medicine, Guy's Hospital, London, U.K.

Derek L.G. Hill Department of Radiological Sciences, Guy's, King's, and St. Thomas' School of Medicine, Guy's Hospital, London, U.K.

Jozef Jarosz   Neuroimaging, King's Healthcare Trust, Denmark Hill, London, U.K.

Mark Jenkinson   Oxford Centre for Functional MRI of the Brain, Oxford University, John Radcliffe Hospital, Oxford, U.K.

Louis Lemieux   Research Group, Institute of Neurology, University College, London, U.K.

Michael I. Miga   Department of Biomedical Engineering, Vanderbilt University, Nashville, Tennessee, U.S.A.

Angela Oatridge   Robert Steiner MR Unit, MRC Clinical Sciences Centre, Imperial College School of Medicine, Hammersmith Hospital, London, U.K.

Keith D. Paulsen   Thayer School of Engineering, Dartmouth College, Hanover, New Hampshire, U.S.A.

Tomáš Paus   McConnell Brain Imaging Center, Montreal Neurological Institute, Montreal, Quebec, Canada

Graeme P. Penney   Department of Radiological Sciences, Guy's, King's, and St. Thomas' School of Medicine, Guy's Hospital, London, U.K.

Uwe Pietrzyk   Forschungszentrum Jülich GmbH, Institut für Medizin, Jülich, Germany

Daniel Rueckert   Department of Computing, Imperial College of Science, Technology, and Medicine, London, U.K.

Stephen M. Smith   Oxford Centre for Functional MRI of the Brain, Oxford University, John Radcliffe Hospital, Oxford, U.K.

Alex P. Zijdenbos   McConnell Brain Imaging Center, Montreal Neurological Institute, Montreal, Quebec, Canada

Contents

Section III   Techniques and Applications of Nonrigid Registration

1

Introduction

Joseph V. Hajnal, Derek L.G. Hill, and David. J. Hawkes

CONTENTS

1.1 Preface

Image registration is the process of aligning images so that corresponding features can easily be related. The term is also used to mean aligning images with a computer model or aligning features in an image with locations in physical space. The images might be acquired with different sensors (e.g., sensitive to different parts of the electromagnetic spectrum) or the same sensor at different times. Image registration has applications in many fields; the one that is addressed in this book is medical imaging. This encompasses a wide range of image usage, but the main emphasis is on radiological imaging.

The past 25 years have seen remarkable developments in medical imaging technology. Universities and industry have made huge investments in inventing and developing the technology needed to acquire images from multiple imaging modalities. Medical images are increasingly widely used in healthcare and biomedical research; a very wide range of imaging modalities is now available. X-ray computed tomography (CT) images are sensitive to tissue density and atomic composition, and the x-ray attenuation coefficient and magnetic resonance imaging (MR) images are related to proton density, relaxation times, flow, and other parameters. The introduction of contrast agents provides information on the patency and function of tubular structures such as blood vessels, the bile duct, and the bowel, as well as the state of the blood-brain barrier. In nuclear medicine, radiopharmaceuticals introduced into the body allow delineation of functioning tissue and measurement of metabolic and pathophysiological processes. Ultrasound detects subtle changes in acoustic impedance at tissue boundaries and diffraction patterns in different tissues, providing discrimination of different tissue types. Doppler ultrasound provides images of flowing blood. Endoscopy and surgical microscopy provide images of visible surfaces deep within the body. These and other imaging technologies now provide rich sources of data on the physical properties and biological function of tissues at spatial resolutions from 5 mm for nuclear medicine down to 1.0 or 0.5 mm for MR and CT, and 20 to 100 μm for optical systems. Each successive generation of image acquisition system has acquired images faster, with higher resolution and improved image quality, and together these have been harnessed for great clinical benefit.

Since the mid 1980s medical image registration has evolved from being perceived as a rather minor precursor to some medical imaging applications to a significant subdiscipline in itself. Entire sessions are devoted to the topic in major medical imaging conferences,[1,2] and workshops have been held on the subject.[3] Image registration has also become one of the more successful areas of image processing, with fully automated algorithms available in a number of applications.

Why has registration become so important? Medical imaging is about establishing shape, structure, size, and spatial relationships of anatomical structures within the patient, together with spatial information about function and any pathology or other abnormality. Establishing the correspondence of spatial information in medical images and equivalent structures in the body is fundamental to medical image interpretation and analysis.

In many clinical scenarios, images from several modalities may be acquired and the diagnostician's task is to mentally combine or "fuse" this information to draw useful clinical conclusions. This generally requires mental compensation for changes in subject position. Image registration aligns the images and so establishes correspondence between different features seen on different imaging modalities, allows monitoring of subtle changes in size or intensity over time or across a population, and establishes correspondence between images and physical space in image guided interventions. Registration of an atlas or computer model aids in the delineation of anatomical and pathological structures in medical images and is an important precursor to detailed analysis.

It is now common for patients to be imaged multiple times, either by repeated imaging with a single modality, or by imaging with different modalities. It is also common for patients to be imaged *dynamically*, that is, to have sequences of images acquired, often at many frames per second. The ever increasing amount of image data acquired makes it more and more desirable to relate one image to another to assist in extracting relevant clinical information. Image registration can help in this task: intermodality registration enables the combination of complementary information from different modalities, and intramodality registration enables accurate comparisons between images from the same modality.

International concern about escalating healthcare costs drives development of methods that make the best possible use of medical images and, once again, image registration can help. However, medical image registration does not just enable better use of images that would be acquired anyway, it also opens up new applications for medical images. These include serial imaging to monitor subtle changes due to disease progression or treatment; perfusion or other functional studies when the subject cannot be relied upon to remain in a fixed position during the dynamic acquisition; and image-guided interventions, in which images acquired prior to the intervention are registered with the treatment device, enabling the surgeon or interventionalist to use the preintervention images to guide his or her work. Image registration has also become a valuable technique for biomedical research, especially in neuroscience, where imaging studies are making substantial contributions to our understanding of the way the brain works. Image registration can be used to align multiple images from the same individual (intrasubject registration) and to compare images acquired from different subjects (intersubject registration).

All the images that we wish to register or manipulate in any other way on a computer must be available in digital form. This means that most medical images are made up of a rectangular array of small square or rectangular elements called *pixels* (an abbreviation of *picture elements*); each pixel has an associated image intensity value. This array provides the coordinate system of the image, and an element in the image can be accessed by its two-dimensional position within this array. A typical CT slice will be formed of 512×512 pixels, and each will correspond to an element of the cut through the patient of about 0.5×0.5 mm^2. This dimension determines the limiting spatial resolution of the image. 2D images are often stacked together to form a 3D volume, and many images are now acquired directly as 3D volumes. Each pixel will now correspond to a small volume element of tissue, or *voxel*. If the slice spacing in high resolution CT is, say, 1.5 mm, the voxel size will be $0.5 \times 0.5 \times 1.5$ mm^3. The number stored in each voxel—the voxel image intensity—will be some average of a physical attribute measured over this volume. In MR, voxels are generally slightly larger, typically $1 \times 1 \times 3$–5 mm^3 in size.

Radiologists have traditionally reviewed medical images by viewing them as film transparencies on a back-illuminated light box. Most imaging modalities involve some digital manipulation and computation, and so these images are now often stored in digital form and displayed on a workstation. Digital storage greatly facilitates further digital manipulation, such as registration of the images and fusion of the information from the different modalities. Subjective judgments of the relative size, shape, and spatial relationships of visible structures and physiology inferred from intensity distributions are used for developing a diagnosis, planning therapy, and monitoring disease progression or response to therapy. A key process when interpreting these images together is the explicit or implicit establishment of correspondence between different points in the images. The spatial integrity of the images can allow very accurate correspondence to be determined. Once correspondence has been established in a verifiable way, multiple images can be interpreted as single unified data sets and conclusions drawn with increased confidence. Creating this single unified data set is the process of "fusion." In many instances, new information becomes available that could not have been deduced from inspection of individual images in loose association with one another.

1.2   Historical Background

Although this is the first book dedicated to medical image registration, it is not a new topic. Image registration has been widely used for many years in x-ray angiography. It is common to acquire x-rays before and after injection of intravascular contrast and then subtract these images in order to visualize the blood vessels in isolation. This technique almost invariably uses digital systems now, but optical subtraction using photographic methods has been extremely effective. A negative of the radiograph taken before the arrival of the contrast material, the "mask," was positioned on a light box over the radiograph taken after the arrival of contrast and an additional film was taken. If the patient moved between the acquisition of the precontrast mask image and the image with contrast, then the subtracted image would contain edge artifacts. Translating and rotating the films prior to optical subtraction greatly reduced these artifacts. Photographic subtraction was also used with MR to correct for patient motion and generate images showing where gadolinium contrast had been taken up.[4]

Image-guided surgery was the first application of medical image registration. Indeed, the very first radiograph acquired for this purpose was reported to have been in Birmingham, U.K., only two weeks after the discovery of x-rays was published in December 1895. A patient had broken a needle in her hand. A radiograph was taken and the casualty officer aligned the plate with the hand in order to successfully guide his scalpel to removal of the needle.[5] Other early examples included battlefield surgery for removal of shrapnel by registering a calibrated pair of x-ray films to the patient so that the x-ray could guide the surgeon precisely to the target in 3D. The stereotactic frame was proposed for image-guided neurosurgery as a means of localizing target structures with respect to anatomical features identified in the patient's radiographs and/or a standard atlas.[6,7] The frame is rigidly fixed to the skull and defines a coordinate system for both imaging and treatment. Stereotactic neurosurgery became more widely used when the technology was computerized and combined with CT,[8,9] and then with multiple preoperative imaging modalities.[10] Stereotactic neurosurgery can only be used for a small proportion of neurosurgical procedures, because the frame has to be attached to the patient prior to imaging and left on until surgery, and the presence of the frame restricts the types of surgery that can be performed, often just to biopsy and electrode implantation. These problems were overcome with the development of more sophisticated registration techniques leading to the introduction of frameless stereotaxy in the mid 1980s,[11] though it was another decade before frameless stereotactic systems obtained the regulatory approval necessary for widespread use in health care.

In image-guided interventions, correspondence is established between image and the physical space of the patient during the intervention. Establishing this correspondence allows the image to be used to guide, direct, and monitor therapy, akin to providing a 3D map for navigation, with the aim of making the intervention more accurate, safer, and less invasive for the patient. In the last few years, image registration techniques have entered routine clinical use in image-guided neurosurgery systems and computer-assisted orthopedic surgery. Systems incorporating image registration are sold by a number of manufacturers.

Stereotactic frames can also be used for intermodality image registration, but their use is restricted to highly invasive surgical procedures because of the need for rigid fixation to the skull. Various relocatable frames were proposed to avoid this invasiveness, but beginning in the mid 1980s, registration algorithms were devised that were "retrospective," that is, did not require special measures to be taken during image acquisition in order for registration to be possible. Various approaches were introduced in the mid 1980s.[12–14] These techniques were devised to make it possible to combine images of the same patient taken with different modalities and they required substantial user interaction.

Another major step forward in image registration came in the first half of the 1990s with the development of retrospective registration algorithms that were fully or virtually fully automated for both intramodality[15,16] and intermodality registration.[17–21] A significant breakthrough in the mid 1990s was the development of image alignment measures and registration algorithms based on entropy and, in particular, mutual information—measures first derived from the information theory developed by Shannon in 1948.[22]

Recently the focus of research in medical image registration has returned to intramodality rather than intermodality registration, and to extending registration algorithms to handle the more complicated transformations needed to model soft tissue deformation and intersubject registration.

Detailed atlases or computer models of anatomy are becoming available, in particular from high resolution sources such as the Visible Human datasets.[4] The Montreal Brain Atlas has been generated by averaging images of the brain across a population. Establishing spatial correspondence between these atlases and an individual's images allows for easier interpretation and, in particular, enables computer assistance in delineation of anatomical structures of interest.

Rapid advances in the power of computer technology and in the performance of new registration algorithms and displays mean that image manipulation deemed impractical or far too computationally expensive only a few years ago can now be undertaken on the PCs available on most people's desks. In our experience, initial work on voxel similarity measures was proving successful in the laboratory in 1994 but took an hour or more to complete.

Between then and late 2000, desktop workstations have increased in speed by nearly two orders of magnitude while their cost has been reduced by an order of magnitude, so the same calculations can now be achieved in a few minutes on desktop PCs. The first algorithms for nonrigid registration required large amounts of interaction or were prohibitively slow, but more recent work has resulted in highly automated algorithms that can run on standard hardware in minutes rather than days.

1.3   Overview of the Book

This book is divided into three sections. Section I, Methodology, introduces the wide variety of techniques used for medical image registration. The concepts behind registration techniques are introduced for a general audience in Chapter 2, and, for those who wish to understand the underlying algorithms or implement registration methods themselves. Behind the techniques are described in more detail in Chapter 3. The necessary additional considerations behind acquiring and preparing data for image registration are discussed in Chapter 4, and correcting errors in the scanners is addressed in Chapter 5. In the final chapter in this section, Chapter 6, the essential problem of detecting when the algorithms have failed is discussed, and how accurately the algorithms have aligned the images is assessed.

Section II describes the relatively mature applications of image registration in which the images can be aligned by global translation and rotation alone—so-called rigid-body registration. The chapters in this section are written by researchers with many years of experience in the applications of serial MR registration (Chapter 7), functional MRI (Chapter 8), registration of PET and MRI (Chapter 9), registration of MRI and CT (Chapter 10), registration in nuclear medicine (Chapter 11), and the use of registration in guided therapeutic procedures (Chapter 12).

Section III focuses on the less mature but rapidly developing field of nonrigid image registration. The topic is introduced in Chapter 13, and alternative approaches are reviewed and examples given of one approach for a variety of applications. The problem of combining images from multiple subjects in cohort studies is examined in detail in Chapter 14, and the rather different approach of using biomechanical models to achieve registration is considered in Chapter 15. Section III tells less of a finished story than Sections I and II, due to the rapid evolution of techniques in this area. The goal of this section is to give insight into some of the applications that drive nonrigid registration and the different approaches being devised.

An observation as this book was prepared (late 2000) was that there are literally hundreds of papers in the literature describing medical image registration methods and applications, and yet this technology is currently used very little in clinical practice, with the exception of image-guided surgery.

Why is this? Maybe the clinical applications are not relevant for day-to-day patient management. This does not appear to be a sustainable view either from the literature or from the view of centers using this technology. It may be that image registration generally forms only one part of a complete image analysis application, and other components, notably image segmentation and labeling, are still not sufficiently robust or automated for routine clinical use. In many applications, this is undoubtedly the case. Perhaps some of the problems with segmentation will be solved by nonrigid atlas registration (see Chapter 14). Another important factor is that to achieve widespread use, the clinical community and the medical imaging industry that supports it must embrace this new technology more effectively. This will require investment in order to: 1) ensure that technical validation and clinical evaluation are effective and timely; 2) proceed rapidly down the path of standardization and integration of information sources in healthcare so that innovative products from small companies can be incorporated earlier and more cheaply into the healthcare environment; 3) ensure that image registration becomes automatic or virtually automatic so that it is robust and transparent to the user; and, finally, 4) ensure that the clinical community, and its scientific and technical support staffs, are made fully aware of the power of this new technology and that medical practice evolves to take full advantage of it.

We hope that this book will go some way in encouraging goals 1, 2, and 3 above by contributing to goal 4.

We are very grateful to the contributing authors for sharing our vision that the time is right for a book on medical image registration, for the effort they have put into their chapters, and, in particular, for responding to our suggestions for making the book a more coherent whole.

References

1. K.M. Hanson, *Medical Imaging 2000: Image Processing*. SPIE 3979, 2000.
2. C. Taylor and A. Colchester, *Medical Image Computing and Computer Assisted Intervention—MICCAI'99*. Lecture Notes in Computer Science 1679, Heidelberg: Springer-Verlag, 1999.
3. F. Pernus, S. Kovacic, H.S. Stiehl, and M.A. Viergever, *Biomedical Image Registration Proc WBIR'99*. Slovenia Pattern Recognition Society, Ljubljana, 1999.
4. G.A.S. Lloyd, P.G. Barker, and P.D. Phelps, Subtraction gadolinium-enhanced magnetic resonance for head and neck imaging, *Br. J. Radiol.*, vol. 66, pp. 12–16, 1993.
5. S. Webb, *The Physics of Medical Imaging*. Institute of Physics Publishing, Bristol, 1988.
6. R.H. Clarke and V. Horsley, On a method of investigating the deep ganglia and tracts of the central nervous system (cerebellum), *Br. Med. J.*, vol. 2, pp. 1799–1800, 1906.
7. E.A. Spiegel, H.T. Wycis, M. Marks, and A.J. Lee, Stereotaxic apparatus for operations on the human brain, *Science*, vol. 106, pp. 349–350, 1947.

8. R.A. Brown, T.S. Roberts, and A.G. Osborn, Stereotaxic frame and computer software for CT-directed neurosurgical localization, *Invest. Radiol.*, vol. 15, pp. 308–312, 1980.

9. L. Leksell and B. Jernberg, Stereotaxis and tomography: a technical note, *Acta Neurochir.*, vol. 52, pp. 1–7, 1980.

10. T.M. Peters, J.A. Clark, A. Olivier, E.P. Marchand, G. Mawko, M. Dieumegarde, L. Muresan, and R. Ethier, Integrated stereotaxic imaging with CT, MR imaging, and digital subtraction angiography, *Radiology*, vol. 161, pp. 821–826, 1986.

11. D.W. Roberts, J.W. Strohbehn, J.F. Hatch, W. Murray, and H. Kettenberger, A frameless stereotaxic integration of computerized tomographic imaging and the operating microscope, *J. Neurosurg.*, vol. 65, pp. 545–549, 1986.

12. G.T.Y. Chen, M. Kessler, and S. Pitluck, Structure transfer between sets of three-dimensional medical imaging data, in *Computer Graphics 1985*, pp. 171–175, Dallas: National Computer Graphics Association, 1985.

13. G.Q. Maguire, Jr., M.E. Noz, E.M. Lee, and J.H. Schimpf, Correlation methods for tomographic images using two- and three-dimensional techniques, in *Information Processing in Medical Imaging 1985*, S. L. Bacharach, Ed., pp. 266–279, Dordrecht: Martinus Nijhoff Publishers, 1986.

14. C.-T. Chen, C.A. Pelizzari, G.T.Y. Chen, M.D. Cooper, and D.N. Levin, Image analysis of PET data with the aid of CT and MR images, in *Information Processing in Medical Imaging 1987*, C. N. de Graaf and M. A. Viergever, Eds., pp. 601–611, New York: Plenum Press, 1988.

15. R.P. Woods, S.R. Cherry, and J.C. Mazziotta, Rapid automated algorithm for aligning and reslicing PET images, *J. Comput. Assist. Tomogr.*, vol. 16, pp. 620–633, 1992.

16. J.V. Hajnal, N. Saeed, E.J. Soar, A. Oatridge, I.R. Young, and G.M. Bydder, A registration and interpolation procedure for subvoxel matching of serially acquired MR images, *J. Comput. Assist. Tomogr.*, vol. 19, pp. 289–296, 1995.

17. R.P. Woods, J.C. Mazziotta, and S.R. Cherry, MRI-PET registration with automated algorithm, *J. Comput. Assist. Tomogr.*, vol. 17, pp. 536–546, 1993.

18. P. Viola and W. Wells, Alignment by maximization of mutual information, in *Proc. 5th Int. Conf. Computer Vision*, pp. 16–23, 1995.

19. A. Collignon, F. Maes, D. Delaere, D. Vandermeulen, P. Suetens, and G. Marchal, Automated multi-modality image registration based on information theory, in *Information Processing in Medical Imaging 1995*, Y. Bizais, C. Barillot, and R. Di Paola, Eds., pp. 263–274, Dordrecht: Kluwer Academic, 1995.

20. C. Studholme, D.L.G. Hill, and D.J. Hawkes, Automated 3D registration of MR and CT images of the head, *Med. Image Anal.*, vol. 1, pp. 163–175, 1996.

21. C. Studholme, D.L.G. Hill, and D.J. Hawkes, Automated 3D registration of MR and PET brain images by multi-resolution optimisation of voxel similarity measures, *Med. Phys.*, vol. 24, pp. 25–35, 1997.

22. C.E. Shannon, The mathematical theory of communication (parts 1 and 2), *Bell Syst. Tech. J.*, vol. 27, pp. 379–423 and 623–656, 1948. Reprint available from *http://www.lucent.com*.

Section I

Methodology

2

Registration Methodology: Introduction

David J. Hawkes

CONTENTS

0-8493-0064-9/01/$0.00+$.50
© 2001 by CRC Press LLC

2.1   Introduction

This chapter presents a descriptive account of methods for image registration. Our intention here is to enable the reader to understand the main concepts behind the different methods without recourse to the underlying mathematics. All equations have been banished! The mathematics and details of implementation are left to the following chapter, which has a very similar structure that will allow the reader to switch between the two for more detailed descriptions when required.

As stated in Chapter 1, medical image registration has a wide range of potential applications. These include:

- Combining information from multiple imaging modalities, for example, when relating functional information from nuclear medicine images to anatomy delineated in high-resolution MR images.
- Monitoring changes in size, shape, or image intensity over time intervals that might range from a few seconds in dynamic perfusion studies to several months or even years in the study of neuronal loss in dementia.
- Relating preoperative images and surgical plans to the physical reality of the patient in the operating room during image-guided surgery or in the treatment suite during radiotherapy.
- Relating an individual's anatomy to a standardized atlas.

To be effective, all these applications require the establishment of spatial correspondence. What we mean by correspondence in image registration is explored in this chapter before presenting, in descriptive terms, the various methods of registration. The process of image registration involves finding transformations that relate spatial information conveyed in one image to those in another or in physical space. We relate the type of transformation to the number of dimensions of the images. We describe the number of parameters, or "degrees of freedom," which are needed to describe this transformation for the different classes of registration algorithm. We introduce the concept of optimization, in which the computer makes a succession of guesses about the correct data before converging to an answer that should be close to the correct one. Issues related to image transformation are discussed, and a few comments on validation conclude the chapter. The following chapter covers the same ground from a more formal mathematical perspective and with more technical details on implementation.

All the images that we wish to register or manipulate in any other way on a computer must be available in digital form. This means that they are stored in coded form with numbers representing the image intensity or color at each location. This is usually achieved with a rectangular array of small square or rectangular elements called *pixels* (an abbreviation of "picture elements"), each pixel having an associated image intensity value. The pixel array provides a natural coordinate system for the images, and an element in each image can be accessed by its two-dimensional (2D) position within this array. A typical CT slice will be formed of 512×512 pixels, and each will correspond to an element of about 0.5×0.5 mm^2 in area. This dimension determines the limiting spatial resolution of the image. 2D slice images are often stacked together to form a 3D volume. Many images are now acquired directly as 3D volumes. Each pixel will now correspond to a small volume element of tissue or *voxel*. If the slice spacing is, say, 1.5 mm, the voxel size will be $0.5 \times 0.5 \times 1.5$ mm^3. The number stored in each voxel, the voxel image intensity, will be some average of the physical attribute measured over this volume. For clinical MR brain images, typical voxels are $0.9 \times 0.9 \times 3$ to 5 mm^3, with 256×256 pixels in a slice. It is also possible to acquire MR images with cubic voxels, e.g., $1.0 \times 1.0 \times 1.0$ mm, and MR images with approximately cubic voxels are often used for registration applications.

2.2 Correspondence

As stated above, image registration establishes spatial correspondence. We should consider carefully what this means. Consider a scenario in which we might have a patient who is imaged with MR and CT over the course of a few hours, or perhaps on subsequent days, as workup for neurosurgery. The process of registration will establish which point on one image corresponds to a particular point on the other. By "correspond" we mean that these points represent a measurement localized to the same small element of tissue within the patient. We can then deduce something about spatial relationships between different structures, each seen by only one modality. The computational process of registration yields the appropriate transformation between the "coordinate systems" of the two sets of scans, which are referenced to the individual scanners. A coordinate system provides a way of describing a position in space.

No measurement is perfectly accurate, and there will always be uncertainty, error, or "tolerance" in this estimate of correspondence. For many clinical applications it is important to know what this tolerance is, so as not to overinterpret the registered datasets. Once correspondence is determined throughout the volume imaged by the two modalities, then one image can be transformed into the coordinate system of the other. This calculation can lead to further approximations or errors. Typically, there will be some blurring of the transformed image. In our simple neurosurgical example, once any scaling errors and geometric distortion produced by the scanners are corrected as described in Chapter 5, the transformation will be very well approximated by that of a "rigid body." A rigid-body transformation, as the name suggests, is one that changes position and orientation without changing shape or size between the two scans.

Finally, we have the process of combining or "fusing" the information in the images in some useful or meaningful way. This process may be left entirely to the clinician in his/her mind's eye, or simple visualization effects may be used, including color or interactive fading in and out of one image's contribution overlaid on the other. Alternatively, two cursors, called "linked cursors," might be used to indicate corresponding points in the two images. Further computation or combined displays of fused information may be generated. Corresponding structures in the two images can be used to check the transformation, while complementary information can be used to deduce useful new information either by qualitative interpretation or by improving the accuracy of measurement. This combination of information is sometimes termed "data fusion," a term originally coined for the combination of information in computing systems for battlefield command and control.

We might wish to use individual 3D images or the combined images for navigation in image-guided surgery. Again, this requires a process of registration, and now correspondence is defined between image and physical space within the patient in the operating room. We require a transformation that for each identified 3D point within the patient allows us to compute the corresponding location of the tissue that occupied that point in the preoperative image. If the tissue has moved as a result of the intervention, then we would like to know by how much and what tissue element now occupies this point.

This process of establishing correspondence becomes more complicated if one of the images represents a projection of physical space, as is the case with most optical images and conventional x-ray radiographs. These images are called "projection" images. One point in a radiograph will correspond to some combination of the x-ray attenuation values along the line in the patient leading from the x-ray source to the imaging plane. This means that one point in the radiograph will correspond to a line of points through a CT or MR image. One point in the CT image will only correspond to a component of the intensity seen at a point in the radiograph. In optical images, only the visible surface will contribute to the image. Establishing correspondence between a pair of points in two projection images that have been calibrated allows the 3D position of that point to be determined. This is the basis of stereo-photogrammetry, used widely outside medicine in robotics, nondestructive testing in industry, analysis of remote or hostile environments, surveillance work, and analysis of satellite images.

What if we are using image registration to monitor change? If the change is only in intensity and we can guarantee that the imaged structure has not changed size, as might be the case in functional neuroimaging of the brain by MRI (fMRI), then the concept of correspondence is straightforward. If, however, change in volume is possible, such as when monitoring atrophic changes in the brain in longterm studies, then the concept of correspondence becomes less well defined. We are using serial MR to monitor neuronal loss, so the tissue corresponding to a certain location in the patient at the first visit may not exist at the later visit. In this case we normally undertake registration and establish correspondence, assuming that the tissue has not changed volume, and change will be inferred from absence of correspondence, often by displacements of boundaries. This may be displayed to good effect by using image subtraction, as explained in more detail in Chapter 7. Detecting a change in boundary location is relatively straightforward. Inferring which particular element of tissue has changed volume is much more difficult. Even in our first example, workup for neurosurgery, changes may occur due to differences in patient positioning, systemic blood pressure, hydration, and imaging at different phases of the breathing or cardiac cycle, although most of these changes are thought to be below the level detectable with current imaging devices.

When tissue changes significantly over time, such as long term monitoring of the breast postmenopause with MR, the concept of correspondence becomes even more difficult to define. Over repeat scans for a year or two, glandular tissue may be replaced by fatty tissue, yet registration to establish anatomical correspondence might have great potential to detect the presence of small focal disease, as described in Chapter 13. In this case the required transformation has to allow the tissue to deform by changing shape and size. This type of transformation is called "nonrigid" and is more appropriate for soft tissues. Over a short time period, for example, a dynamic acquisition of 3D MR images taken over a few tens of minutes, tissue will obey the laws of physical motion associated with elasticity and viscosity; during longer periods of time, tissue may grow or be destroyed. When monitoring surgery or therapeutic response, tissue will, by definition, be removed, and therefore correspondence in the excised or ablated region cannot exist. Conversely, the growth of a tumor adds tissue and structure. Anesthetics and drugs to control edema may also change tissue volumes.

Finally, we need to consider correspondence when combining images from multiple subjects or images between an individual and an atlas derived from one or more other individuals. Is correspondence defined in anatomical terms, e.g., the most anterior pole of the occipital cerebral cortex? Or is it defined in geometric terms, e.g., the portion of cerebral cortex in this region with the highest surface curvature? Is it defined in functional terms, e.g., the region of the cerebral cortex associated with vision that exhibits the greatest change in blood flow when the subject observes a flashing checkerboard pattern? Or is it defined by a particular histological appearance? On a coarse scale these may all correspond in normal subjects

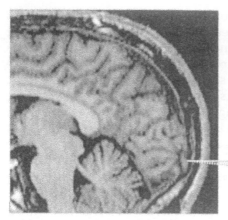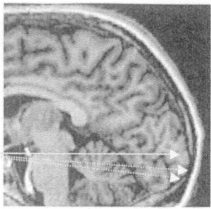

FIGURE 2.1

A pair of near mid sagittal slices of MR images of different individuals that have been scaled and registered assuming a rigid-body transformation. The solid line gives the transformation derived from the registration process while either of the two dotted lines might be more plausible from an anatomical perspective, within the constraints of this simple 2D example.

but on a fine scale, still within the spatial resolution of current imaging devices, and certainly when including pathology, they may not. These distinctions are illustrated in Figure 2.1, which shows three possible correspondences on a pair of MR slices from two individuals that have been aligned with one another and scaled so that the heads are the same size. Of course, correspondence is defined in 3D, not 2D as in this example, but nevertheless the figure illustrates the problem. In many applications reported in the literature, correspondence is implicitly defined as the points resulting from arbitrary transformations derived using algorithms that plausibly "morph" one image into another. Morphing is a term used to describe a process in computer graphics in which one image is transformed seamlessly into another, for example, a photograph of Tony Blair transformed into a photograph of Margaret Thatcher. There is an infinite number of possible transformations that can morph one image into another, including those that lead to creation or destruction of complete structures. Medical imaging applications usually require deformations of the images that maintain correspondence (nose to nose, eye to eye, etc.). Registration of images from different individuals requires the use of deformations that can accommodate biological variations, and is discussed in Chapter 14. Where the images are related by a physical process, the transformation may be modeled or constrained by those processes that result in the differences between imaged structures. In practice, we generally do not have sufficient information to do this. Algorithms based on physical models of elasticity or viscosity provide plausible transformations but do not model the real physical processes that lead to individual variability. These issues are explored in more detail in Chapter 14.

2.3   Types of Transformation

2.3.1   Dimensionality Transformations

The process of registration involves computation of a transformation between the coordinate systems of the images or between an image and physical space. We are three-dimensional beings who move, so in principle, registration should be four-dimensional. In practice, we usually make some approximations and assumptions so that the body can be represented with fewer dimensions.

2.3.1.1   2D-to-2D

If the geometry of image acquisition is tightly controlled, 2D images may be registered purely via a rotation and two orthogonal translations. It may also be necessary to correct for differences in scaling from the real object to each of the images. However, computationally straightforward, clinically relevant examples of this are rare, as controlling the geometry of image acquisition is usually very difficult. One example is the registration of x-ray radiographs of the hand with ^{99m}Tc methyl-diphosphonate planar nuclear medicine images for the diagnosis of suspected scaphoid injury.[1] Color Figure 2.2* shows a nuclear medicine image overlaid in color on the radiograph, confirming a scaphoid fracture. In this example, a purpose-built holding device constrained the hand to be in identical positions in the two images.

2.3.1.2   3D-to-3D

Of more widespread applicability is the accurate registration of multiple 3D images such as MR and CT volumes. The assumption is usually made that the internal anatomy of the patient has not distorted or changed in spatial relationships between organs, so that the imaged part of the body behaves as a "rigid body." In this case three translations and three rotations will bring the images into registration. Careful calibration of each scanning device is required to determine image scaling, i.e., the size of the voxels in each modality. 3D-to-3D registration is the most well developed and widely used method and is the primary emphasis of this book.

2.3.1.3   2D-to-3D

2D-to-3D registration may be required when establishing correspondence between 3D volumes and projection images such as x-ray or optical images. Another class of 2D-to-3D registration arises when the position of one or

---

* Color Figures follow page 22.

more slices from tracked B-mode ultrasound, interventional CT, or interventional MRI are to be established relative to a 3D volume. The main application of these methods is in image-guided interventions, as described in more detail in Chapter 12.

2.3.1.4   Time

Another class of registration problem concerns registration of image sequences that follow some process that changes with time. An obvious example is imaging of the heart, where images are acquired in synchrony with the heartbeat, monitored by the ECG or blood pressure waveform. Synchronized or "gated" acquisitions allow averaging of images over multiple cardiac cycles to reduce image noise in nuclear medicine and MR imaging. In a similar way, temporal registration of x-ray images of the heart before and after injection of contrast material allows synchronous subtraction of mask images. All these methods assume that the heart cycle does not change from beat to beat. The same principle can be applied to images acquired at different stages of the breathing cycle, although the breathing cycle is less reproducible and therefore registration errors will be greater. Acquisition of images over time and subsequent registration can be used to study dynamic processes such as tissue perfusion, blood flow, and metabolic or physiological processes.

2.3.2   Degrees of Freedom of the Transformation

The number of parameters needed to describe a registration transformation is referred to as the number of "degrees of freedom." This depends on the dimensionality of the images and the constraints of the imaged structures. The simplest transformation corresponds to the motion of a rigid body. For 2D-to-2D registration, there will be three degrees of freedom: two translations and one rotation. Figure 2.3 provides an example of two images related by a rigid transformation. The middle image also shows that a transformation will lead to the loss of some data from the original image and to

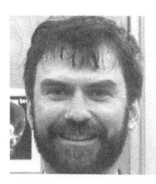 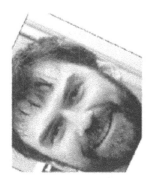 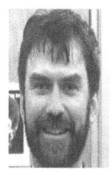

FIGURE 2.3
Three 2D images related by a rigid rotation (left and middle) and horizontal scaling (left and right).

some regions where there is missing data. For 3D-to-3D registration, as stated above, two positions of a rigid body can always be related to one another in terms of three translations and three rotations, giving six degrees of freedom. The particular conditions of imaging may mean that we do not know the pixel or voxel sizes or the fields of view, in which case the registration algorithm may need to determine these. This will lead to an extra two degrees of freedom in 2D or three degrees of freedom in 3D, equating to scaling in each direction, also illustrated in Figure 2.3. A particular distortion in 3D images generated from CT results from a gantry tilt, often used to reduce x-ray dose to the eyes. Without correction this will result in a 3D volume that is skewed, akin to a leaning stack of sliced bread (see Chapter 10, Figure 10.2). If gantry angle is unknown, we have another degree of freedom. This is a special case of the "affine" transformation. In the affine transformation, any straight line in one image will transform to a straight line in the other and parallel lines are preserved, allowing a combination of rigid body motion, scaling, and skew about any of the three axes. The affine transformation has 12 degrees of freedom. A mathematical definition is given in the next chapter.

In 2D-to-3D rigid-body registration, matching a perspective projection such as an optical image or x-ray image to a volume results in up to ten degrees of freedom. Usually four of these can be determined from a one-off calibration of the camera or x-ray set, provided the focal length of the camera or the distance between the x-ray set and imaging device is fixed, leaving the six parameters of the rigid-body transformation to be determined in the registration process.

In nonrigid registration, many more degrees of freedom are required. Two general categories of nonrigid registration occur: registration of images to an atlas or images from another individual, so called "intersubject registration" or registration of tissue that deforms over time, sometimes called "intrasubject registration." Figure 2.4 provides a 2D example of intersubject registration.

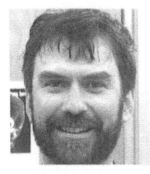 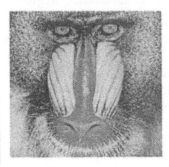 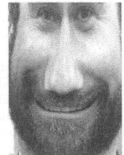

FIGURE 2.4
An example of interindividual, nonrigid registration (in 2D) of a professor (left) to a mandrill (center), resulting in the warped image (right). The transformation was achieved by identifying a number of corresponding point landmarks and transforming with the thin-plate spline function described in Chapter 3.

Constraints on the allowed deformation must be applied to make the problem computationally tractable and physically plausible. These constraints will depend on the application. Examples range from the addition of a relatively small number of extra degrees of freedom (typically five to ten) where the variation across a population can be described by parameters derived from principal component analysis as used in the active shape model[2] to the many tens of thousands implicit in the algorithm of Rueckert et al.[3] In studies of soft tissue deformation, understanding the physics of the deformation process might reduce the number of degrees of freedom of the transformation (see Chapter 15). Models based on the laws of physics have also been used to reduce the degrees of freedom of the matching process in intersubject registration. The example in Figure 2.4 was generated using a "thin-plate spline" deformation, a well known algorithm described in Chapter 3, that calculates the deformation expected in a thin plate that is anchored at a number of tie points or points of correspondence. As stated above, these quasi-physical models, unlike the biomechanical models discussed in Chapter 15, do not represent any real physical process within the patient.

2.4   Image Registration Algorithms

Registration algorithms compute image transformations that establish correspondence between points or regions within images, or between physical space and images. This section briefly introduces some of these methods. Broadly, these divide into algorithms that use corresponding points or corresponding surfaces, or operate directly on the image intensities.

2.4.1   Corresponding Landmark-Based Registration

One of the most intuitively obvious registration procedures is based on identification of corresponding point landmarks or "fiducial markers" in the two images. For a rigid structure, identification and location of three landmarks will be sufficient to establish the transformation between two 3D image volumes, provided the fiducial points are not all in a straight line. In practice it is usual to use more than three. The larger the number of points used, the more any errors in marking the points are averaged out. The algorithm for calculating the transformation is well known and straightforward.[4] It involves first computing the average or "centroid" of each set of points. The difference between the centroids in 3D tells us the translation that must be applied to one set of points. This point set is then rotated about its new centroid until the sum of the squared distances between each corresponding point pair is minimized. The square root of the mean of this squared distance is often recorded by the registration algorithm. It is also referred to as the root mean square (RMS) error, residual error or fiducial registration error (FRE). The mathematical solution for calculating this transformation has been known for many years, and is known as the solution to the orthogonal Procrustes problem after the unpleasant practice of Procrustes, a robber in Greek mythology, fitting his guests with extreme prejudice to a bed of the wrong size. The mathematics of the solution are provided in Chapter 3 together with the full story of the fate of Procrustes.

Many commercial image registration packages and image guided-surgery systems quote the FRE. Although this can be useful as a quick check of gross errors in correspondence, FRE is not a direct measure of the accuracy with which features of interest in the images are aligned. Indeed, it can be misleading, as changing the positions of the registration landmarks in order to reduce FRE can actually increase the error in correspondence between other structures in the images. A more meaningful measure of registration error is the accuracy with which a point of interest (such as a surgical target) in the two images can be aligned. This error is normally position-dependent in the image, and is called the target registration error (TRE). In practical terms, TRE, and how it varies over the field of view, is the most important parameter determining image registration quality. Fitzpatrick[5] has derived a formula to predict TRE based on corresponding point identification. The formula computes TRE from the distribution of fiducial points and the estimate of error in identifying correspondence at each point, the fiducial localization error (FLE). This formula has been verified by computer simulation and predicts experimental results accurately (see Chapter 3).

The point landmarks may be pins or markers fixed to the patient and visible on each scan. These may be attached to the skin or screwed into bone. The latter can provide very accurate registration but are more invasive and cause some discomfort and a small risk of infection or damage to underlying tissue. Skin markers, on the other hand, can easily move by several millimeters due to the mobility of the skin, and are difficult to attach firmly. Care must be taken to ensure that the coordinate of each marker is computed accurately and that the coordinate computed in each modality corresponds to the same point in physical space. Subvoxel precision is possible, for example, by using the intersection of two tubes containing contrast material visible in each modality,[6] the apex of a "V,"[7] or the center of gravity of spherical or cylindrical markers with a volume much larger than the voxel sizes.[8] Markers like these can be identified automatically in the images. Each of these systems was also designed so that the corresponding point in physical space could be accurately located. These are used widely in image-guided surgery as described in Chapter 12.

Alternatively, corresponding internal anatomical landmarks may be identified by hand on each image. These must correspond to truly point-like anatomical landmarks at the resolution of the images (such as the apical turn of the cochlea), structures in which points can be unambiguously defined (such as bifurcations of blood vessels or the center of the orbits of the eyes), or surface curvature features that are well defined in 3D. Several methods have been reported to register clinical images using corresponding anatomical landmarks that have been identified interactively by a skilled user.[9–11] Assuming all markers are identified with the same accuracy, registration error as measured by TRE can be reduced by increasing the number of fiducial markers. If the error in landmark identification or FLE is randomly distributed about the true landmark position, the TRE reduces as the square root of the number of points identified, for a given spatial distribution of points. TRE values of about 2 mm at the center rising to about 4 mm at the periphery are to be expected when registering MR and PET images of the head using 12 anatomical landmarks well distributed over the image volume. For registering MR and CT images, including the skull base, typical misregistration errors (TRE values) will be about 1 mm at the center, rising to about 2 mm at the periphery for 12 to 16 landmarks.[11] Finding these landmarks automatically and reliably is difficult and remains a research issue.

Figure 2.5 shows an example of aligned and combined CT and MR volumes of a patient with a large acoustic neuroma extending into the internal auditory meatus. These images are useful for planning skull base surgery.[10] Figure 2.6 depicts an aligned MR and PET image of the head showing that a suspicious bright region seen on contrast-enhanced MR does not correspond to a region

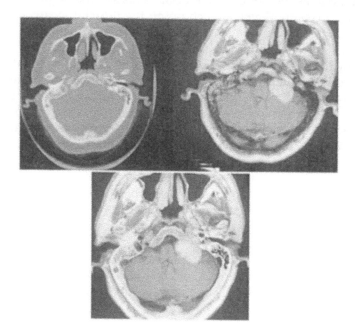

FIGURE 2.5
Slice (bottom) through a 3D volume formed by aligning and combining CT (top left) and MR (top right) volumes. CT intensity is displayed when this corresponds to bone otherwise the MR intensity is shown. This type of display has been useful in planning skull base surgery.[10]

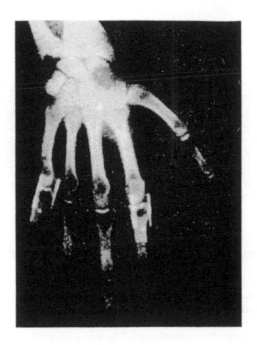

COLOR FIGURE 2.2

A planar nuclear medicine image overlaid in color on the corresponding radiograph indicating a scaphoid fracture.[1] Red corresponds to the highest radioisotope concentration.

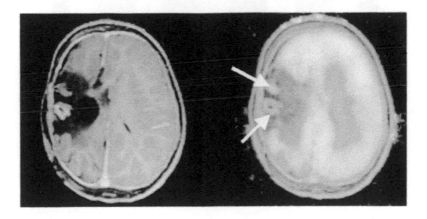

COLOR FIGURE 2.6

A slice from an MR volume (left) with the corresponding slice (right) of the PET [18]FDG volume aligned in 3D and overlaid on the MR using a "hot-body" intensity scale. This image shows that the suspicious bright region (lower arrow) is unlikely to be recurrence of the astrocytoma that had previously been surgically removed and treated with radiotherapy. The small bright region (upper arrow) anterior to this corresponds to normally functioning cortex with the expected [18]FDG uptake.

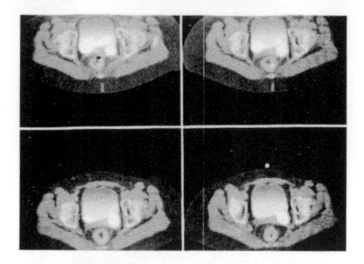

COLOR FIGURE 2.7
Four consecutive slices through the pelvis from a CT volume, with aligned [18]FDG PET images overlaid, showing concentration of isotope both in the bladder and in a region of dense tissue near the cervix. This indicated that the dense mass was recurrent tumor rather than fibrotic changes associated with previous radiotherapy. This was confirmed at surgery.

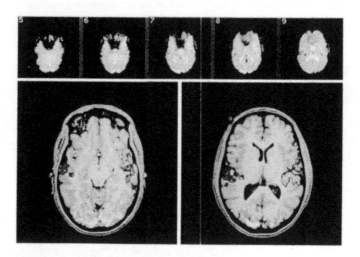

COLOR FIGURE 8.6
Activation from visual (red-yellow) and auditory (blue) stimulation. The top row shows statistically significant areas of activation rendered in color on top of the raw functional low resolution data. A typical raw functional image was then registered to a structural scan of the same subject, and the resulting transformation applied to the activation images. The resampled activation images were then overlaid as color on top of the high resolution image; two example slices are shown in the bottom row — the left image corresponds approximately to slice 6 in the low resolution data, and the right image lies somewhere between slices 8 and 9.

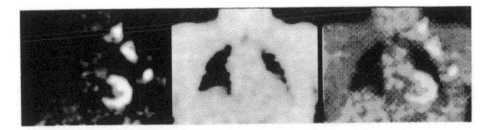

COLOR FIGURE 9.3
Example of a PET study of the thorax showing an emission image (left), a transmission image (middle), and a fusion of both images (right). The emission image provides rather coarse anatomical information. The addition of the transmission images provides a first step towards the interpretation of focal uptake sites with respect to morphological structures, but it cannot replace high resolution MR images.

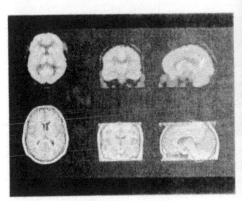

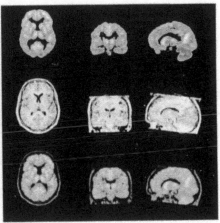

COLOR FIGURE 9.5A
Unregistered PET and MR images of the brain. A contour has been extracted from the PET images and superimposed on both sets. The contour provides clear delineation of the brain in the PET image and reveals an obvious misalignment with the MRI, because the PET contour does not describe the outer circumference of the brain in the latter images. This is a typical display as used during interactive registration procedures.

COLOR FIGURE 9.5B
Registered PET and MR images for the same study as shown in Figure 9.5A. The third row shows a combined image display as obtained after checkerboard fusion has been applied on both sets. Now a direct spatial relationship between function and morphology can be appreciated in a single display.

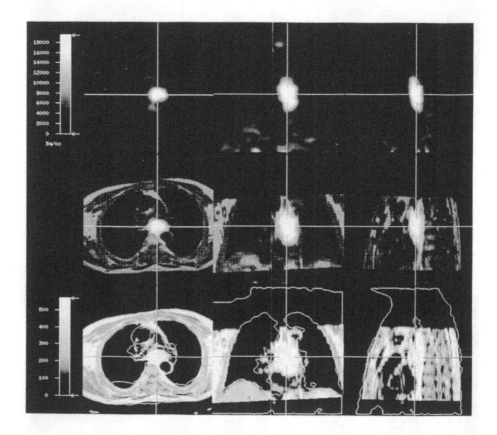

COLOR FIGURE 9.8

Registered PET and MR images in the case of an extracranial study of the thorax (esophageal carcinoma). PET emission images (top), fusion of PET (emission) and MR images (middle) and MR images (bottom) with a contour, which was extracted from PET transmission images (not shown). It can be seen that the axial coverage of the PET images is larger than that of the MRI. However, it was possible to align both the outer shape and internal structures of the lung with an interactive registration technique. During image data acquisition, special care was taken to position the patient's arms in the same way in both scanners. (Data: courtesy of Dr. Theissen, Nuclear Medicine, University of Cologne.)

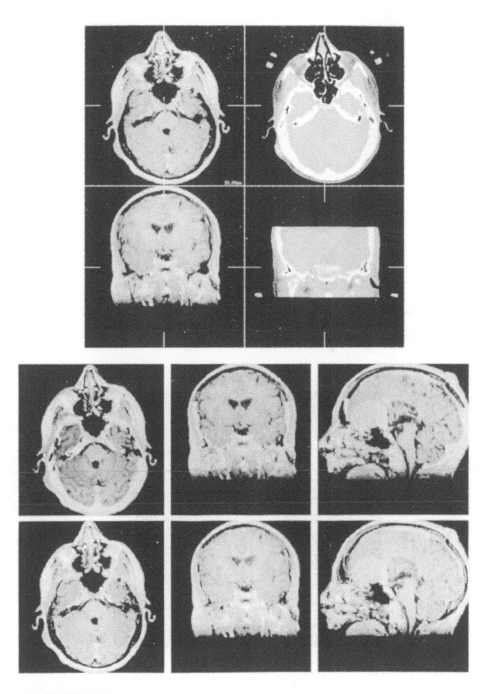

COLOR FIGURE 10.4
Example displays of registered MR and CT images. Adjacent display of corresponding axial and coronal views, with cursor indicating correspondence (top), color overlay of bone from CT on soft tissue from MR (middle), and overlay of the boundary of bone from CT on MR (bottom).

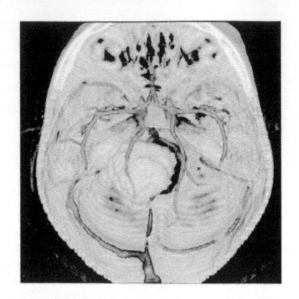

COLOR FIGURE 10.5
A volume-rendered image incorporating bone detail from CT (gray), the lesion from contrast-enhanced MRI (green), and blood vessels from MRA (red).

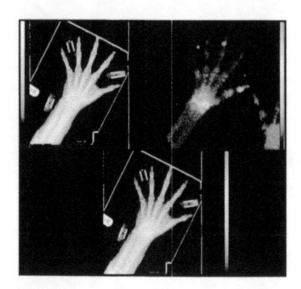

COLOR FIGURE 11.2
An example of planar registration is shown. The bone scan and planar x-ray are both performed with the hand in a rigid frame. The scan shows increased uptake in the scaphoid, indicative of a fine fracture. The markers used to register the two studies are visible between the 4th and 5th fingers and between thumb and forefinger. Slightly increased uptake is also visible in the joint of the thumb.

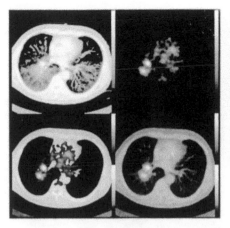

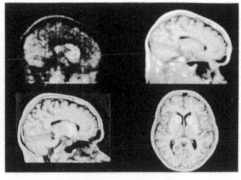

COLOR FIGURE 11.3

Two examples of PET co-registration are shown. The images on the left show PET [18F]-DG and x-ray CT scans of the thorax of a patient with primary lung cancer. From top left clockwise the images are: CT, PET, CT/PET interlaced, and CT/PET showing the PET data above a predetermined threshold (10% of maximum) substituted for the CT data. The images on the right show the normal distribution pattern in a PET DOPA scan together with an MRI scan. The images from top left clockwise are: PET DOPA scan, MRI, and co-registered studies in transverse and sagittal orientations. Both the PET-CT and PET-MRI data were co-registered with the same algorithm (Woods' AIR [automated image realignment] program[17] described in Chapter 3). In the thoracic example, the subject's PET attenuation images were co-registered to the CT scan, as the emission [18F]-DG scan bears little resemblance to the CT. (The PET DOPA scans and MRI are courtesy of Dr. Paola Piccini and Dr. Michele Hu, MRC Cyclotron Unit, Hammersmith Hospital). MR-PET registration is discussed in greater detail in Chapter 8.

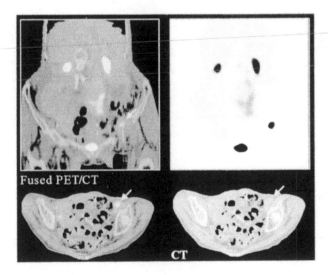

COLOR FIGURE 11.6

[18F]-DG PET-CT scan on a patient with recurrent ovarian carcinoma. The images from top right clockwise are the PET coronal image, x-ray CT transverse image, and co-registered and overlaid ("fused") transverse and coronal PET-CT images. The areas of highest uptake bilaterally at the top of the coronal section of the PET image (upper right) are the renal pelvic drainage areas, and the bladder is seen at the bottom of the image. This is normal physiological distribution for [18F]-DG. There is a large abnormal area of diffuse uptake adjacent to the midline, and a small abnormal focus in the left side of the pelvis. This uptake (arrowed in the CT and fusion images) corresponds to an enlarged lymph node on the CT scan. Without the fused image it would be difficult to be certain that the uptake was localized to the node rather than the underlying bone, which drastically alters the patient's management. (Images courtesy of Professor David Townsend, University of Pittsburgh Medical Center.)

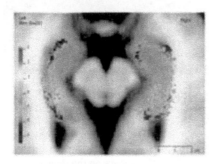 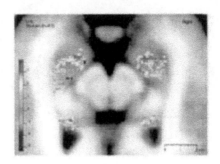

COLOR FIGURE 14.7
This image is a transverse slice through the long axis of the hippocampus showing the results from the voxel-based regression analysis for the female (left) and male (right) groups.

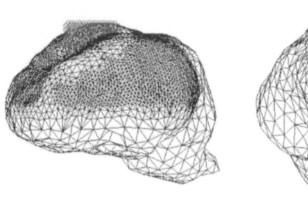 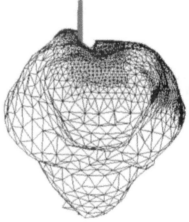

COLOR FIGURE 15.10
Example of a 3D retraction computation which follows the process outlined conceptually in Figure 15.9.

of high uptake of ^{18}FDG (2-[^{18}F]–fluoro-2-deoxy-D-glucose) on PET and therefore is unlikely to represent recurrent tumor. Figure 2.7 shows a sequence of CT axial slices, with the corresponding aligned ^{18}FDG PET images overlaid in pale green, taken through the pelvis of a patient who had received previous radiotherapy for cervical carcinoma. The images clearly show increased uptake in the denser mass shown on CT. This is likely to represent recurrent tumor rather than radiation-induced fibrotic changes, and this was confirmed at surgery. Figure 2.5 and Color Figures 2.6 and 2.7* were aligned using manually identified landmarks assuming that the part of the patient imaged could be represented as a rigid body. Now this process is almost completely replaced by the fully automated registration method based on voxel similarity and described in Section 2.4.3.

2.4.2 Surface-Based Registration

Corresponding surfaces may be identified and used for registration. In these algorithms, corresponding surfaces are delineated in the two imaging modalities and a transformation computed that minimizes some measure of distance between the two surfaces.[12–15] At registration this measure should be minimum. The first widely used method was the "head and hat" algorithm,[13] but most methods are now based on the iterative closest point algorithm.[15]

2.4.2.1 The "Head and Hat" Algorithm

In the "head and hat" algorithm, the contours of the surface are drawn on a series of slices from one modality. This is called the head. A set of points that correspond to the same surface in the other modality are identified. This set is called the hat. The computer then attempts a series of trial fits of the hat points on the head contours. The process of progressively refining these trial fits is known as *iteration*. At each iteration the sum of the squares of the distances between each hat point and the head is calculated, and the process continues until this value is minimized. The hat now fits on the head. As its name implies, this was first used on images of the head and, in particular, the alignment of MR and PET images. Unfortunately, just as there are many ways of placing a real hat on a head, this algorithm can be prone to choosing the wrong solution. These types of algorithms tend to fail when the surfaces show symmetries to rotation, which is often the case for many anatomical structures. The head can be rotated cranio-caudally (nodding) with minimal displacement of the skin surface in a direction perpendicular to the surface. This problem is illustrated diagrammatically in 2D in Figure 2.8. Figure 2.9 provides orthogonal cuts of an MR image and an overlaid PET image of the head that are grossly misregistered, yet the surfaces of the brain are surprisingly well aligned over much of the volume.

---

* Color Figures follow page 22.

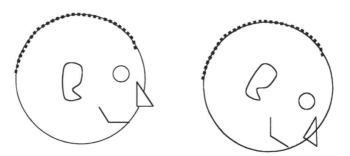

FIGURE 2.8
This illustrates in 2D how a contour-based method of alignment can produce multiple solutions if the contour exhibits axes of symmetry, in this case cranio-caudal tilt. Both alignments of the thick dotted line and thin continuous line will produce very similar mean distances between the two contours. The same arguments apply to surfaces in 3D.

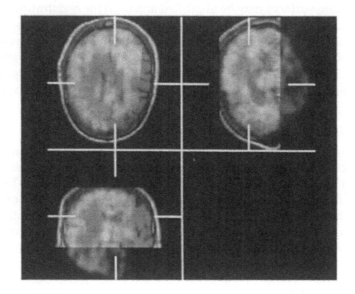

FIGURE 2.9
An example of three orthogonal slices through a 3D MR volume overlaid with the PET[18]FDG volume. The volume is grossly misregistered, yet the outline of the brain is surprisingly well aligned. (C. Studholme, Ph.D. Thesis, University of London, 1997.)

2.4.2.2 *Distance Transforms*

Surface matching was made more computationally efficient by precomputing the distance from every point in space to one of the surfaces to be registered. This is called a distance transform and makes the computation at each iteration much faster.

2.4.2.3 The Iterative Closest Point Algorithm

The iterative closest point algorithm,[15] although originally devised for other purposes, has been widely applied to surface-based registration of medical images. In the most usual form of this algorithm, one surface is represented by a set of points while the other is represented by a surface made up of many triangular patches or "facets." The algorithm proceeds by finding the closest point on the appropriate triangular patch to each of the points in turn. The closest points form a set, and these are registered using the corresponding landmark-based registration and the residual error is calculated. The closest points are found from this new position and the process is repeated until the residual error drops by less than a preset value.

These methods are described in more detail in the next chapter. They use more of the available data than landmark identification, and robust and accurate methods have been reported for some applications. Unfortunately, the technique is highly dependent on identification of corresponding surfaces, yet different imaging modalities can provide very different image contrast between corresponding structures. The process of delineation is hard to do accurately. Computer-assisted segmentation currently almost always requires some manual editing or adjustment. The surface may also exhibit natural symmetries to certain rotations, leading to poorly constrained transformations.

Other features, such as lines and tubes, as well as combinations of features, have also been used.[16] In principle, adjacent surfaces may be used for registration incorporating knowledge of the spatial relationships of different surfaces.[17]

2.4.3 Registration Based on Voxel Intensities Alone — Voxel Similarity Measures

In recent years a number of robust and accurate algorithms have been devised that use the intensities in the two images alone without any requirement to segment or delineate corresponding structures. These are often collectively referred to as voxel similarity-based registration. As these algorithms have been so successful, it is worth spending a few words to describe their historical development and to introduce a way of representing the image intensities of a pair of images that are to be registered. This representation is called the joint histogram or joint probability distribution. These terms will be described shortly. Unlike the algorithms described above, these methods use all (or a large proportion of) the data in each image and so tend to average out any errors caused by the noise or random fluctuations of image intensity. The simplest and earliest purely intensity-based registration method was applied to images from the same modality and therefore the images are unlikely to have changed very much.

2.4.3.1 Registration of Multiple Images of the Same Patient Acquired Using the Same Imaging Modality

There can be considerable clinical benefit in accurately aligning images of the same subject acquired with the same modality at different times in order to detect subtle changes in intensity or shape of a structure. This technique is most widely used for aligning serial MR images of the brain, as discussed in Chapter 7. Because the images are acquired using the same modality, an approximately linear relationship will exist between the voxel intensities in one image and voxel intensities in the other. In these cases the correlation coefficient (CC)[18] is a good measure of alignment. The formula for the correlation coefficient is presented in the next chapter, but it basically involves multiplication of corresponding image intensities. One image is moved with respect to the other until the largest value of the correlation coefficient is found. Statistically speaking, this is where there is the strongest linear relationship between the intensities in one image and the intensities at corresponding locations in the other. Instead of multiplying corresponding intensities, we may subtract them, which leads to another measure, the sums of squared intensity differences (SSD). In this case, alignment is adjusted until the smallest SSD is found.[19] That which can be subtracted or multiplied can also be divided. If two images are very similar, their ratio will be most uniform at registration. This is the basis of Woods[2] ratio image uniformity (RIU) algorithm in which the variance of this ratio is calculated.[20] Alignment is adjusted until the smallest variance is found. In early publications this was referred to as the variance of intensity ratios (VIR) algorithm. While the details of the formulae used are different, these algorithms are conceptually very similar. Performance, too, is similar except when the underlying assumptions are violated due to changes in overall image brightness, shading, etc.

As the small differences in very similar images may have clinical significance, care must be taken to ensure that the computation of the transformation neither removes nor masks this important information. Rescaling of either size or intensity, for example, must not mask real changes in volume. This danger can be avoided if all images are rescaled and intensities normalized by reference back to an image of a standard object or calibration phantom.[21] The most common technique for aligning these images is to find a rigid-body transformation. Prior to carrying out the rigid-body registration, it is advisable to correct for any scaling or intensity errors in the images (discussed in Chapter 5), and it may be necessary to carry out additional preprocessing such as segmentation (discussed in Chapter 4). A promising alternative approach is to register the images using a nonrigid transformation. In this case, the images after alignment should look virtually identical, and the calculated registration transformation provides quantitative information on the parts of the images that have changed size between images.

2.4.3.2   Voxel Similarity Measures Applied to Images from Different Modalities—Entropy as a Measure of Alignment

In the past five years there has been significant progress, worldwide, in using statistical relationships between voxel intensity values to align images acquired from different modalities. This work stems from the observation that while images from different modalities exhibit complementary information, there is usually also a high degree of shared information between images of the same structures. For example, the human observer is able to fuse stereoscopically very different images such as MR and CT of the same structure provided the images' brightness and contrast are adjusted appropriately.

Any algorithm that is used to register images from two different modalities must be insensitive to modality-specific differences in image intensity associated with the same tissue, and also accommodate differences in relative intensity from tissue to tissue. The first successful application of a voxel similarity-based algorithm to the registration of images from different modalities was that proposed by Woods for MR-to-PET registration.[22] We refer to this algorithm as partitioned intensity uniformity (PIU). The algorithm assumes that at each intensity in the MR image the range of the corresponding PET intensities is small. Implementation involved an almost trivial change to the original source code of the program for VIR but proved to be robust for the registration of MR and PET images of the head, provided the scalp was first removed from the MR images. Van den Elsen[23] proposed another algorithm, this time specific to MR-to-CT registration, in which the CT intensities were remapped or transformed so that soft tissue was bright, while both bone and air were dark. This had the effect of making a CT scan look a little like an MR image so linear correlation of intensities could be used as a measure of alignment. While effective in certain circumstances for aligning images of the head and spine, it never really caught on.

The initial success of these algorithms in specific applications inspired the search for a more general registration algorithm that would work with multimodality data. The required breakthrough came when a new way of looking at the intensities of the two images was suggested.[24] Each point in one image will correspond to a point in the other, and these two points each have an image intensity associated with them. We can generate a scatter plot of these image intensities, point by point. These are two-dimensional plots of image intensity of one image against corresponding image intensity of the other. The resulting plot is a type of two-dimensional histogram. This is sometimes called a joint intensity histogram and, when divided by the number of contributing pixels, is equal to the joint probability distribution. For each pair of image intensities in the two images, the joint probability distribution provides a number equal to the probability that those intensities occur together at corresponding locations in the two images. Examples of this for a pair of registered MR and PET images are given in Figure 2.9 (left). Interesting things

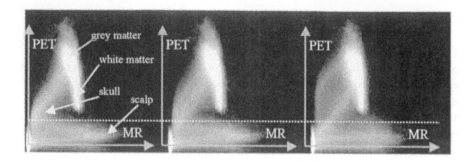

FIGURE 2.10
The joint probability distributions of intensities for aligned MR and [18]FDG PET volumes (left), misaligned with a 2 mm translation (middle) and misaligned with a 5 mm translation (right).[24] Also indicated are the regions of the plot approximately corresponging to the scalp, skull, gray matter, and white matter. The intensity values of the scalp will lie below the dotted line.

happen if we now repeat these plots at different alignments. The distinctive pattern in these two images starts to diffuse and disperse, as seen in Figure 2.10 (middle and right). Examples for two MR volumes and an MR and CT volume of the head are provided in Chapter 3, Figure 3.1. We can see from the plots in Figure 2.10 why the PIU algorithm works for MR and PET registration. If we remove the scalp, i.e., everything below the dotted line on Figure 2.10, then at registration there is only a narrow band of PET intensities for each MR intensity. This band broadens with misregistration, thus increasing the PIU measure. Likewise, we can see from the MR and CT plots in the next chapter how the remapping of the CT intensity will produce a strong linear relationship between MR and the remapped CT image intensities that will reduce with misalignment. This linear relationship was exploited in the method proposed by Van den Elsen.[23] Of more importance, however, these plots provide insight into an entirely new concept of image registration that is based on image entropy and information theory.

Information theory dates back to the pioneering work of Shannon in the 1940s.[25] Working at Bell Laboratories on how information is transmitted along a noisy telephone line or radio link, he devised a theory around a new measure of information. Its mathematical form was the same as the entropy defined in statistical mechanics, so he called this measure entropy. Entropy is a measure of disorder; a value for Shannon's entropy can be calculated directly from the joint probability distribution. Disorder (and entropy) increases with increasing misregistration in both the joint probability distribution (the plots in Figure 2.10 become more diffuse) and the visual appearance of the images when overlaid with one another. This suggests entropy as a possible measure of image alignment. Minimizing the joint entropy, calculated from the joint intensity histogram, was proposed by Studholme et al.[26] and Collignon[27] as a basis for a registration method.

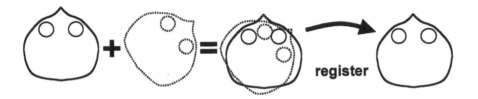

FIGURE 2.11
Diagrammatic explanation in 2D that the superimposition of an aligned image pair contains less information than a misaligned pair.

Unfortunately, joint entropy on its own does not provide a robust measure of image alignment, as it is often possible to find alternative (mis)alignments that result in much lower joint entropy. As an example, an alignment which results in just the overlap of air surrounding the patient, with the image data of the patient completely separated, will often produce a global minimum of entropy. It seems plausible that an appropriate measure might be the difference between the information in the overlapping volume of the combined or overlaid images and the information in the corresponding volumes of the two original images. Such a measure is provided by mutual information, which was proposed independently by Collignon et al.[27] and the MIT group.[28] Mutual information is given by the difference between the sum of the entropies of the individual images at overlap and the joint entropy of the combined images. As an illustrative example, consider two images of the same individual, each containing two eyes. Misaligned, the combined images will contain four eyes, while at alignment there will only be two. There is, therefore, less "information" in the conventional sense of the word in the combined images at registration. The extra information at misalignment is purely artifactual. This concept is explained diagrammatically in Figure 2.11.

At alignment we postulate that the joint entropy is minimized with respect to the entropy of the overlapping part of the individual images, so that the mutual information is maximized. Mutual information is a measure of how one image "explains" the other. It makes no assumption of the functional form or relationship between image intensities in the two images. Shannon first presented the functional form of mutual information in 1948.[25] He defined it as the "rate of transmission of information" in a noisy communication channel between source and receiver.

The mutual information measure with modifications associated with normalization[29] has proved very robust[30,31] and has resulted in fully automated 3D-to-3D rigid-body registration algorithms that are now in widespread use. The mathematical description of these measures is provided in the next chapter.

2.4.4 2D-3D Registration

Registration of x-ray or video images to a 3D-volume image involves establishing the pose of the x-ray or video image in relation to a previously acquired CT or MR volume. This has potential applications in image-guided interventions in the spine, pelvis, or head, or in endoscopic or microscopic surgery. More details of potential applications are provided in Chapter 12.

The two main classes of methods for 2D-3D registration are feature-based and direct intensity-based. In feature-based methods of x-ray image alignment, silhouettes of bony structures are delineated in the x-ray image, and the algorithm aligns the projections of these silhouettes with the surface of the same structure delineated from a CT (or MR) volume. One algorithm makes use of geometric properties of tangent lines of projected silhouettes and tangent planes of 3D surfaces.[32] This type of algorithm is fast, but is highly dependent on the integrity of the segmentation in both images.

An alternative method is to match the pixel and voxel intensities directly. The method is based on digitally reconstructed radiographs (DRRs), first proposed for stereotactic neurosurgical applications.[18] DRRs are computed by integrating (summing intensities) along rays through the CT volume to simulate the process of perspective projection in x-ray imaging. New DRRs can readily be calculated for trial poses and then compared with the true x-ray image using an appropriate measure of similarity.[33,34] The confounding effect of soft tissue movement is minimized by removing the soft tissue from the CT image by intensity thresholding.

Video images may be used to register visible surfaces to MR or CT volumes. Again there are two methods for establishing registration, those based on matching a reconstructed surface and those that are intensity based. In the first, a pattern of light (lines, random dots, etc.) is projected onto the visible surface. Correspondence of the pattern in the two calibrated video images is used to reconstruct the surface in 3D. This surface is then registered to the corresponding MR or CT derived surface using an appropriate surface registration method such as the iterative closest point algorithm. Recently, alternative methods have been proposed which do not rely on the initial step of reconstructing a surface. In these methods the voxel intensities are used directly to match to the 3D surface derived from MR or CT. Viola has proposed using the mutual information between optical image intensities and directions of the MR or CT surface normals.[35] An alternative approach uses the observation that intensities of a given point on a surface appear very similar or "photoconsistent" when viewed under the same lighting conditions with two or more cameras.[36] Trial registrations are iteratively tested until an appropriate photoconsistency criterion is satisfied.

2.5 Nonrigid Registration Algorithms

As already stated, the two main application areas where nonrigid registration algorithms are required are when establishing correspondence between an image of one individual and atlas, computer model, or image of another individual (intersubject registration), and when establishing correspondence between images of tissues that have deformed, shrunk, or grown over time (intrasubject registration). As described above, the issues of correspondence are rather different.

2.5.1 Intersubject Registration

Establishing correspondence of an atlas with a set of images or a number of images from a cohort of individuals requires a transformation that reflects the variation in anatomy between the atlas and the individual patient. There will be changes in shape and size as well as grosser changes in topology. This remains an area of active research with several approaches under investigation. Approaches include extending the rigid-body method to incorporate deformations that follow quadratic and higher order polynomial curves, or a wide range of other, more complicated functions such as Fourier or wavelet basis functions and splines, including radial basis functions such as the thin-plate spline and B-splines. These methods are described in Chapter 13.

Registration algorithms have been devised based on some approximation to the physical process inducing the deformation, including the elastic properties of solids and the dynamics of viscous fluids. These transformations produce physically plausible transformations and are possible to compute, although they take some time. Such algorithms, however, do not directly model the underlying causes for the differences in shape, and hence results should be interpreted with care.

In the optimization process used in all nonrigid algorithms, the goodness of match is balanced against some constraint prohibiting implausible deformations. This constraint may be provided by some estimate of the energy required to physically induce the deformation, as if the structures to be registered were made of elastic material, or may be couched in probabilistic terms. Multiscale approaches may be used in which a rigid-body transformation is computed for a coarse or blurry image, followed by multiple rigid-body transformations for arrays of volume elements at progressively finer detail with interpolation between these elements.[37] One intriguing algorithm, aptly named the "Demons" algorithm, models the deformation on the physical process of diffusion.[38] The mathematics are analogous to Maxwell's demons in statistical physics.

The problem might be made easier by using statistical shape models based on principal component analysis of the variations observed across a population of individuals.[2] In these models the variation in shape of a structure between one individual and another is captured by a small number of parameters or so called "modes of variation." In the original paper by Cootes et al.,[2] the outline of the hand is used as an example and the different modes correspond to the individual movements of each finger. While somewhat contrived, this shows how a very small number of parameters can capture quite complex variations in shape. In a study of fetal liver shape, only five modes are required to capture 89% of the variation in shape.[39]

In principle, a tissue growth model might be used to model differences between different individuals. Study of tissue growth and links with gene expression and environmental factors is an exciting area of research, but it is likely to be many years before such models can be used to align images from different subjects.

2.5.2 Intrasubject Registration

Almost all registration work so far has been applied to the brain, which is assumed to be held rigid by the confines of the skull, or to other bony structures. We are beginning to see extension of registration algorithms to other structures that deform over time. These deformations may either be due to natural involuntary motion (e.g., the heartbeat) or voluntary motion (e.g., change in body position within the scanner), or may be induced by an intervention. In the former, we need to align images to establish correspondence point by point. In image-guided interventions, tissue can distort and deform between preoperative scans and the intervention. Anatomical structures may move in relation to each other. Intraoperative data in the form of point coordinates, optical images from microscopes or endoscopes, ultrasound, or x-ray may provide updated information on location and deformation of anatomical structures. This new information might be used as a basis for predicting deformation of adjacent tissues. The general problem, as in matching to an atlas described above, is often poorly constrained, but in this case we may use the physical constraints of the tissues involved. For example, bony structures will usually remain rigid, and soft tissues will obey the laws of physics when deforming. Known information about the tissue such as volume preservation or local rigidity might be incorporated to constrain what would otherwise be a wide range of possible solutions. For example, the breast is unlikely to change in volume over the course of a 20-minute dynamic, contrast-enhanced MR sequence of acquisitions.

While devising effective nonrigid registration methods remains a research topic, there are a number of algorithms undergoing evaluation that show great promise, e.g., Rueckert et al.[3] Perhaps surprisingly, it appears that the transformation mapping one individual's anatomy to another might obey rather similar smoothness constraints to that which occurs naturally in soft tissue deformations. Algorithms tend to fall into two classes: those based on modeling, if only approximately, some physical process such as viscous fluid flow or elastic deformation, and those based on some interpolating or approximating function. These issues are discussed in more detail in Chapter 13 along with an introduction to the mathematics involved in the more successful approaches.

2.6   Optimization

Only two regularly used algorithms directly calculate a transformation to establish correspondence. The first is the Procrustes method based on point correspondence, described earlier. The other is when two images have very similar intensities and the transformation required to establish correspondence is small. In this case, the transformation can be approximated by the first term in an expansion of the function relating one image to the other as a series of terms, i.e., the Taylor series. An approximate transformation can be calculated directly.[40] These algorithms are described in more detail in Chapter 3.

In all other algorithms, a process of optimization is required. This means that the algorithm takes a series of guesses from an initial starting position. The starting position has to be sufficiently close for the algorithm to converge to the correct answer, i.e., it has to be within what is known as its "capture range." This first guess can be set automatically or with a simple user interaction. The algorithm computes a number, known as the cost function or similarity function, relating to how well the two images are registered. Mutual information, correlation coefficient, and sum-of-squared-intensity differences are all examples of cost functions. Some cost functions (e.g., the correlation coefficient) increase as the images come into alignment; others (e.g., sum-of-squared-intensity-differences) decrease. The registration algorithm proceeds by taking another guess and recalculating the cost function. Progression towards an optimal registration is then achieved by seeking transformations that increase (or decrease) the cost function until a maximum (or minimum) of the cost function is found. The best registration that can be achieved is defined by this maximum (or minimum). The strategy for "optimization", i.e., guessing subsequent alignment transformations, is an important subdiscipline in the area of computing known as numerical methods. The next chapter contains a more detailed treatment of optimization of cost functions.

2.7 Transformation of Images

Registration algorithms are designed to establish correspondence. In many applications this is sufficient. All that is required is an indication of what point in one image corresponds to a particular point in the other. In some applications, however, we need to transform an image into the space of the other. This process requires resampling one image on the grid corresponding to the voxels or pixels in the other. To do this, interpolation is required. The accuracy with which this interpolation is done depends on the motivation for registering the images in the first place. In most applications simple nearest neighbor or trilinear interpolation will suffice. In nearest neighbor interpolation, as the name suggests, the location of each voxel in the transformed image is transformed back to the appropriate location in the original image and the nearest voxel value is copied into the transformed voxel. In trilinear interpolation the linearly weighted average of the eight nearest voxels is taken. For the highest accuracy, sampling theory tells us that a sinc $((\sin x)/x)$ weighting function applied to all voxels should be used.[19] This is particularly important when studying very subtle changes in the intensities or sizes of structures from images taken over a period of time. Interpolation errors can easily exceed the original image noise and can swamp subtle changes that would otherwise be detectable in subtraction images. The mathematics of these issues are addressed in Chapter 3, with applications described in Chapter 7. Unfortunately, accurate sinc interpolation can be extremely time consuming even on very fast computers, and can, therefore, limit applicability. Recent innovations in this area such as shear transformations are making high quality interpolation much faster.

Some consideration needs to be given to the spatial resolution and pixel or voxel sizes of the two images. Transforming from a high resolution modality such as CT or MR with voxel sizes of perhaps $1 \times 1 \times 1$ mm or finer onto a voxel grid from, for example, PET with a voxel size of $3 \times 3 \times 3$ mm will result, inevitably, in loss of information. On the other hand, transforming a PET image onto the grid of an MR or CT image will dramatically increase the memory required to store the PET image (by a factor of 27 in this example), unless some form of data compression is used. The choice of the final transformed image-sampling grid will depend on the specific application.

2.8   Validation

Complex software has to be verified and validated. This is particularly important in medical applications, where erroneous results can risk a patient's health or even life. Verification is the process by which the software is shown to do what it is specified to do (e.g., maximize mutual information). The software industry has developed standards, protocols, and quality procedures for verification. This is an important topic, but beyond the scope of this book.

Validation is the process whereby the software is shown to satisfy the needs of the application with accuracy and other performance criteria (e.g., register two images within a certain tolerance, within a certain processing time, and with less than a certain rate of failure). Validation of image registration algorithms will usually follow a sequence of measurements using computer-generated models (software phantoms), images of physical phantoms of accurately known construction and dimensions, and images of patients or volunteers. The process must demonstrate both high robustness and high accuracy. Robustness implies a very low failure rate and, if failure does occur, that this is communicated to the user. Assessment of accuracy requires knowledge of a "gold standard" or "ground truth" registration. This is difficult to achieve with clinical images, but several methods have recently been reported. These are described in more detail in Chapter 6.

Finally, in any new technology applied to medicine we must evaluate whether there is a clear benefit to the patient and, if so, that it is achieved in a cost-effective manner. This is the topic of health technology assessment. It is touched on in application chapters but is largely beyond the scope of this book. It is clear that image registration is invaluable in neurosciences research and the clinical application of image-guided surgery. Many other applications will undoubtedly be accepted as the technology matures.

2.9 Summary and Conclusion

This chapter has introduced the basic ideas that underlie image registration. The concept of correspondence was discussed in some detail. A clear definition of correspondence is required in any new application (and many new applications are being suggested all the time). This is particularly important as the development of applications in nonrigid and intersubject registration gathers pace. The chapter proceeds with a discussion of the dimensionality of the data to be registered and the number of degrees of freedom of the transformation. This book is primarily concerned with registering 3D images assuming that the part of the body imaged can be treated as if it were a rigid body. Image registration has also been successfully applied to 2D images, between 2D and 3D images, and to time series. We are also beginning to see progress in devising useful and practical algorithms that allow images to be aligned in cases where the structure that is imaged deforms, or when aligning images from different individuals.

A descriptive account of the more successful image registration algorithms is provided. The intention in this chapter is to provide insight into the concepts behind the algorithms, not to provide mathematical, algorithmic, or implementation details. Our focus is on an understanding of how these algorithms work that the nontechnical individual can understand. The description of the algorithms for the more mathematically inclined is left to the next chapter. We describe the well known point-based and surface-based algorithms, and, in more detail, the highly successful voxel intensity or voxel similarity approaches. We touch on recent work on nonrigid registration algorithms, which are dealt with in more detail in Chapter 13.

Very few registration algorithms provide a direct calculation of the transformation. The computer has to search iteratively for the best solution. This is the process of optimization described conceptually in Section 2.6. Finally, we usually need to transform one of the images into the coordinate system or "space" of the other. Some of the issues and pitfalls in transformation are discussed in Section 2.7.

Finally, all complex computations must be validated. This is particularly important in medical applications. This topic is introduced in Section 2.8 and expanded throughout this book.

References

1. D.J. Hawkes, L. Robinson, J.E. Crossman, H.B. Sayman, R. Mistry, and M.N. Maisey, Registration and display of the combined bone scan and radiograph in the diagnosis and management of wrist injuries. *Eur. J. Nucl. Med.* vol. 18, 752–756, 1991.
2. T.F. Cootes, C.J. Taylor, D.H. Cooper, and J. Graham, Training models of shape from sets of examples. *British Machine Vision Conference 1992* (D. Hogg and R. Boyle, Eds.), pp. 9–18. London: Springer, 1992.
3. D. Rueckert, L.I. Sonoda, C. Hayes, D.L.G. Hill, M.O. Leach, and D.J. Hawkes, Non-rigid registration using free-form deformations: application to breast MR images. *IEEE Trans. Med. Imaging,* vol. 18, no. 8, 712–721, 1999.
4. K.S. Arun, T.S. Huang, and S.D. Bostein, Least squares fitting of two 3D point sets. *IEEE Trans. Pattern Anal. Machine Intell.,* vol. 9, 698–700, 1987.
5. M.J. Fitzpatrick, J. West, and C. Maurer, Jr., Predicting error in rigid-body, point-based registration. *IEEE Trans. Med. Imaging,* vol. 17, pp. 694–702, 1998.
6. A.C.F. Colchester, J. Zhao, K.S. Holton-Tainter, C.J. Henri, N. Maitland, and P.T.E Roberts, A surgical planning and guidance system using intraoperative video imaging. *Med. Image Anal.* vol. 1, 73–90, 1996.
7. P.A. Van den Elsen and M.A. Viergever, Marker guided registration of electo-magnetic dipole data with tomographic images. In *Information Processing in Medical Imaging* (A.C.F. Colchester and D.J. Hawkes, Eds.), pp. 142–153. Heidelburg: Springer-Verlag, 1991.
8. C.R. Maurer, J.M. Fitzpatrick, R.L. Galloway, M.L. Wang, R.J. Macuinas, and G.S. Allen, The accuracy of image-guided neurosurgery using implantable fiducial markers, in *Computer Assisted Radiology 1995* (H. Lemke, Ed.), pp. 1197–1202 Berlin: Springer, 1995.
9. A.C. Evans, S. Marret, L. Collins, and T.M. Peters, Anatomical-functional correlative analysis of the human brain using three-dimensional imaging systems. *SPIE* vol. 1092, pp. 264–274, 1989.
10. D.L.G. Hill., D.J. Hawkes, J.E. Crossman, M.J. Gleeson, T.C.S. Cox, E.E.C.M.L. Bracey, et al., Registration of MR and CT images for skull base surgery using point-like anatomical features. *Br. J. Radiol.* vol. 64, pp. 1030–1035, 1991.
11. D.L.G. Hill, D.J. Hawkes, M.J. Gleeson, T.C.S. Cox, A.J. Strong, W.L. Wong, et al. Accurate frameless registration of MR and CT images of the head: applications in planning surgery and radiation therapy. *Radiology* vol. 191, pp. 447–454, 1994.
12. G. Borgefors, Distance transformations in digital images. *Comput. Vision, Graphics Image Process.* vol. 34, pp. 344–371, 1986.
13. C.A. Pelizzari, G.T.Y. Chen, D.R. Spelbring, R.R. Weichselbraum, and C. Chen, Accurate three-dimensional registration of CT, PET and/or MR images of the brain. *J. Comput. Assist. Tomogr.* vol. 13, pp. 20–26, 1989.
14. H. Jiang, R.A. Robb, and K.S. Holton, New approach to 3-D registration of multimodality medical images by surface matching. *SPIE,* vol. 1808, pp. 196–213, 1992.
15. P.J. Besl and N.D. McKay, A method for registration of 3D shapes. *IEEE Trans. Pattern Anal. Machine Vision.* vol. 14, pp. 239–256, 1992.
16. C.R. Meyer, G.S. Leichtman, J.A. Brunsberg, R.L. Wahl, and L.E. Quint, Simultaneous usage of homologous points, lines and planes for optimal 3-D linear registration of multimodality imaging data. *IEEE Trans. Med. Imaging,* vol. 14, pp. 1–11, 1995.

17. D.L.G. Hill and D.J. Hawkes, Medical image registration using knowledge of adjacency of anatomical structures. *Image Vision Computing,* vol. 12, pp. 173–178, 1994.
18. L. Lemieux, N.D. Kitchen, S. Hughes, and D.G.T. Thomas. Voxel based localisation in frame-based and frameless stereotaxy and its accuracy. *Med. Physics,* vol. 21, pp. 1301–1310, 1994.
19. J.V. Hajnal, N. Saeed, A. Oatridge, E.J. Willimas, I.R. Young, and G.M. Bydder, Detection of subtle brain changes using subvoxel registration and subtraction of serial MR images. *J. Comp. Assist. Tomogr.* vol. 19, pp. 677–691, 1995.
20. R.P. Woods, S.R. Cherry, and J.C. Mazziotta, Rapid automated algorithm for aligning and reslicing PET images. *J. Comput. Assist. Tomogr.,* vol. 16, pp. 620–633, 1992.
21. D.L.G. Hill, C.R. Maurer, Jr., C. Studholme, R.J. Maciunas, J.M. Fitzpatrick, and D.J. Hawkes, Correcting scaling errors in tomographic images using a nine degree of freedom registration algorithm. *J. Comput. Assist. Tomogr.* vol. 22, pp. 317–323, 1998.
22. R.P. Woods, J.C. Mazziotta, and S.R. Cherry, MRI PET registration with automated algorithm. *J. Comput. Assist. Tomogr.* vol. 17, pp. 536–546, 1993.
23. P.A. van den Elsen, E.J.D. Pol, T.S. Sumanaweera, P.F. Hemler, S. Napel, and J.R. Adler, Grey value correlation techniques used for automatic matching of CT and MR volume images of the head. *SPIE* vol. 2359, pp. 227–237, 1994.
24. D.L.G. Hill, C. Studholme, and D.J. Hawkes, Voxel similarity measures for automated image registration. *SPIE* vol. 2359, pp. 205–216, 1994.
25. C.E. Shannon, The mathematical theory of communication (parts 1 and 2). *Bell Syst. Tech J.* vol. 27, pp. 379–423 and 623–656, 1948. Reprint available from *http://www.lucent.com.*
26. C. Studholme, D.L.G Hill, and D.J. Hawkes, Multiresolution voxel similarity measures for MR-PET registration, in *Information Processing in Medical Imaging (IPMI'95)* (Y. Bizais, C. Barillot, and R. Di Paola, Eds.), pp. 287–298. Dordrecht: Kluwer, 1995.
27. A. Collignon, F. Maes, D. Delaere, D. Vandermeulen, P. Suetens, and G. Marchal, Automated multimodality image registration using information theory, in *Information Processing in Medical Imaging (IPMI '95)* (Y. Bizais, C. Barillot, and R. Di Paola, Eds.), pp. 263–274. Dordrecht: Kluwer, 1995.
28. W.M. Wells, P. Viola, H. Atsumi, S. Nakajima, and R. Kikinis, Multi-modal volume registration by maximization of mutual information. *Med. Image Anal.,* vol. 1, pp. 35–51, 1996.
29. C. Studholme, D.L.G. Hill, and D.J. Hawkes, An overlap invariant entropy measure of 3D medical image alignment. *Pattern Recogn.* vol. 32, pp. 71–86, 1999.
30. C. Studholme, D.L.G. Hill, and Hawkes D.J., Automated 3D registration of MR and CT images of the head. *Med. Image Anal.,* vol. 1, pp. 163–175, 1996.
31. C. Studholme, D.L.G. Hill, and D.J. Hawkes, Automated 3D registration of MR and PET brain images by multi-resolution optimisation of voxel similarity measures. *Med. Physics,* vol. 24, pp. 25–36, 1997.
32. S. Lavallee and R. Szeliski, Recovering the position and orientation of free-form objects from image contours using 3D distance maps. *IEEE Trans. Pattern Anal. and Machine Intell.,* vol. 17, pp. 378–390, 1995.
33. G.P. Penney, J. Weese, J.A. Little, P. Desmedt, D.L.G. Hill, and D.J. Hawkes. A comparison of similarity measures for use in 2D-3D medical image registration. *IEEE Trans. Med. Imaging,* vol. 17, pp. 586–595, 1998.

34. J. Weese, G.P. Penney, P. Desmedt, T.M. Buzug, D.L.G. Hill, and D. J. Hawkes, Voxel-based 2D/3D registration of fluoroscopy images and CT scans for image guided surgery. *IEEE Trans. Biomedi. Eng.*, vol. 1, pp. 284–293, 1997.
35. P.A. Viola, Alignment by maximization of mutual information. Ph.D. thesis, Massachusetts Institute of Technology, 1995.
36. M.J. Clarkson, D. Rueckert, D.L.G. Hill, and D.J. Hawkes, A multiple 2D video –3D medical image registration algorithm. *SPIE Medical Imaging 2000: Image Processing*, vol. 3979, pp. 342–352.
37. D.L. Collins, T.M. Peters, and A.C. Evans, An automated 3D non-linear image deformation procedure for determination of gross morphometric variability in human brain. *Visualization in Biomed. Comput. 1994, SPIE* vol. 2359, pp. 180–190, 1994.
38. J-P. Thirion, Image matching as a diffusion process: an analogy with Maxwell's demons. *Med. Image Anal.*, vol. 2, pp. 243–260, 1998.
39. C.F. Ruff, S.W. Hughes, and D.J. Hawkes, Volume estimation from sparse planar images using deformable models. *Image Vision Computing*, vol. 17, pp. 559–565, 1999.
40. K.J. Friston, C.D. Frith, P.F. Liddle, and R.S.J. Fracowiak, Comparing functional (PET) images: The assessment of significant change. *J. Cerebr. Blood Flow Metab.* vol. 11, pp. 690–699, 1997.

3

Registration Methodology: Concepts and Algorithms

Derek L.G. Hill and Philipe Batchelor

CONTENTS

3.1   Introduction

In the previous chapter, the concepts behind image registration were introduced in a nonmathematical way. The aim of this chapter is to describe some of the main algorithms used in image registration in greater detail, and to compare their applicability. This requires a more mathematical approach.

This chapter uses three-dimensional (3D) rigid-body registration as an exemplar. The algorithms described in most detail are those used for rigid-body registration of 3D tomographic images of the same subject. Many of the concepts and algorithms introduced here are also applicable to other registration applications including registration of 2D and 3D images, image-physical space registration, nonrigid intrasubject registration, and intersubject registration.

The field of nonrigid registration for both intrasubject and intersubject applications is an area of active current research, and is the topic of the third part of this book.

3.2   Notation and Terminology

In order to align two images, we need to know the transformation that relates the *position* of features in one image or coordinate space with the *position* of the corresponding feature in another image or coordinate space. We use the symbol $\mathbf{T}$ to represent this registration transformation.

Using the language of geometry, this transformation is a spatial mapping. We can consider the mapping $\mathbf{T}$, that transforms a position x from one image to another, or from one image to the coordinate system of a treatment device (image to physical registration).

$$\mathbf{T} : x_B \mapsto x_A \Leftrightarrow \mathbf{T}(x_B) = x_A \qquad (3.1)$$

It is sometimes useful to also consider the inverse mapping $\mathbf{T}^{-1}$ that maps x_A to x_B.* With image data we have to consider intensity values as well as positions, and we refer to $A(x_A)$ as the intensity value at the location x_A, and similarly for image B. It is important to remember that the medical images A and B are derived from a real object, i.e., the patient. The images have a limited field of view that does not normally cover the entire patient. Furthermore, this field of view is likely to be different for the two images.

---

* Although rigid-body and affine transformations that form the focus of this chapter are invertible, not all more complicated transformations are.

We can usefully think of the two images as mappings of points in the patient within their field of view (or *domain*, Ω) to intensity values.

$$A : \mathbf{x}_A \in \Omega_A \mapsto A(\mathbf{x}_A)$$
$$B : \mathbf{x}_B \in \Omega_B \mapsto B(\mathbf{x}_B)$$

Because the images are likely to have different fields of view, the domains Ω_A and Ω_B will be different. This is a very important factor, which accounts for a good deal of the difficulty in devising accurate and reliable registration algorithms. We will return to this issue later in this section.

As the images A and B represent one object X, imaged with the same or different modalities, there is a relation between the spatial locations in A and B. Image A is such that position $\mathbf{x} \in X$ is mapped to $\mathbf{x}_A$, and images B maps $\mathbf{x}$ to $\mathbf{x}_B$. The registration process involves recovering the spatial transformation $\mathbf{T}$ which maps $\mathbf{x}_B$ to $\mathbf{x}_A$ over the entire domain of interest, i.e., that maps from Ω_A to Ω_B within the overlapping portion of the domains. We refer to this overlap domain as $\Omega_{A,B}^{\mathbf{T}}$. This notation makes it clear that the overlap domain depends on the domains of the original images A and B, and also on the spatial transformation $\mathbf{T}$. The overlap domain can be defined as:

$$\Omega_{A,B}^{\mathbf{T}} = \{\mathbf{x}_A \in \Omega_A | \mathbf{T}^{-1}(\mathbf{x}_A) \in \Omega_B\} \tag{3.2}$$

Registration algorithms that make use of geometrical features in the images involve identifying features such as sets of image points $\{\mathbf{x}_A\}$ and $\{\mathbf{x}_B\}$ that correspond to the same physical entity visible in both images, and calculating $\mathbf{T}$ for these features.

Registration algorithms that work directly on image intensity values work differently. These algorithms nearly always iteratively determine the image transformation $\mathbf{T}$ that optimizes some measure of the similarity between the voxel intensities in the two images (a *voxel similarity measure*). At each iteration, they transform the image using the current estimate of $\mathbf{T}$ and recalculate a voxel similarity measure. Unless $\mathbf{T}$ is simply a translation by an integer number of pixels or voxels, the transformation carried out at each iteration involves interpolation between sample points. For these algorithms, it is useful to introduce new notation for the transformation $\mathcal{T}$ that maps both the position and the associated intensity value at that position. In this chapter, we use the notation $\mathbf{T}$ when mapping of position is all that is required, and $\mathcal{T}$ when the intensity at a position is also taken into account. Any time that $\mathcal{T}$ is used, the type of interpolation used by the algorithm is likely to alter the solution obtained. For example, throughout this chapter, we treat image A as the reference, or target, image and image B as the iteratively transformed, or source, image. We use the notation B^T to represent image B transformed, using the current transformation estimate $\mathbf{T}$. This image B^T is defined at the voxel coordinates of image A. The voxel values in B^T, of course, depend on the type of interpolation used, hence the use of $\mathcal{T}$ rather than **T** as the superscript.

Many of these voxel similarity measures involve analyzing level sets, or isointensity sets, within the images. For a single image A, an isointensity set with intensity value a is the set of voxels in A, such that:

$$\Omega_a = \{\mathbf{x}_A \in \Omega_A | A(\mathbf{x}_A) = a\} \tag{3.3}$$

Some algorithms do not work on isointensity sets corresponding to a single intensity value but on isointensity sets corresponding to small groups, or bins, of intensities. For example, a 12-bit image may have its intensities grouped into 256 four-bit bins. We use a to mean either individual intensities or intensity bins, as appropriate.

It is important to remember that Ω_a is the isointensity set within all of image A that is within the domain Ω_A. As stated above, for registration using voxel similarity measures, we work within the overlap domain $\Omega_{A,B}^{\mathsf{T}}$. The level set within this overlap domain is, of course, a function of **T**. To emphasize this **T** dependence, we define the isointensity set in image A with value a within $\Omega_{A,B}^{\mathsf{T}}$ as:

$$\Omega_a^{\mathsf{T}} = \{\mathbf{x}_A \in \Omega_{A,B}^{\mathsf{T}} | A(\mathbf{x}_A) = a\} \tag{3.4}$$

Similarly, we can consider an isointensity set in image B. Image B is always the image that we consider transformed, so the definition is slightly different than for image A. We consider the isointensity set to be the set of voxels in the overlap domain $\Omega_{A,B}^{\mathsf{T}}$ that have intensity b in image $B^{\mathcal{T}}$.

$$\Omega_b^{\mathsf{T}} = \{\mathbf{x}_A \in \Omega_{A,B}^{\mathsf{T}} | B^{\mathcal{T}}(\mathbf{x}_A) = b\} \tag{3.5}$$

3.2.1   Image Field of View

For intrasubject registration, the object being studied is the same for both images, but the domains Ω_A and Ω_B may be different in extent, and are always different in position and/or orientation. The domain over which the transformation $\mathcal{T}$ is valid is $\Omega_{A,B}^{\mathsf{T}}$. This domain is, in general, smaller than either Ω_A or Ω_B, and also is a function of the transformation **T**. The latter point is important and sometimes overlooked. It is true even if the images A and B have identical fields of view, since any translation or rotation of image B with respect to image A will alter the overlap domain. For registration algorithms that make use of corresponding geometrical features, the difference in field of view of images A and B can cause difficulties, as features identified in one image may not be present in the second. The dependence of $\Omega_{A,B}^{\mathsf{T}}$ on **T** is, however, not especially important in these algorithms. For registration algorithms that make use of image intensity values to iteratively determine **T**, greater difficulties arise. The isointensity sets used by these algorithms are the sets of fixed intensities within $\Omega_{A,B}^T$. Since $\Omega_{A,B}^T$ changes with **T**, algorithms that are too sensitive to changes in $\Omega_{A,B}^T$ may be unreliable.

The difficulty caused by the different fields of views of images *A* and *B* is further illustrated by considering an approach to rigid-body registration called the method of moments.[1] When applying this to images of a part of the body, e.g., the head, that part of the body is first delineated from images *A* and *B* using a segmentation algorithm, giving the binary volumes O_A and O_B. The images can then be registered by first aligning the centroids (from the first order moment) of O_A and O_B, and then aligning the principal axes of O_A and O_B (from the second order moment). This approach is, however, unsatisfactory for most medical image registration applications because the first and second order moments are highly sensitive to change in image field of view. In order for this method to work accurately, the object used for the calculations must be entirely within $\Omega_{A,B}^T$, and it is frequently difficult to delineate structures with this property.

3.2.2   The Discrete Nature of the Images

Another important property of the medical images with which we work is that they are discrete. That is, they sample the object at a finite number of voxels. In general, this sampling is different for images *A* and *B*, and while the sampling is commonly uniform in a given direction, it may be anisotropic; that is, it varies along the different axes of the images. Discretization has important consequences for image registration, so it is useful to build this concept into our notational framework.

We can define our domain Ω in the following way.

$$\Omega =: \tilde{\Omega} \cap \Gamma_\varsigma \tag{3.6}$$

where $\tilde{\Omega}$ is a *bounded* continuous set defining the volume of the patient imaged, and Γ is an infinite discrete grid. Γ is our *sampling* grid, which is characterized by the anisotropic sample spacing $\varsigma = (\varsigma^x, \varsigma^y, \varsigma^z)$. The sampling is normally different for the images *A* and *B* being registered, and we denote this by introducing sampling grids Γ_{ς_A} and Γ_{ς_B} for the domains Ω_A and Ω_B.

For any given **T**, the intersection of the discrete domains Ω_A and Ω_B is likely to be the empty set, because no sample points will exactly overlap. In order, therefore, to compare the images *A* and *B* for any estimate of **T** it is necessary to interpolate between sample positions and to take account of the differences in sample spacing ς_A and ς_B. This introduces two problems. First, fast interpolation algorithms are imperfect, introducing blurring or ringing into the image. This changes the image histograms and hence alters the isointensity sets discussed above. Second, we must be careful when the image *B* being transformed has higher resolution sampling than the reference image *A*, or we risk aliasing when we resample *B* from Ω_B to generate B^T in Ω_A. In this case, we should first blur *B* with a filter of resolution ς_A or lower before resampling.

Because the transformation $\mathcal{T}$ maps both positions and intensities at these positions, $\mathcal{T}$ (unlike the spatial mapping $\mathbf{T}$) has to take account of the discrete sampling.

3.3   Types of Transformation

The spatial mapping $\mathbf{T}$ describes the relationship between locations in one image and corresponding locations in a second image. The images could be two-dimensional (2D) or three-dimensional (3D), so the mapping may be from 2D space to 2D space, from 3D space to 3D space, or between 3D and 2D space. In all cases, the object being imaged—all or part of a human subject—is three-dimensional. There are consequently very few situations in which a 2D–2D mapping adequately aligns two images. The most common applications of image registration involve aligning pairs of 3D images. Another important application is aligning 2D images with 3D images (2D–3D registration). In 2D–3D registration, $\mathbf{T}$ involves a 3D–3D mapping followed by projection of the 3D object onto a 2D plane.

If the images registered are of the same object that is merely in a different position, then we can describe the required registration transformation using just translations and rotations. This gives us a rigid-body transformation. In three dimensions, this has six degrees of freedom which can be defined as translation in the x, y, and z directions, and rotations α, β, and γ about these three axes. From these unknowns, we can construct a *rigid-body* transformation matrix $\mathbf{T}_{rigid}$ that will map any point in one image to a transformed point in the second. This transformation can be represented as a rotation $\mathbf{R}$ followed by a translation $\mathbf{t} = (t_x, t_y, t_z)^T$ that can be applied to any point $\mathbf{x} = (x, y, z)^T$ in the image:

$$\mathbf{T}_{rigid}(\mathbf{x}) = \mathbf{R}\mathbf{x} + \mathbf{t} \qquad (3.7)$$

where the rotation matrix $\mathbf{R}$ is constructed from the rotation angles as follows:

$$\mathbf{R} = \begin{pmatrix} \cos\beta\cos\gamma & \cos\alpha\sin\gamma + \sin\alpha\sin\beta\cos\gamma & \sin\alpha\sin\gamma - \cos\alpha\sin\beta\cos\gamma \\ -\cos\beta\sin\gamma & \cos\alpha\cos\gamma - \sin\alpha\sin\beta\sin\gamma & \sin\alpha\cos\gamma + \cos\alpha\sin\beta\sin\gamma \\ \sin\beta & -\sin\alpha\cos\beta & \cos\alpha\cos\beta \end{pmatrix} \quad (3.8)$$

For a 2D–3D rigid-body registration, we need to consider both the rigid-body transformation and a projection of the transformed 3D object onto a plane.

When combining rigid-body transformations with projections, it can be useful to combine the translational and rotational components of the rigid-body transformation into a single 4×4 matrix using homogeneous coordinates:

$$T_{rigid}(x) = \begin{pmatrix} \cos\beta\cos\gamma & \cos\alpha\sin\gamma + \sin\alpha\sin\beta\cos\gamma & \sin\alpha\sin\gamma - \cos\alpha\sin\beta\cos\gamma & t_x \\ -\cos\beta\sin\gamma & \cos\alpha\cos\gamma - \sin\alpha\sin\beta\sin\gamma & \sin\alpha\cos\gamma + \cos\alpha\sin\beta\sin\gamma & t_y \\ \sin\beta & -\sin\alpha\cos\beta & \cos\alpha\cos\beta & t_z \\ 0 & 0 & 0 & 1 \end{pmatrix} \begin{pmatrix} x \\ y \\ z \\ 1 \end{pmatrix}$$

(3.9)

It is common to consider projection of an object defined in (x, y, z) space along the z axis onto the u, v plane. The projection can be characterized by the intrinsic parameters of the imaging system (u_0, v_0, k_u, k_v). For projection x-ray, we can interpret these as follows: u_0 and v_0 define the ray-piercing point (the point in the (u, v) imaging plane from which a normal vector goes through the x-ray source), and k_u and k_v equal the pixel sizes in the horizontal (u) and vertical (v) directions, respectively, divided by the imaging-plane-to-focal-spot distance. These intrinsic parameters can often be determined by calibration of the imaging system. Alternatively, they can be considered as unknowns, adding four degrees of freedom to the registration algorithm. This transformation $T_{projection}$ can be represented as a 4×3 matrix which projects the 3D object along the z axis:

$$T_{projection} = \begin{pmatrix} k_u & 0 & u_0 & 0 \\ 0 & k_v & v_0 & 0 \\ 0 & 0 & 1 & 0 \end{pmatrix}$$

(3.10)

A 3D point in homogeneous coordinates $(x, y, z, 1)^T$ is multiplied by this matrix, giving a vector $(\lambda u, \lambda v, \lambda)^T$, and the resulting 2D point on the projection plane $(u, v)^T$ is obtained by dividing the first and second elements of the vector by the third element λ, which is a scaling factor.

The transformation required for rigid-body 2D–3D registration, T_{2D-3D} is the composition of the projection and rigid-body transformations:

$$T_{2D-3D} = T_{projection} T_{rigid}$$

(3.11)

Further details about projection transformations and homogeneous coordinates can be obtained from many books on graphics and computer vision, including Foley et al.[2]

When we are considering structures made of bone or enclosed in bone, this rigid-body transformation (or rigid-body transformation followed by projection) can correctly align images of the same object in different positions. This assumption works remarkably well for images of the brain, as the bone of the skull restricts the movement of the brain to less than 1 mm.[3*] Unfortunately, repositioning patients often results in changes in the position of objects that cannot simply be described using translations and rotations. We can extend the transformation a little, while still maintaining a single matrix that will transform all points in the image, if we restrict the additional changes to stretches and skews. This gives an *affine transformation*. Unfortunately, soft tissue in the body tends to deform in more complicated ways, so an affine transformation does not add greatly to the number of registration problems that can be solved. Whereas the rigid-body transformation preserves the distance between all points in the object transformed, an affine transformation preserves parallel lines. Two areas where affine transformations are useful are in correcting for scanner errors (which can be errors in scale or skew) and in approximate alignment of brain images from different subjects. These applications are discussed in Chapters 5 and 14, respectively.

For most organs in the body, and for accurate intersubject registration, many more degrees of freedom are necessary to describe the tissue deformation with adequate accuracy. These nonrigid (perhaps more correctly termed nonaffine) registration transformations are discussed further in Chapter 13.

Linear transformations: Many authors refer to affine transformations as linear. This is not strictly true, as a linear map is a special map **L** which satisfies:

$$\mathbf{L}(\alpha \mathbf{x}_A + \beta \mathbf{x}'_A) = \alpha \mathbf{L}(\mathbf{x}_A) + \beta \mathbf{L}(\mathbf{x}'_A) \quad \forall \mathbf{x}_A, \mathbf{x}'_A \in \mathbb{R}^D \qquad (3.12)$$

The translational part of affine transformations violates this. An affine map is more correctly described as the composition of linear transformations with translations.

Furthermore, reflections are a linear transformation, but they are normally undesirable in medical image registration. For example, if a registration algorithm used in image-guided neurosurgery calculated a reflection as part of the transformation, it might result in a patient having a craniotomy on the wrong side of his head. If there is any doubt about whether an algorithm might have calculated a reflection, this should be checked prior to use. Since affine transformations can be represented in matrix form, a reflection can be detected simply from a negative value of the determinant of this matrix.

The term *nonlinear* transformation is often used interchangeably with *nonrigid*. Both terms are used in this book to refer to a transformation with more degrees of freedom than an affine transformation. As stated previously, these types of transformations are discussed in detail in Chapters 13 through 15.

One-to-one transformations: For intrasubject registration, the object imaged with the same or different modalities is one patient. It would at first seem likely that the desired transformation **T** should be one to one. This means that

---

* This is only valid provided the skull remains closed. In neurosurgery, for example, deformation can be much greater.

each point in image A gets transformed to a single point in image B, and vice versa. There are several situations in which this does not happen. First, if the dimensionality of the images is different such as in the registration of a radiograph to a CT scan, a one-to-one transformation is impossible. Second, the issues of image field of view and sampling discussed above mean that parts of the patient sampled in one image may not be present in the second image, even if the patient has not changed.

For various types of nonaffine registration, a one-to-one transformation is not desirable. For example, in registration of images from different subjects, or of the same subject before and after surgery, there may be structures in image A that are absent from image B, or vice versa.

3.4   Registration Algorithms

The algorithms that find **T** given two images are called registration algorithms. In this section we describe algorithms that use points identified in the images (Section 3.4.1), surfaces delineated from the images (Section 3.4.2), and voxel intensity values (Section 3.4.3).

As stated at the start of this chapter, we are using 3D rigid-body registration as the exemplar application. All these algorithms can straightforwardly be extended to the case of affine transformations. These approaches can also be extended to nonaffine registration transformations, but the extension is quite different when using points, surfaces, or voxel intensity values. These nonaffine approaches are discussed in Chapter 13.

3.4.1   Points and the Procrustes Problem

Point-based registration involves identifying corresponding 3D points in the images to be aligned, registering the points, and inferring the image transformation from the transformation determined from the points. The 3D points used for registration are often called *fiducial markers* or *fiducial points*. Using the notation introduced in section 3.2, we want to find points $\{x_A\}$ in image A and $\{x_B\}$ in image B corresponding to the set of features $\{x\}$ in the object. The corresponding points are sometimes called homologous landmarks, to emphasize that they should represent the same feature in the different images. The most common approach is then to find the least square rigid-body or affine transformation that aligns the points. This transformation can subsequently be used to transform any arbitrary point from one image to the other.

3.4.1.1   *The Orthogonal Procrustes Problem*

The orthogonal Procrustes problem draws its name from the Procrustes area of statistics. Procrustes was a robber in Greek mythology. He would offer travelers hospitality in his roadside house and the opportunity to stay the night in a bed that would perfectly fit each visitor. As the visitors discovered to their cost, however, it was the guest who was altered to fit the bed, rather than the bed to fit the guest. Short visitors were stretched to fit, and tall visitors had suitable parts of their bodies cut off so they would fit. The result, it seems, was invariably fatal. The hero Theseus put a stop to this unpleasant practice by subjecting Procrustes to his own method. The term "Procrustes" became a criticism for the practice of unjustifiably forcing data to look like they fit another set. More recently, Procrustes statistics has lost its negative associations and is used in shape analysis.

The Procrustes problem is an optimal fitting problem of least square type: given two configurations of N points in D dimensions $P = \{\mathbf{p}_i\}$ and $Q = \{\mathbf{q}_i\}$, one seeks the transformation $\mathbf{T}$ which minimizes $G(\mathbf{T}) = |\mathbf{T}(P) - Q|^2$. The notation is P, Q are the N-by-D matrices whose rows are the coordinates of the points $\mathbf{p}_i, \mathbf{q}_i$, and $\mathbf{T}(P)$ is the corresponding matrix of transformed points. The standard case is when $\mathbf{T}$ is a rigid-body transformation.[4,5] One can additionally consider scaling, i.e., look for the minimum of similarity transformations.[4] If $\mathbf{T}$ is affine, we are faced with a standard least square.[6]

Solutions: The classical Procrustes problem, i.e., $\mathbf{T} \in \{$rigid-body transformations$\}$ has known solutions. A matrix representation of the rotational part can be computed using Singular Value Decomposition (SVD).[4,6-9]

First replace P and Q by their demeaned versions

$$\mathbf{p}_i \rightarrow \mathbf{p}_i - \bar{\mathbf{p}}$$

$$\mathbf{q}_i \rightarrow \mathbf{q}_i - \bar{\mathbf{q}}$$

This reduces the problem to the orthogonal Procrustes problem in which we wish to determine the orthogonal rotation $\mathbf{R}$. Central to the problem is the D-by-D correlation matrix $K := P^T Q$, as this matrix quantifies how much the points in Q are "predicted" by points in P. If $P = [\mathbf{p}_1^T, ..., \mathbf{p}_N^T]^T$ is a matrix of row vectors (and the same for Q), $K = \Sigma_i K_i$ where $K_i := \mathbf{p}_i \mathbf{q}_i^T$, then:

$$K = UDV^t \Rightarrow \mathbf{R} = V \Delta U^T \qquad \Delta := \mathrm{diag}(1, 1, \det(VU^T))$$

where $K = UDV^T$ is the SVD of K.

It is essential for most medical registration applications that $\mathbf{R}$ does not include any reflections. This can be detected from the determinant of VU^T, which should be $+1$ for a rotation with no reflection, and will be -1 if there is a reflection. In the above equation, Δ takes this into account.

Finally the translation $\mathbf{t} = \bar{\mathbf{q}} - \mathbf{R}\bar{\mathbf{p}}$.

This approach has been widely used in medical image registration, first for intermodality registration,[10,11] and more recently in image–guided surgery.[12] The theory of errors has been advanced in the medical application domain through the work of Fitzpatrick and colleagues.[5,13]

The Procrustes algorithm is used for determining rigid-body or affine transformations. Point landmarks can also be used to determine nonaffine transformations using algorithms such as the thin-plate spline described in Chapter 13.

3.4.1.2 Errors in Rigid-Body Point Registration

It is clear that the localization of the fiducial points is never perfect. This is what Fitzpatrick et al.[5] call the fiducial localization error (FLE). The least square residual itself is called the fiducial registration error (FRE), and this has a distribution described by Sibson.[14] Fitzpatrick et al. stress that what really matters is not the value of FRE, as the fiducials are not the points of interest, but what they defined as the target registration error (TRE), i.e., the error induced by FLE at a given target. Explicitly, if the FLE is ε, the rotation and translations which solve the Procrustes problem are going to be dependent on ε: $\mathbf{T}_\varepsilon := (\mathbf{R}_\varepsilon, \mathbf{t}_\varepsilon)$. The TRE at the target x is then $|\mathbf{T}_\varepsilon(\mathbf{x}) - \mathbf{T}(\mathbf{x})|$, and to first order in ε, this decreases as in $1/\sqrt{N}$, where N is the number of fiducial points.[5] This result can be summarized as follows. The squared expectation value of TRE at position x, (coordinates $(x_1,\ldots, x_D)$ in D dimensions) is going to be (to first order)

$$\langle \text{TRE}(\mathbf{x})^2 \rangle \cong \langle \text{FLE} \rangle^2 \left(\frac{1}{N} + \frac{1}{D} \sum_{i}^{D} \sum_{j \neq i}^{D} \frac{x_i^2}{\Lambda_i^2 + \Lambda_j^2} \right)$$

where Λ are the singular values of the marker locations, and are related to the distribution of markers with respect to the principal axes of the point distribution.

3.4.2 Surface Matching

Boundaries, or surfaces, in medical images are frequently more distinct than landmarks, and various segmentation algorithms can successfully locate high contrast surfaces. This is especially true of the skin surface—the boundary between tissue and air—which is high contrast in most imaging modalities, with the important exception of certain tracers in nuclear medicine emission tomography. If equivalent surfaces can be automatically segmented from two images to be combined, then rigid-body registration can be achieved by fitting the surfaces together. The surface matching algorithms described below are normally only used for rigid-body registration. An alternative approach that does not require automatic segmentation but which can be thought of as an interactive version of surface matching, is to provide the user with an interactive image transformation package that allows the user to translate and rotate one image with respect to the other, while displaying the edge-map from the image being transformed on top of the intensity values of the reference image.[15]

3.4.2.1   The Head and Hat Algorithm

Pelizzari and colleagues[16,17] proposed a surface fitting technique for registration of images of the head that became known as the "head and hat" algorithm. Two equivalent surfaces are identified in the images. The first, from the higher resolution modality, is represented as a stack of disks and is referred to as the head. The second surface is represented as a list of unconnected 3D points. The registration transformation is determined by iteratively transforming the (rigid) hat surface with respect to the head surface, until the closest fit of the hat onto the head is found. The measure of closeness of fit used is the square of the distance between a point on the hat and the nearest point on the head, in the direction of the centroid of the head. The iterative optimization technique used is the Powell method.[18] The Powell optimization algorithm performs a succession of one dimensional optimizations, finding in turn the best solution along each of the six degrees of freedom, and then returning to the first degree of freedom. The algorithm stops when it is unable to find a new solution with a significantly lower cost (as defined by a tolerance factor) than the current best solution. This algorithm has been used with considerable success for registering images of the head,[17] and has also been applied to the heart.[19] As first described, the head surface was derived from MR data, and the hat surface from PET data. The surfaces most commonly used are the skin surface (from MR and PET transmission images) or the brain surface (from MR images and PET emission images).

3.4.2.2   Distance Transforms

The performance of the head and hat algorithm was improved by using a distance transform to preprocess the head images. A distance transform is applied to a binary image in which object pixels (or voxels) have the value 1, and other voxels have the value 0. All voxels in this image are labeled with their distance from the surface of the object. By prelabeling all image voxels in this way, the computational cost per iteration can be substantially reduced (potentially to a single address manipulation and accumulation for each transformed hat surface point). A widely used distance transform is the chamfer filter proposed by Borgefors.[20] This approach was used for rigid-body medical image registration, e.g. by Jiang[21] and van Herk.[22] More recently, exact Euclidean distance transforms have been used in place of the chamfer transform.[23]

Given estimates for the six degrees of freedom of the rigid-body transformation, the hat points are transformed and their distances from the head surface are calculated from the values in the relevant voxels in the distance transform. These values are squared and summed to calculate the cost associated with the current transformation estimate. The risk of finding local optima can be reduced by starting out registration at low resolution and gradually increasing the resolution to refine the accuracy, combined with outlier rejection to ignore erroneous points.[21]

3.4.2.3   Iterative Closest Point (ICP)

The ICP algorithm was proposed by Besl and McKay in 1992[24] for the registration of 3D shapes. It was not designed with medical images in mind, but has subsequently been applied to medical images with considerable success, and is now probably the most widely used surface matching algorithm in medical imaging applications.[25-27] The original paper is written in terms of registration of collected data to a model. The collected data, $\mathcal{P}$, could come from any sensor that provides 3D surface information, including laser scanners, stereo video, and so forth. The model data, χ, could come from a computer-aided design model. In medical imaging applications, both sets of surface data might be delineated from radiological images, or the model might be derived from a radiological image and the data from stereo video acquired during an operation. The algorithm is designed to work with seven different representations of surface data: point sets, line segment sets (polylines), implicit surface, parametric curves, triangle sets, implicit surfaces, and parametric surfaces. For medical image registration the most relevant representations are likely to be point sets and triangle sets, as algorithms for delineating these from medical images are widely available.

The algorithm has two stages and iterates. The first stage involves identifying the closest model point for each data point, and the second involves finding the least square rigid-body transformation relating these point sets. The algorithm then redetermines the closest point set and continues until it finds the local minimum match between the two surfaces, as determined by some tolerance threshold.

Whatever the original representation of the data surface $\mathcal{P}$, it is first converted to a set of points $\{\mathbf{p}_i\}$. The model data remain in their original representation. The first stage involves identifying, for each point $\mathbf{p}_i$ on the data surface $\mathcal{P}$, the closest point on the model surface χ. This is the point $\mathbf{x}$ in χ for which the distance d between $\mathbf{p}_i$ and $\mathbf{x}$ is minimum.

$$d(\mathbf{p}_i, \chi) = \min_{\mathbf{x} \in \chi} \|\mathbf{x} - \mathbf{p}_i\|$$

The resulting set of closest points (one for each $\mathbf{p}_i$) is $\{\mathbf{q}_i\}$. For a triangulated surface, which is the most likely model representation from medical image data, the model χ comprises a set of triangles $\{t_i\}$. The closest model point to each data point is found by linearly interpolating across the facets. If triangle t_i has vertices $\mathbf{r}_1$, $\mathbf{r}_2$, and $\mathbf{r}_3$, then the smallest distance between the point $\mathbf{p}_i$ and the triangle t_i is

$$d(\mathbf{p}_i, t_i) = \min_{u+v+w=1} \|u\mathbf{r}_1 + v\mathbf{r}_2 + w\mathbf{r}_3 - \mathbf{p}_i\|$$

where $u \in [0, 1]$, $v \in [0, 1]$ and $w \in [0, 1]$. The closest model point to the data point $\mathbf{p}_i$ is, therefore, $\mathbf{q}_i = (u\mathbf{r}_1, v\mathbf{r}_2, w\mathbf{r}_3)$.

A least squares registration between the points $\{\mathbf{p}_i\}$ and $\{\mathbf{q}_i\}$ is then carried out using the method* described in Section 3.4.1. The set of data points $\{\mathbf{p}_i\}$ is then transformed to $\mathbf{p}_i'$ using the calculated rigid-body transformation, and then the closest points once again identified. The algorithm terminates when the change in mean square error between iterations falls below a defined threshold.

The optimization can be accelerated by keeping track of the solutions at each iteration. If there is good alignment between the solutions (to within some tolerance), then both a parabola and straight line are fitted through the solutions, and the registration estimate is updated using one of these estimates based on a slightly ad-hoc method to be "on the safe side."

As the algorithm iterates to the local minimum closest to the starting position, it may not find the correct match. The solution proposed by Besl and McKay[24] is to start the algorithm multiple times, each with a different estimate of the rotation alignment, and choose the minimum of the minima obtained.

3.4.3 Voxel Similarity Measure

Registration using voxel similarity measure involves calculating the registration transformation T by optimizing some measure calculated directly from the voxel values in the images rather than from geometrical structures such as points or surfaces derived from the images. As stated in Section 3.2, with voxel similarity measures we are iteratively determining T, whereas in the case of point registration or surface matching we first identify corresponding features, determine $\mathbf{T}$ directly or iteratively from these, and finally infer T.

In Sections 3.4.1 and 3.4.2, we did not distinguish between registration where images A and B are of the same modality and registration of A and B when they are of different modalities. For registration using voxel similarity measures this is an important distinction, as seen from the following example. A common reason for carrying out same modality, or intramodality, registration is to compare images from a subject taken at slightly different times in order to ascertain whether there have been any subtle changes in anatomy or pathology. If there has been no change in the subject, we might expect that after registration and subtraction there will be no structure in the difference image, just noise. Where there is a small amount of change in the structure, we would expect to see noise in most places in the images, with a few regions visible in which there has been some change. If there were a registration error, we would expect to see artifactual structure in the difference image resulting from the poor alignment. In this application, various voxel similarity measures suggest themselves. We could, for example, iteratively calculate T while minimizing the structure in the difference image on the grounds that at correct registration there will be either

---

* In fact, the authors used the equivalent quaternion method.[24]

no structure or a very small amount of structure in the difference image, whereas with increasing misregistration, the amount of structure would increase. The structure could be quantified, for example, by the sum of squares of difference values, the sum of absolute difference values, or the entropy of the difference image. An alternative intuitive approach (at least for those familiar with signal processing techniques) would be to find T by cross-correlation of images A and B.

With intermodality registration, the situation is quite different. There is, in general, no simple relationship between the intensities in the images A and B. No simple arithmetic operation on the voxel values is, therefore, going to produce a single derived image from which we can quantify misregistration.

There have been some interesting attempts to overcome this difficulty by preprocessing the images to make them more alike. One approach is to make one of the images being registered look like the other. This has been applied to MR-CT registration by remapping the high CT intensities to low intensities to make the CT images look more like MR images,[28] and to MR and PET registration by simulating a PET image from the MR image.[33] A second approach is to generate similar derived images from each modality, e.g., by applying scale-space derivatives to both images in order to identify intensity ridges, which, at an appropriate scale, should be similar between modalities.[29]

Recent algorithm developments have, perhaps surprisingly, resulted in techniques applicable to both intermodality and intramodality registration, and which work well for a wide variety of applications without the need for modality-specific preprocessing. The most successful of the current approaches are based on ideas that come from information theory.

In Sections 3.4.4 to 3.4.8 we describe some of the most widely used voxel similarity measures for medical image registration. With all these similarity measures it is necessary to use an optimization algorithm to iteratively find the transformation T that maximizes or minimizes the value of the measure, as appropriate. It is also necessary to implement appropriate resampling and interpolation techniques for use in each iteration, taking into account the issues raised in Section 3.2.

3.4.4 Minimizing Intensity Difference

One of the simplest voxel similarity measures is the sum of squared intensity differences (SSD) between images which is minimized during registration. For voxel locations x_A in image A, within an overlap domain $\Omega_{A,B}^T$ comprising N voxels:

$$\text{SSD} = \frac{1}{N} \sum_{x_A \in \Omega_{A,B}^T} |A(x_A) - B^T(x_A)|^2 \tag{3.13}$$

The measure, like other voxel similarity measures, needs to be normalized so that it is invariant to the number of voxels N in the overlap domain $\Omega_{A,B}^T$.

It can be shown that this is the optimum measure when two images only differ by Gaussian noise.[30] For intermodality registration, this will never be the case. This strict requirement is seldom true for intramodality registration either, as noise in medical images such as modulus MRI scans is frequently not Gaussian, and also because there has likely been change in the object being imaged between acquisitions or there would be little purpose in registering the images!

The SSD measure is widely used for serial MR registration, for example by Hajnal et al.,[31,32] and by Friston's statistical parametric mapping (SPM) software.[33,34] The SPM approach uses a linear approximation (often with iterative refinement) based on the assumption that the starting estimate is close to the correct solution and the image is smooth, rather than the iterative approach used by other researchers.

The SSD measure is very sensitive to a small number of voxels that have very large intensity differences between images A and B. This might arise, for example, if contrast material is injected into the patient between the acquisition of images A and B, or if the images are acquired during an intervention and instruments are in different positions relative to the subject in the two acquisitions. The effect of these "outlier" voxels can be reduced by using the sum of absolute differences, SAD rather than SSD:

$$\text{SAD} = \frac{1}{N} \sum_{x_A \in \Omega_{A,B}^T} |A(x_A) - B^T(x_A)| \tag{3.14}$$

3.4.5 Correlation Techniques

The SSD measure makes the implicit assumption that after registration the images differ only by Gaussian noise. A slightly less strict assumption would be that at registration there is a linear relationship between the intensity values in the images. In this case, the optimum similarity measure is the correlation coefficient CC

$$\text{CC} = \frac{\sum_{x_A \in \Omega_{A,B}^T} (A(x_A) - \bar{A}) \cdot (B^T(x_A) - \bar{B})}{\left\{ \sum_{x_A \in \Omega_{A,B}^T} (A(x_A) - \bar{A})^2 \cdot \sum_{x_A \in \Omega_{A,B}^T} (B^T(x_A) - \bar{B})^2 \right\}^{1/2}} \tag{3.15}$$

where $\bar{A}$ is the mean voxel value in image A within the domain $\Omega_{A,B}^T$, and $\bar{B}$ is the mean of B^T within $\Omega_{A,B}^T$. The correlation coefficient can be thought of as a normalized version of the widely used cross correlation measure C.

$$C = \frac{1}{N} \sum_{x_A \in \Omega_{A,B}^T} A(x_A) \cdot B^T(x_A) \tag{3.16}$$

One interesting property of correlation techniques is that correlation can be carried out in either the spatial domain or the spatial frequency domain (k-space).

In k-space, rigid-body transformations have special properties due to the properties of the Fourier transform.[35] In particular, a spatial domain translation becomes a phase change in k-space. The modulus of k-space or power spectrum of the image does not contain any phase information and is, therefore, invariant to translation. Rotations in the spatial domain are rotations by the same angle in k-space. Rotation can be decoupled from translation by computing the modulus of the data. By converting to a polar representation of k-space, the rotation becomes a simple shift of angular coordinate, which can be solved by correlation of the polar representation of the magnitude of k-space. Once the rotation has been found, the translation can be determined from the phase difference in the Cartesian k-space. This approach is not iterative, so it can be fast. This type of approach has been applied to medical images,[36,37] but the applicability appears to be limited by the implicit assumption that the objects of interest are in the fields of view of both images being registered, i.e., that all image features are contained in the overlap domain $\Omega_{A,B}^T$. Since medical images almost invariably only sample part of the patient, segmentation of features of interest that lie within $\Omega_{A,B}^T$ is necessary before this approach can be reliably used.[37]

3.4.6 Ratio Image Uniformity (RIU)

This algorithm was originally introduced by Woods[38] for the registration of serial PET studies, but has more recently been widely used for serial MR registration.[39] The algorithm can be thought of as working with a derived ratio image calculated from images A and B. An iterative technique is used to find the transformation T that maximizes the uniformity of this ratio image, which is quantified as the normalized standard deviation of the voxels in the ratio image. The RIU acronym was not introduced when the algorithm was first published, and it is also frequently referred to as the variance of intensity ratios algorithm (VIR). The RIU algorithm is most easily thought of in terms of an intermediate ratio image R comprising N voxels within the overlap domain $\Omega_{A,B}^T$.

$$R(\mathbf{x}_A) = \frac{A(\mathbf{x}_A)}{B^T(\mathbf{x}_A)} \ \forall \mathbf{x}_A \in \Omega_{A,B}^T, \qquad \bar{R} = \frac{1}{N} \sum_{\mathbf{x}_A \in \Omega_{A,B}^T} R(\mathbf{x}_A) \qquad (3.17)$$

$$\mathrm{RIU} = \frac{\sqrt{\frac{1}{N} \sum_{\mathbf{x}_A \in \Omega_{A,B}^T} (R(\mathbf{x}_A) - \bar{R})^2}}{\bar{R}} \qquad (3.18)$$

3.4.7 Partitioned Intensity Uniformity (PIU)

The first widely used intermodality registration algorithm that used a voxel similarity measure was proposed by Woods for MR-PET registration soon after he proposed his RIU algorithm.[40] Here, we refer to this intermodality algorithm as partitioned intensity uniformity (PIU). This algorithm involved a fairly minor change to the source code of his previously published RIU technique (see section 3.4.6), but transformed its functionality. The RIU algorithm is based on an idealized assumption that "all pixels with a particular MR pixel value represent the same tissue type so that values of corresponding PET pixels should also be similar to each other." The algorithm therefore partitions the MR image into 256 separate bins (or isointensity sets) based on the value of the MR voxels, then seeks to maximize the uniformity of the PET voxel values within each bin. Once again, uniformity within each bin is maximized by minimizing the normalized standard deviation.

In the discussion above, we have described the algorithm in terms of MR and PET registration only. We can now formulate the algorithm more generally in terms of images A and B. It is important to note that the two images are treated differently, so there are two different versions of the algorithm, depending on whether image A or image B is partitioned.

For registration of the images A and B, the PIU can be calculated in two ways: either as the sum of the normalized standard deviation of voxel values in B for each intensity a in A (PIU_B) or the sum of the normalized standard deviation of voxel values in A for each intensity b in B (PIU_A).

$$\text{PIU}_B = \sum_a \frac{n_a}{N} \frac{\sigma_B(a)}{\mu_B(a)} \quad \text{and} \quad \text{PIU}_A = \sum_b \frac{n_b}{N} \frac{\sigma_A(b)}{\mu_A(b)} \qquad (3.19)$$

where:

$$n_a = \sum_{\Omega_a^T} 1 \qquad\qquad\qquad n_b = \sum_{\Omega_a^T} 1$$

$$\mu_B(a) = \frac{1}{n_a} \sum_{\Omega_a^T} B^T(\mathbf{x}_A) \qquad \mu_A(b) = \frac{1}{n_b} \sum_{\Omega_b^T} A(\mathbf{x}_A)$$

$$\sigma_B(a) = \frac{1}{n_a} \sum_{\Omega_a^T} (B^T(\mathbf{x}_A) - \mu_B(a))^2 \qquad \sigma_A(b) = \frac{1}{n_b} \sum_{\Omega_b^T} (A(\mathbf{x}_A) - \mu_A(b))^2$$

The PIU algorithm was widely used for MR-PET registration. It requires the scalp to be first removed from the MR image to avoid a breakdown of the idealized assumption described above. The technique was never widely used for registration of other modalities, but its success inspired considerable research activity aimed at identifying alternative voxel similarity measures for intermodality registration.

3.4.8 Information Theoretic Techniques

Image registration can be described as trying to maximize the amount of shared information in two images. In a very qualitative sense, we might say that if two images of the head are correctly aligned, then corresponding structures will overlap so that we will have two ears, two eyes, one nose, and so forth. When the images are out of alignment, however, we will have duplicate versions of these structures from A and B.

Using this concept, registration can be thought of as reducing the amount of information in the combined image, which suggests the use of a measure of *information* as a registration metric. The most commonly used measure of information in signal and image processing is the Shannon-Wiener entropy measure H, originally developed as part of communication theory in the 1940s.[41, 42]

$$H = -\sum_i p_i \log p_i \qquad (3.20)$$

H is the average information supplied by a set of i symbols whose probabilities are given by $p_1, p_2, p_3, \ldots, p_i$.

This formula, except for a multiplicative constant, is derived from three conditions that a measure of uncertainty in a communication channel should satisfy. These are

1. The functional should be continuous in p_i;

2. If all p_i equal $\frac{1}{n}$, where n is the number of symbols, then H should be monotonically increasing in n; and

3. If a choice is broken down into a sequence of choices, then the original value of H should be the weighted sum of the constituent H. That is $H(p_1, p_2, p_3) = H(p_1, p_2 + p_3) + (p_2 + p_3)H\left(\frac{p_2}{p_2 + p_3}\frac{p_3}{p_2 + p_3}\right)$.

Shannon proved that the $-\Sigma p_i \log p_i$ form was the only functional form satisfying all three conditions.

Entropy will have a maximum value if all symbols have equal probability of occurring (i.e., $p_n = \frac{1}{n} \forall i$), and have a minimum value of zero if the probability of one symbol occurring is one, and the probability of all the others occurring is zero.

Any change in the data that tends to equalize the probabilities of the symbols $p_1, p_2, p_3, \ldots, p_i$ (i.e., that makes the histogram more uniform) increases the entropy. Blurring the data reduces noise, and so sharpens the histogram and results in reduced entropy. Registration algorithms often iteratively transform images, and the interpolation algorithms used for these transformations blur the data (as described more fully in Section 3.5). The consequences of interpolation-induced entropy changes need to be carefully considered.

3.4.8.1 *Joint Entropy*

In image registration we have two images, A and B, to align. We therefore have two symbols at each voxel location for any estimate of the transformation T. Joint entropy measures the amount of information we have in the combined images.[41] If A and B are totally unrelated, then the joint entropy will be the sum of the entropies of the individual images. The more similar (i.e., less independent) the images are, the lower the joint entropy compared to the sum of the individual entropies.

$$H(A, B) \leq H(A) + H(B) \tag{3.21}$$

The concept of joint entropy can be visualized using a joint histogram calculated from images A and B, examples of which are shown in Figure 3.1. For all

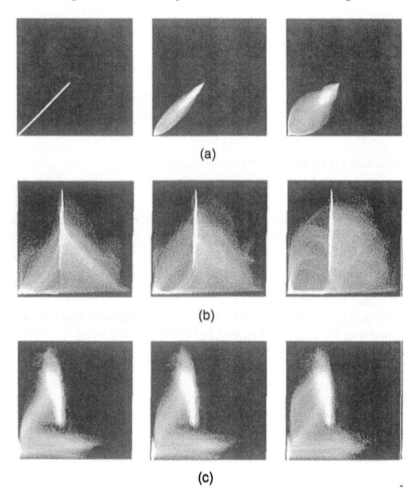

FIGURE 3.1
Example 2D histograms from Hill et al.[43] for (a) identical MR images of the head, (b) MR and CT images of the head, and (c) MR and PET images of the head. For all modality combinations, the left panel is generated from the images when aligned, the middle panel when translated by 2 mm, and the right panel when translated by 5 mm. Note that, while the histograms are quite different for the different modality combinations, misregistration results in a dispersion or blurring of the signal. Although these histograms are generated by lateral translational misregistration, misregistration in other translation or rotation directions has a similar effect.

voxels x_A in the overlapping regions of the images $\Omega^{T}_{A,B}$, we plot the intensity of this voxel in image A, $A(x_A)$ against the intensity of the corresponding voxel in image B, $B^{T}(x_A)$. The joint histogram can be normalized by dividing by the total number of voxels N in $\Omega^{T}_{A,B}$, and regarded as a joint probability distribution function (PDF) p^{T}_{AB} of images A and B. We use the superscript T to emphasize that p^{T}_{AB} changes with T. Due to the quantization of image intensity values, the PDF is discrete, and the values in each element represent the probability of pairs of image values occurring together. The joint entropy $H(A, B)$ is therefore given by:

$$H(A, B) \;=\; -\sum_{a}\sum_{b} p^{T}_{AB}(a, b)\log p^{T}_{AB}(a, b) \tag{3.22}$$

The number of elements in the PDF can either be determined by the range of intensity values in the two images or from a reduced number of intensity "bins." For example, MR and CT images registered could have up to 4096 (12 bits) intensity values, leading to a very sparse PDF with 4096 by 4096 elements. The use of 32 to 256 bins is more common. In the above equation, a and b represent either the original image intensities or the selected intensity bins.

As seen in Figure 3.1, as misregistration increases the brightest regions of the histogram get less bright, and the number of dark regions is reduced. If we interpret the joint histogram as a joint probability distribution, then misregistration involves reducing the highest values in the PDF and reducing the number of zeros in the PDF; this will increase the entropy. Conversely, when registering images we want to find a transformation that will produce a small number of PDF elements with very high probabilities and give us as many zero probability elements in the PDF as possible, which will minimize the joint entropy.

The simple form of the equation for joint entropy (Equation 3.22) can hide an important limitation of this measure. As we have emphasized with the T superscript on the joint probabilities, joint entropy is dependent on T. In particular, p^{T}_{AB} is very dependent on $\Omega^{T}_{A,B}$ which is undesirable, and also on the interpolation algorithm used to transform the image B^{T} at each iteration. The overlap dependence can be made clear by the following example. A change in T may alter the amount of air surrounding the patient overlapping in the images A and B. Since the air region contains noise that will tend to occupy the lowest value intensity bins (e.g., $a = 0$, $b = 0$), changing this overlap will alter the joint probability $p^{T}_{AB}(0, 0)$. If the overlap of air increases, $p^{T}_{AB}(0, 0)$ will increase, reducing the joint entropy $H(A, B)$. If the overlap of air decreases, $p^{T}_{AB}(0,0)$ will reduce, increasing $H(A, B)$. A registration algorithm that seeks to minimize joint entropy will tend, therefore, to maximize the amount of air in $\Omega^{T}_{A,B}$, which may result in an incorrect solution. The interpolation dependence of p^{T}_{AB} is clear if we remember that interpolation algorithms will tend to blur images, which sharpens the corresponding image histogram, changing the joint histogram and consequently joint probability distribution p^{T}_{AB}.

3.4.8.2   *Mutual Information*

A solution to the overlap problem from which joint entropy suffers is to consider the information contributed to the overlapping volume by each image registered as well with the joint information. The information contributed by the images is simply the entropy of the portion of the image that overlaps with the other image volume:

$$H(A) = -\sum_a p_A^T(a) \log p_A^T(a) \tag{3.23}$$

$$H(B) = -\sum_b p_B^T(b) \log p_B^T(b) \tag{3.24}$$

where p_A^T and p_B^T are the marginal probability distributions, which can be thought of as the projection of the joint PDF onto the axes corresponding to intensities in images A and B, respectively. It is important to remember that the marginal entropies are not constant during the registration process. Although the information content of the images being registered is constant, the information content of the portion of each image that overlaps with the other image will change with each change in estimated registration transformation $\mathbf{T}$. Furthermore, with each iteration, image B is transformed to B^T, which involves interpolation, further altering the probabilities. The superscripts on the formulae for the marginal probability distributions reflect this dependence of the probability distribution on $\mathbf{T}$ (i.e., the change in overlap) for image A and on T for image B, which is resampled at each iteration.

Communication theory provides a technique for measuring the joint entropy with respect to the marginal entropies. This measure, introduced as "rate of transmission of information" by Shannon in his 1948 paper that founded information theory,[41] has become known as mutual information $I(A, B)$, and was independently and simultaneously proposed for intermodality medical image registration by researchers in Leuven, Belgium,[44,45] and at Massachusetts Institute of Technology in the U.S.[30,46]

$$I(A, B) = H(A) + H(B) - H(A, B) = \sum_a \sum_b p_{AB}^T(a, b) \log \frac{p_{AB}^T(a, b)}{p_A^T(a) \cdot p_B^T(b)} \tag{3.25}$$

Mutual information can qualitatively be thought of as a measure of how well one image explains the other, and is maximized at the optimal alignment. We can make our description more rigorous if we think more about probabilities. The conditional probability $p(b|a)$ is the probability that B will take the value b given that A has the value a. The conditional entropy is therefore the average of the entropy of B for each value of A, weighted according to the probability of getting that value of A.

$$H(B|A) = -\sum_{a,b} p_{AB}^T(a, b) \log p^T(b|a) = H(A, B) - H(A) \tag{3.26}$$

Using Equation 3.26, we can rewrite the equation for mutual information as:

$$I(A, B) = H(A) - H(B|A) = H(B) - H(A|B) \tag{3.27}$$

The conditional entropy term in Equation 3.27 will be zero if knowing the intensity $A(x_A)$ enables us to perfectly predict the corresponding intensity value in B^T. Registration by maximization of mutual information, therefore, involves finding the transformation that makes image A the best possible predictor for image B^T, within the region of overlap.

Knowing the value of a voxel in image A reduces the uncertainty (and hence entropy) for the value of the corresponding location in image B when the images of the same object are correctly aligned. This can be thought of as a generalization of the assumption made by Woods in his PIU measure. The PIU measure assumes that, at registration, the uniformity of values in B corresponding to a given value a in A should be maximum. The information theoretic approaches assume that, at alignment, the value of a voxel in A is a good predictor of the value at the corresponding location in B. As misregistration increases, one image becomes a less good predictor of the second.

3.4.8.3   Normalized Mutual Information

Mutual information does not entirely solve the overlap problem described above. In particular, changes in overlap of very low intensity regions of the image (especially noise around the patient) can disproportionately contribute to the mutual information. Alternative normalizations of joint entropy have been proposed to overcome this problem.

Three normalization schemes have so far been proposed in journal articles. Equations 3.28 and 3.29 were mentioned in passing in the discussion section of Maes et al.[45]

$$\tilde{I}_1(A, B) = \frac{2I(A, B)}{H(A) + H(B)} \tag{3.28}$$

$$\tilde{I}_2(A, B) = H(A, B) - I(A, B) \tag{3.29}$$

Studholme has proposed an alternative normalization devised to overcome the sensitivity of mutual information to change in image overlap.[47]

$$\tilde{I}_3(A, B) = \frac{H(A) + H(B)}{H(A, B)} \tag{3.30}$$

The third version of normalized mutual information has been shown to be considerably more robust than standard mutual information.[47] Furthermore, it can be shown that the versions of normalized mutual information in Equations 3.28 and 3.30 are closely related.

$$\tilde{I}_3(A, B) = \frac{H(A) + H(B)}{H(A, B)} = \frac{I(A, B)}{H(A, B)} + 1 = \frac{1}{\tilde{I}_1(A, B) - 2} \quad (3.31)$$

3.4.9   Optimization and Capture Ranges

With the exception of registration using the Procrustes technique described in section 3.4.1, and, under certain circumstances, the registration algorithm in the SPM software,[33] all the registration algorithms reviewed in this chapter require an iterative approach in which an initial estimate of the transformation is gradually refined by trial and error. In each iteration, the current estimate of the transformation is used to calculate a similarity measure. The optimization algorithm then makes another (better, we hope) estimate of the transformation, evaluates the similarity measure again, and continues until the algorithm converges, at which point no transformation can be found that results in a better value of the similarity measure, to within a preset tolerance. A review of optimization algorithms can be found in Press et al.[18]

One of the difficulties with optimization algorithms is that they can converge to an incorrect solution called a "local optimum." It is sometimes useful to consider the parameter space of values of the similarity measure. For rigid-body registration, there are six degrees of freedom, giving a six-dimensional parameter space, and for an affine transformation with twelve degrees of freedom, the parameter space has twelve dimensions. Each point in the parameter space corresponds to a different estimate of the transformation. Nonaffine registration algorithms have more degrees of freedom (often many hundreds or thousands), in which case the parameter space has correspondingly more dimensions. The parameter space can be thought of as a high dimensionality image in which the intensity at each location corresponds to the value of the similarity measure for that transformation estimate. If we consider dark intensities as good values of similarity and high intensities as poor ones, an ideal parameter space image would contain a sharp low intensity optimum with monotonically increasing intensity with distance away from the optimum position. The job of the optimization algorithm would then be to find the optimum location given any possible starting estimate.

Unfortunately, parameter spaces for image registration are frequently not this simple. There are often multiple optima within the parameter space, and registration can fail if the optimization algorithm converges to the wrong optimum. Some of these optima may be very small, caused either by interpolation artifacts (discussed further in Section 3.5), or a local good match between features or intensities. These small optima can often be removed from the parameter space by blurring the images prior to registration. In fact, a hierarchical approach to registration is common: the images are first registered at low resolution, then the transformation solution obtained at this resolution is used as the starting estimate for registration at a higher resolution, and so on.[48]

Multiresolution approaches do not entirely solve the problem of multiple optima in the parameter space. It might be thought that the optimization problem involves finding the globally optimal solution within the parameter space, and that a solution to the problem of multiple optima is to start the optimization algorithm with multiple starting estimates, resulting in multiple solutions, and choose the solution which has the best value of the similarity measure. This sort of approach, called "multistart" optimization, can be effective for surface-matching algorithms. For voxel similarity measures, however, the problem is more complicated. The desired optimum when registering images using voxel similarity measures is frequently *not* the global optimum, but is one of the local optima. The following example serves to illustrate this point. When registering images using joint entropy, an extremely good value of the similarity measure can be found by transforming the images such that only air in the images overlaps. This will give a few pixels in the joint histogram with very high probabilities, surrounded by pixels with zero probability. This is a very low entropy situation and will tend to have lower entropy than the correct alignment. The global optimum in parameter space will, therefore, tend to correspond to an obviously incorrect transformation. The solution to this problem is to start the algorithm within the "capture range" of the correct optimum; that is, within the portion of the parameter space in which the algorithm is more likely to converge to the correct optimum than the incorrect global one. In practical terms, this requires that the starting estimate of the registration transformation is reasonably close to the correct solution. The size of the capture range depends on the features in the images and cannot be known *a priori*, so it is difficult to know in advance whether the starting estimate is sufficiently good. This is not, however, a very serious problem, as visual inspection of the registered images can easily show convergence outside the capture range. In this case, the solution is clearly and obviously wrong (e.g., relevant features in the image do not overlap at all). If this sort of failure of the algorithm is detected, the registration can be restarted with a better starting estimate obtained, for example, by interactively transforming one image until it is approximately aligned with the other.

3.5 Image Transformation

Image registration involves determining the transformation **T** that relates the domain of image *A* to image *B*. This transformation can then be used to transform one image into the coordinates of the second within the region of overlap of the two domains $\Omega_{A,B}^{T}$. As discussed in section 3.2, this process involves interpolation and needs to take into account the difference in sample spacing in image *A* and *B*.

3.5.1   A Consideration of Sampling and Interpolation Theory

The origins of the sampling theorem remain a matter of debate. According to conventional wisdom, Shannon showed in 1949[42] that a band-limited signal sampled with an infinite periodic sampling function can be perfectly interpolated using the sinc function interpolant previously proposed by the mathematician Whittaker.[49] According to Butzer and Stens,[50] Shannon had first written down this theorem in 1940, but the Russian Kotel'nikov had discovered it independently in 1933. Furthermore, it appears that Ogura had formulated the theorem even earlier, in 1920 in a Japanese publication, and erroneously attributed his result to Whittaker.[50] Many medical images are, however, not band limited. For example, multislice datasets are not band limited in the through-slice direction, as the field of view is truncated with a top hat function. Even in MR image volumes reconstructed using a 3D Fourier transform, the condition is not usually satisfied because the image data provided by the scanner are often truncated to remove slices at the periphery of the field of view. Also, data provided are modulus, and taking the modulus is a nonlinear operation that can increase the spatial frequency content.*

Even if the images being transformed were band limited, it would not be possible to carry out perfect interpolation using a sinc function, because a sinc function is infinite in extent.

For many purposes, this problem is entirely ignored during medical image analysis. The most widely used image interpolation function is probably trilinear interpolation, in which a voxel value in the transformed coordinates is estimated by taking a weighted average of the nearest eight neighbors in the original dataset. The weightings, which add up to one, are inversely proportional to the distance of each neighbor from the new sample point. For accurate comparison of registered images, for example by subtracting one image from another, the errors introduced by trilinear interpolation become important. It can be shown that trilinear interpolation applies a low-pass filter to the image and introduces aliasing.[52] For transformations that contain rotations, the amount of low-pass filtering varies with position in the image. If subtracting one image from another to detect small change, for example in serial MR imaging, the low-pass filtering in this process can lead to substantial artifacts. Subtracting a low-pass filtered version of an image from the original is a well known edge enhancement method, so even in the case of identical images differing only by a rigid-body transformation, using linear interpolation followed by subtraction does not result in the expected null result, but instead results in an edge-enhanced version of the original.

Hajnal recently brought this issue to the attention of the MR image analysis community[31] and proposed that the solution is to interpolate using a sinc function truncated with a suitable window function such as a Hamming window.

---

* According to Butzer[50] and Unser,[51] more general versions of the sampling theory for functions that are not necessarily band limited were published even earlier than the theorem for the classic band-limited case; in 1927 by Whittaker, and even in 1908 by de la Vallée Poussin.

Care must be taken when truncating the interpolation kernel to ensure that the integral of the weights of the truncated kernel is unity, or an artifactual intensity modulation can result.[51,53]

Various modifications to sinc interpolation have recently been proposed. These fall into three categories: first, the use of sinc functions with various radii truncated with various window functions;[54] second, approximations to windowed sinc functions such as cubic or B-spline interpolants;[54,55] and third, the shear transform, which involves transforming the image using a combination of shears.[56,57] This third approach is fast, though it does result in artifacts in the corners of the image which must be treated with caution.

An assumption implicit in the discussion above is that the original data being interpolated are uniformly sampled. This is not always the case in medical images. MR physics researchers are used to the problem of nonuniform sampling in the acquisition, or k-space domain,[58,59] but this problem is less often considered in the spatial domain. The most common circumstances when nonuniform sampling arises are in free-hand 3D ultrasound acquisition, as discussed in Chapter 5, and in certain types of CT acquistion where the slice spacing changes during the acquisition. The correct way of interpolating from nonuniformly sampled data onto a uniform grid is the reverse of sinc interpolation. This methodology, sometimes used in k-space regridding,[60,61] involves calculating the sinc coefficients to go from the desired uniform sampling points to the nonuniform locations acquired, and inverting the matrix of coefficients in order to do the correct interpolation. In the cases of 3D ultrasound and CT with variable slice spacing, the data are a long way from being band limited, so the benefits of inverse sinc interpolation may be small in any case.

3.5.2 Interpolation during Registration

Many registration algorithms involve iteratively transforming image B with respect to image A while optimizing a similarity measure calculated from the voxel values. Interpolation errors can introduce modulations in the similarity measure with T. This is most obvious for transformations involving pure translations of datasets with equal sample spacing, where the period of the modulation is the same as the sample spacing.[62] This periodic modulation of the similarity measure introduces local optima that can lead to the incorrect registration solution being determined.

The computational cost of "correct" interpolation is far too high for this approach to be used in each iteration, so lower cost interpolation techniques must be used. There are several possible approaches. The first is to use low-cost interpolation, such as trilinear or nearest neighbor, until the transformation is close to the desired solution, then carry out the final few iterations using more expensive interpolation. An alternative strategy is to take advantage of the spatial-frequency dependence of interpolation errors. Trilinear interpolation low-pass filters the data, and therefore, if the images are blurred prior to registration (high spatial frequency components are removed), the interpolation errors are smaller, so errors in the registration are less. Although the loss of resolution that results from blurring is a disadvantage, registration errors caused by interpolation errors can be greater than the loss of precision resulting from blurring.

3.5.3   Transformation for Intermodality Image Registration

It should be emphasized that these interpolation issues are more critical for intramodality registration, where accuracy of considerably better than a voxel is frequently desired, than for intermodality image registration. In intermodality registration, one image is frequently of substantially lower resolution than the other, and the desired accuracy is of the order of a single voxel at the higher resolution. Furthermore, it is common for the final registration solution to be used to transform the lower resolution image to the sample spacing of the higher resolution modality. Interpolation errors are still likely to be present if trilinear interpolation is used without care, and may slightly reduce the registration accuracy or degrade the quality of the transformed images.

3.6   Conclusions

In this chapter, notation for the image registration problem has been introduced, emphasizing the importance of change in image overlap and image resampling in the registration problem. Various image registration algorithms based on corresponding features or image intensity values were then described. Until recently, the great majority of image registration algorithms was restricted to rigid-body or affine transformations, and the algorithms described here reflect that emphasis. Recently, nonaffine registration to compensate for tissue deformation or differences between subjects has become an area of active research. Many of the similarity measures described in Section 3.4.3 can also be applied to nonaffine registration problems by increasing the number of dimensions in the search space. A more thorough treatment of nonaffine registration is given in Chapter 13.

For image-to-physical registration, points and surfaces are widely used for registration because these can easily be identified on the patient in the operating room using a tracked localizer system (discussed in more detail in Chapter 12). For image-to-image registration, the great majority of registration algorithms use intensity information. The most generally applicable of these algorithms are currently based on information theory.

One appeal of these information theoretic approaches, apart from their success, is the mystique that surrounds the word entropy. An interesting anecdote to emphasize this point comes from a conversation between Shannon and Von Neumann (quoted in Applebaum[63]). Apparently Shannon asked Von Neumann which name he should give to his measure of uncertainty. Von Neumann answered, "You should call it 'entropy,' and for two reasons: first, the function is already in use in thermodynamics under that name; second, and more importantly, most people don't know what entropy really is, and if you use the word 'entropy' in an argument, you will win every time!"

References

1. T.L. Faber and E.M. Stokely, Orientation of 3-D structures in medical images, *IEEE Trans. Pattern Anal. Mach. Intell.*, vol. 10, pp. 626–633, 1988.
2. J.D. Foley, A. van Dam, S.K. Feiner, and J.F. Hughes, *Computer Graphics: Principles and Practice*, Addison-Wesley, Reading, MA, 2nd ed., 1996.
3. B.P. Poncelet, V. J. Wedeen, R. M. Weisskoff, and M.S. Cohen, Brain parenchyma motion: measurement with cine echoplanar MR imaging, *Radiology*, vol. 185, pp. 645–651, 1992.
4. I. Dryden and K. Mardia, *Statistical Shape Analysis*, John Wiley and Sons, NY, 1998.
5. J. Fitzpatrick, J. West, and C. Maurer, Jr., Predicting error in rigid-body, point-based registration, *IEEE Trans. Medical Imaging*, vol. 17, pp. 694–702, 1998.
6. G.H. Golub and C.F. van Loan, *Matrix Computations*, Johns Hopkins University Press, Baltimore, 3rd ed., 1996.
7. K. Kanatani, Analysis of 3-D rotation fitting, *IEEE Trans. Pattern Anal. Mach. Intell.*, vol. 16, pp. 543–549, 1994.
8. P.H. Schönemann, A generalized solution of the orthogonal Procrustes problem, *Psychometrika*, vol. 31, pp. 1–10, 1966.
9. S. Umeyama, Least-squares estimation of transformation parameters between two point patterns, *IEEE Trans. Pattern Anal. Mach. Intell.*, vol. 13, pp. 376–380, 1991.
10. A.C. Evans, C. Beil, S. Marrett, C.J. Thompson, and A. Hakim, Anatomical-functional correlation using an adjustable MRI-based region of interest atlas with positron emission tomography, *J. Cereb. Blood Flow Metab.*, vol. 8, pp. 513–530, 1988.
11. D.L.G. Hill, D.J. Hawkes, J.E. Crossman, M.J. Gleeson, T.C.S. Cox, E.E.C.M.L. Bracey, A.J. Strong, and P. Graves, Registration of MR and CT images for skull base surgery using point-like anatomical features, *Br. J. Radiol.*, vol. 64, pp. 1030–1035, 1991.
12. C.R. Maurer, Jr., J.M. Fitzpatrick, M.Y. Wang, R.L. Galloway, Jr., R.J. Maciunas, and G.S. Allen, Registration of head volume images using implantable fiducial markers, *Medical Imaging 1997: Image Processing*, vol. Proc. SPIE 3034, pp. 561–579, 1997.
13. J. West, J. Fitzpatrick, M. Wang, B. Dawant, C. Maurer, Jr., R. Kessler, R. Maciunas, C. Barillot, D. Lemoine, A. Collignon, F. Maes, P. Suetens, D. Vandermeulen, P. van den Elsen, S. Napel, T. Sumanaweera, B. Harkness, P. Hemler, D. Hill, D. Hawkes, C. Studholme, A. Maintz, M. Viergever, G Malandain, X. Pennex, M. Noz, G. Maguire, Jr., M. Pollack, C. A. Pelizzari, R. Robb, D. Hanson, and R. Woods, Comparison and evaluation of retrospective intermodality brain image registration techniques, *J. Computer Assisted Tomogr.*, vol. 21, no. 4, pp. 554–566, 1997.

14. R. Sibson, Studies in the robustness of multidimensional scaling: perturbational analysis of classical scaling, *J. R. Statist. Soc. B*, vol. 41, pp. 217–229, 1979.
15. U. Pietrzyk, K. Herholz, and W.-D. Heiss, Three-dimensional alignment of functional and morphological tomograms, *J. Comput. Assist. Tomogr.*, vol. 14, pp. 51–59, 1990.
16. C.A. Pelizzari, G.T.Y. Chen, D.R. Spelbring, R.R. Weichselbaum, and C.-T. Chen, Accurate three-dimensional registration of CT, PET, and/or MR images of brain, *J. Comput. Assist. Tomogr.*, vol. 13, pp. 20–26, 1989.
17. D.N. Levin, C.A. Pelizzari, G.T.Y. Chen, C.-T. Chen, and M.D. Cooper, Retrospective geometric correlation of MR, CT, and PET images, *Radiology*, vol. 169, pp. 817–823, 1988.
18. W.H. Press, S.A. Teukolsky, W.T. Vetterling, and B.P. Flannery, *Numerical Recipes in C: The Art of Scientific Computing*, Cambridge University Press, Cambridge, England, 2nd ed., 1992.
19. T.L. Faber, R.W. McColl, R.M. Opperman, J.R. Corbett, and R.M. Peshock, Spatial and temporal registration of cardiac SPECT and MR images: methods and evaluation, *Radiology*, vol. 179, pp. 857–861, 1991.
20. G. Borgefors, Distance transformations in arbitrary dimensions, *Comput. Vision Graph. Image Process.*, vol. 27, pp. 321–345, 1984.
21. H. Jiang, R.A. Robb, and K.S. Holton, A new approach to 3-D registration of multimodality medical images by surface matching, *Visualization in Biomed. Computing 1992*, vol. Proc. SPIE 1808, pp. 196–213, 1992.
22. M. van Herk and H.M. Kooy, Automated three-dimensional correlation of CT-CT, CT-MRI and CT-SPECT using chamfer matching, *Med. Phys.*, vol. 21, pp. 1163–1178, 1994.
23. C.T. Huang and O.R. Mitchell, A Euclidean distance transform using grayscale morphology decomposition, *IEEE Trans. Pattern Anal. Mach. Intell.*, vol. 16, pp. 443–448, 1994.
24. P.J. Besl and N.D. McKay, A method for registration of 3-D shapes, *IEEE Trans. Pattern Anal. Mach. Intell.*, vol. 14, pp. 239–256, 1992.
25. E. Cuchet, J. Knoplioch, D. Dormont, and C. Marsault, Registration in neurosurgery and neuroradiotherapy applications, *J. Image Guided Surg.*, vol. 1, pp. 198–207, 1995.
26. J. Declerck, J. Feldmar, M.L. Goris, and F. Betting, Automatic registration and alignment on a template of cardiac stress and rest reoriented SPECT images, *IEEE Trans. Med. Imaging*, vol. 16, pp. 727–737, 1997.
27. C.R. Maurer, Jr., R.J. Maciunas, and J.M. Fitzpatrick, Registration of head CT images to physical space using multiple geometrical features, *Med. Imaging 1998: Image Process.*, vol. Proc. SPIE 3338, pp. 72–80, 1998.
28. P. A. van den Elsen, E.-J.D. Pol, T.S. Sumanaweera, P.F. Hemler, S. Napel, and J. R. Adler, Grey value correlation techniques used for automatic matching of CT and MR brain and spine images, *Visualization Biomed. Computing 1994*, vol. Proc. SPIE 2359, pp. 227–237, 1994.
29. P.A. van den Elsen, J. B. A. Maintz, E.-J. D. Pol, and M.A. Viergever, Automatic registration of CT and MR brain images using correlation of geometrical features, *IEEE Trans. Med. Imaging*, vol. 14, pp. 384–396, 1995.
30. P.A. Viola, *Alignment by Maximization of Mutual Information*, PhD thesis, Massachusetts Institute of Technology, 1995.

31. J.V. Hajnal, N. Saeed, E.J. Soar, A. Oatridge, I.R. Young, and G.M. Bydder, A registration and interpolation procedure for subvoxel matching of serially acquired MR images, *J. Comput. Assist. Tomogr.*, vol. 19, pp. 289–296, 1995.

32. J.V. Hajnal, N. Saeed, A. Oatridge, E.J. Williams, I.R. Young, and G.M. Bydder, Detection of subtle brain changes using subvoxel registration and subtraction of serial MR images, *J. Comput. Assist. Tomogr.*, vol. 19, pp. 677–691, 1995.

33. K.J. Friston, J. Ashburner, J.B. Poline, C.D. Frith, J.D. Heather, and R.S.J. Frackowiak, Spatial registration and normalization of images, *Human Brain Mapping*, vol. 2, pp. 165–189, 1995.

34. J. Ashburner and K.J. Friston, Nonlinear spatial normalization using basis functions, *Human Brain Mapping*, vol. 7, pp. 254–266, 1999.

35. R.C. Gonzalez and R.E. Woods, *Digital Image Processing*, Addison Wesley, Reading, MA, 1992.

36. A. Apicella, J.S. Kippenhan, and J.H. Nagel, Fast multi-modality image matching, *Med. Imaging III: Image Process.*, vol. Proc. SPIE 1092, pp. 252–263, 1989.

37. A. Kassam and M.L. Wood, Fourier registration of three-dimensional brain MR images: exploiting the axis of rotation, *J. Magn. Reson. Imaging*, vol. 6, pp. 894–902, 1996.

38. R.P. Woods, S.R. Cherry, and J.C. Mazziotta, Rapid automated algorithm for aligning and reslicing PET images, *J. Comput. Assist. Tomogr.*, vol. 16, pp. 620–633, 1992.

39. R.P. Woods, S.T. Grafton, C.J. Holmes, S.R. Cherry, and J.C. Mazziotta, Automated image registration: I. General methods and intrasubject, intramodality validation, *J. Comput. Assist. Tomogr.*, vol. 22, pp. 139–152, 1998.

40. R.P. Woods, J.C. Maziotta, and S.R. Cherry, MRI-PET registration with automated algorithm, *J. Comput. Assist. Tomogr.*, vol. 17, pp. 536–546, 1993.

41. C.E. Shannon, The mathematical theory of communication (parts 1 and 2), *Bell Syst. Tech. J.*, vol. 27, pp. 379–423 and 623–656, 1948. Reprint available from http://www.lucent.com.

42. C.E. Shannon, Communication in the presence of noise, *Proc. IRE*, vol. 37, pp. 10–21, 1949. Reprinted in *Proc. IEEE* 86:447–457, 1998.

43. D.L.G. Hill and D.J. Hawkes, Voxel similarity measures for automated image registration, *Visualization Biomed. Computing 1994*, vol. Proc. SPIE 2359, pp. 205–216, 1994.

44. A. Collignon, F. Maes, D. Delaere, D. Vandermeulen, P. Suetens, and G. Marchal, Automated multi-modality image registration based on information theory, in *Information Process. Med. Imaging 1995*, Y. Bizais, C. Barillot, and R. Di Paola, Eds., pp. 263–274, Dordrecht, Kluwer Academic, The Netherlands, 1995.

45. F. Maes, A. Collignon, D. Vandermeulen, G. Marchal, and P. Suetens, Multimodality image registration by maximization of mutual information, *IEEE Trans. Med. Imaging*, vol. 16, pp. 187–198, 1997.

46. W.M. Wells, III, P. Viola, H. Atsumi, S. Nakajima, and R. Kikinis, Multi-modal volume registration by maximization of mutual information, *Med. Image Anal.*, vol. 1, pp. 35–51, 1996.

47. C. Studholme, D.L.G. Hill, and D.J. Hawkes, An overlap invariant entropy measure of 3D medical image alignment, *Pattern Recognition*, vol. 32, pp. 71–86, 1999.

48. C. Studholme, D.L.G. Hill, and D.J. Hawkes, Automated 3D registration of MR and PET brain images by multi-resolution optimisation of voxel similarity measures, *Med. Phys.*, Vol. 24, pp. 25–35, 1997.

49. J.M. Whittaker, Interpolatory function theory, in *Cambridge Tracts in Mathematics and Mathematical Physics No. 33*, ch. 4, Cambridge University Press, 1935.

50. P. Butzer and R. Stens, Sampling theory for not necessarily band-limited functions: a historical overview, *SIAM Rev.*, vol. 34, no. 1, pp. 40–53, 1992.

51. M. Unser, Sampling—50 years after Shannon, *Proc. IEEE*, vol. 88, no. 4, pp. 569–587, 2000.

52. J. Parker, R.V. Kenyon, and D. Troxel, Comparision of interpolating methods for image resampling, *IEEE Trans. Med. Imaging*, vol. 2, pp. 31–39, 1983.

53. N.A. Thacker, A. Jackson, D. Moriarty, and E. Vokurka, Improved quality of re-sliced MR images using re-normalized sinc interpolation, *J. Magn. Reson. Imag.*, vol. 10, pp. 582–588, 1999.

54. T.M. Lehmann, C. Gonner, and K. Spitzer, Survey: interpolation methods in medical image processing, *IEEE Trans. Med. Imaging*, vol. 18, pp. 1049–1075, 1999.

55. M. Unser, Splines: a perfect fit for signal an image processing, *IEEE Signal Process. Mag.*, vol. 16, pp. 22–38, Nov. 1999.

56. W.F. Eddy, M. Fitzgerald, and D.C. Noll, Improved image registration by using Fourier interpolation, *Magn. Reson. Med.*, vol. 36, pp. 923–931, 1996.

57. R.W. Cox and A. Jesmanowicz, Real-time 3D image registration for functional MRI, *Magn. Reson. Med.*, vol. 42, pp. 1014–1018, 1999.

58. J. O'Sullivan, A fast sinc function gridding algorithm for Fourier inversion in computer tomography, *IEEE Trans. Med. Imaging*, vol. 4, pp. 200–207, 1985.

59. C.H. Mayer, B.S. Hu, D.G. Nishimura, and A. Macovski, Fast spiral coronary artery imaging, *Magn. Reson. Med.*, vol. 28, pp. 202–213, 1992.

60. M.D. Robson, A.W. Anderson, and J. Gore, Diffusion-weighted multiple shot echo planar imaging of humans without navigation, *Magn. Reson. Med.*, vol. 38, pp. 82–88, 1997.

61. D. Atkinson, D. Porter, D. Hill, F. Calamante, and A. Connelly, Sampling and reconstruction effects due to motion in diffusion-weighted interleaved echo planar imaging, *Magn. Reson. Med.*, vol. 44, pp. 101–109, 2000.

62. J. Pluim, J.B.A. Maintz, and M.A. Viergever, Interpolation artefacts in mutual information-based image registration, *Comp. Vision Image Understanding*, vol. 77, pp. 211–232, 2000.

63. D. Applebaum, *Probability and Information: An Integrated Approach*, Cambridge University Press, 1996.

4

Preparation and Display of Image Data

Joseph V. Hajnal

CONTENTS

4.1 Introduction

Image registration entails combining information from two or more images. Once images are no longer viewed in isolation, new constraints and requirements arise. Appropriate data must be acquired; various properties of the data that are not normally prominent have consequences for subsequent data processing and the results that can be achieved. Once the data have been acquired they will frequently have to be transferred from the scanning system (MRI, CT, US, etc.) to a separate computer for subsequent processing. This may include data format conversion, coordinate transformation, distortion correction, intensity correction, and so on, in order to achieve consistent input data for the registration process. Finally, it may be necessary to preprocess the data in some way, for example by image segmentation, to provide the registration algorithms with appropriate input information.

These preparation steps form an essential prerequisite to successful comparison or fusion of image data. The purpose of this chapter is to introduce the necessary concepts and terminology and provide information that can help in resolving difficulties in implementation of image registration. The considerations of image acquisition and data preparation described here are pertinent irrespective of the quality, calibration, state of repair, etc., of the imaging hardware employed. In addition, it is also frequently necessary to take account of errors introduced in images as a result of deficiencies in the image acquisition process. These scanner errors are the subject of Chapter 5.

Once the images have been registered and so share a common coordinate system, they will usually need to be assessed or analyzed together, as well as individually. Display of the images to facilitate comparison can present challenges, and a number of methods have been devised. Some common display techniques are also reviewed.

4.2   Image Acquisition

In general, registration of data representing a three-dimensional (3D) object, such as a brain, requires full 3D data coverage. However, many imaging modalities produce individual 2D images analogous to slices through the object, or projections of the 3D object onto a 2D plane (e.g., plain x-ray images). When individual 2D image slices are acquired, these can readily be registered with one another, but the information they contain may be irreconcilably mismatched because of movement of critical structures out of the plane. When registering two 2D projection images, satisfactory registration is often impossible because structures overlapping in one view do not overlap in the second. Modalities such as MRI, CT, SPECT, and PET are frequently used to provide 3D coverage, but this is often in the form of discrete slices which may only provide partial information in the through-slice direction. Such multislice data may deliberately be obtained with gaps between slices to increase acquisition efficiency and/or minimize cross talk between slices. When such data are resliced to a new set of image planes, the missing information at the edges of the original slices results in errors in the final data. Thus, the resliced images are different from those that would have been obtained if a direct image acquisition had been performed at the final slice location. The impact of these errors depends critically on the application and on their magnitude and location. For example, in multimodal registration, where CT or MR images are being used to provide contextual anatomical information, errors in intensity or incorrect resolution of fine structural detail may be of little or no consequence. By contrast, in single modality serial studies using rigid-body registration, such as fMRI, small local intensity errors produced by reslicing incomplete data may be as large as the effects being studied and so may mask true effects or produce false positive results.

A key feature of errors introduced by reslicing incomplete data is that such errors are local in the sense that individual pixels or groups of pixels get corrupted, and the nature of the errors is related to the underlying structure and the missing information. To provide an objective assessment of the nature of the coverage supported by the image data, it is instructive to follow the Fourier space treatment by Noll et al.[1] This analysis is targeted at MRI data but is applicable more generally to other medical images. The key concept is sampling density in the through-slice direction.

We consider the object being imaged (brain, breast, leg, etc.) and examine its Fourier domain representation, which is a spectrum of spatial frequencies. Since the object exists in 3D, its Fourier domain representation also has three dimensions. For simplicity, we will look in detail at one spatial direction, namely the through-slice direction (see Figure 4.1a). Because the object has structure down to microscopic scales, its native spatial frequency spectrum extends over a large range (Figure 4.1b).

We now consider the process of slice definition, for example, by a selective excitation in MRI, the beam of x-rays used in CT, or sonic beam profile in ultrasound, etc. (Figure 4.1c, d). Selection of a single slice may be viewed as multiplication of the object by the slice sensitivity profile and summation or projection in the through-slice direction. Slices can in principle be acquired at any location, so to formulate the problem more generally we may consider replacing each point on the object with the signal that would be achieved for a slice centered at that point. The result is called a convolution of the slice profile with the object (Figure 4.1e). Selection of any given slice is then simply a delta function sample of the convolved distribution. Viewed from the Fourier domain, convolution of the slice profile with the object is equivalent to multiplication of the object spectrum by the slice profile spectrum (Figure 4.1f). In general, the slice spectrum has a more limited frequency content than the object spectrum, so the process reduces available spectral content (Figure 4.1f). Selection of a set of regularly spaced slices with separation d can now be seen as acquisition of a set of samples up to a frequency $\frac{2\pi}{d}$ in the Fourier representation (Figures 4.1g, h). The frequency content not sampled by the process is lost and results in aliasing of information in the slice direction. The process of reslicing resamples the data and redistributes the aliased signals along with the correctly sampled signals to produce corrupted signal intensities (Figure 4.1i, j).

To control the degree of aliasing requires choice of a slice profile, which determines the bandwidth that must be sampled, and sampling with sufficient density in real (object) space to cover the necessary frequency range. This always necessitates overlapping slices, and the degree of overlap is determined by the slice profile. An idealized top hat profile would have a large, potentially infinite spectrum, necessitating sampling at very closely spaced intervals. The implication is extensively overlapped slices and not the intuitive starting point of contiguous slices. Use of softer slice profiles (e.g., Gaussian profiles) degrades slice definition, but requires less dense sampling.[1]

Many medical images are not acquired with uniform sampling; perhaps the most striking example is freehand ultrasound. However, the concepts discussed above provide guiding principles for image acquisition with clear conclusions as to the results of undersampling. If data such as freehand ultrasound

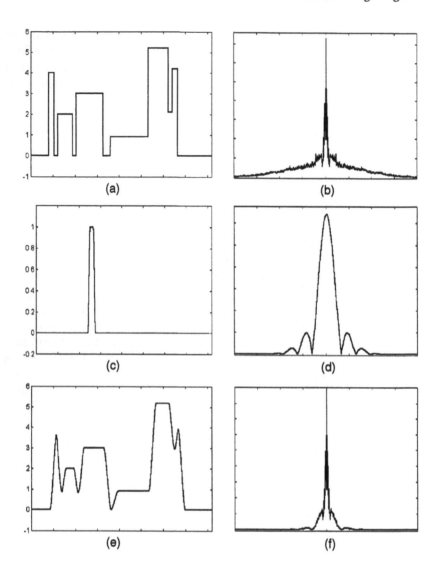

FIGURE 4.1

(a) Real space profile through the object to be imaged. (b) Frequency spectrum obtained from (a) by Fourier transformation. Note the broad wings of the spectrum, reflecting the very wide range of frequencies required to characterize the object. (c) Slice profile used to select a single slice from (a). Within the slice the sensitivity of the imaging system is unity, whereas far from the slice there is zero sensitivity to the object. Gradual transitions exist at the edges of the slice profile. (d) The frequency spectrum obtained for the slice profile by Fourier transformation. Note that although the central maximum is broader than in (b), the full spectrum occupies a much narrower frequency range. (e) The object profile convolved with the slice profile. Selecting a slice corresponds to obtaining a point sample of this profile. (f) The frequency spectrum obtained by Fourier transformation of (e), and equivalent to the product of (b) and (d). Note that the broad wings in (b) have been suppressed, thus narrowing the frequency range that must be sampled.

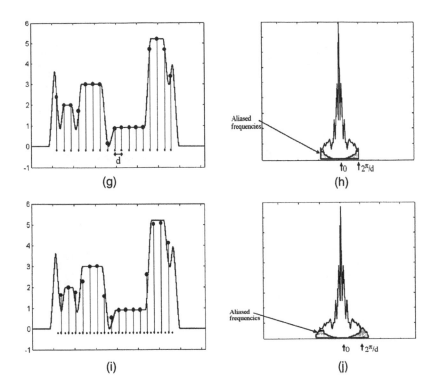

FIGURE 4.1 (continued)
(g) The convolved object sampled at regular intervals with spacing d. The sampled values lie exactly on the convolved object profile. (h) Selection of slices at spacing d results in sampling of the spectrum in (f) up to a frequency of $2\pi/d$. Frequencies outside this range get folded back, resulting in aliasing (shaded regions). Note that the frequency scale (horizontal axis) has been expanded for clarity. (i) Resampling the slices from the originally acquired slice positions results in local signal intensity errors (The calculated sample values no longer lie on the convolved object profile). (j) The process of resampling the slices alters the frequency spectrum because the aliased frequencies interact with the interpolation algorithm. (Note that the spectrum now extends beyond $2\pi/d$. The horizontal frequency scale is the same as in (h)). (Adapted from Noll[1] with thanks to Dr. C. Triantyfallou).

are being deliberately acquired for the purposes of image registration, it may be valuable to monitor spatial coverage and take steps to fill in sparsely sampled regions. When insufficient sampling has been achieved, this can be detected and the final results judged accordingly. A feature of sampling in the real object space, as in slice selection, is that local undersampling results in local vulnerability to intensity errors upon reslicing.

Slice overlap naturally comes at a price, which may be time and/or dose for CT and ultrasound but is further complicated by saturation effects in MRI.[2] Conventional multislice MRI is not obtained with overlapping slices and so is highly vulnerable to data corruption due to aliasing when resliced (Figure 4.2). However, true 3D MRI data, in which Fourier encoding is applied in all three spatial directions, are intrinsically adequately sampled, so are amenable to reslicing without aliasing errors.

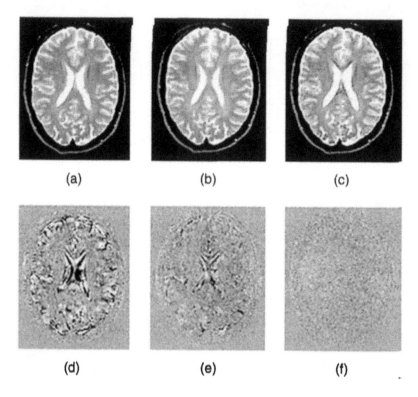

FIGURE 4.2

Transverse T_2 weighted multislice MRI images of the brain of a normal volunteer acquired with a Gaussian slice profile and contiguous slices. (a) First examination; (b) second examination displaced by approximately half the separation between adjacent slices; (c) image (b) resliced after rigid-body registration to match (a); (d) subtraction image (c) minus (a); (e) as (d) but using slices overlapped by 25%; (f) as (d), but using a 50% slice overlap. There are substantial residual signals in (c) arising from incorrectly resliced pixel values because of undersampling in the slice direction. These artifacts are reduced in (d) and virtually absent in (e).

When two datasets with different degrees of undersampling are to be aligned, it may be valuable to consider keeping the least well sampled dataset static and reslicing the other to match the former. Related issues of missing data concern the edges of the region of support of the data, where otherwise adequately sampled images will nevertheless suffer from intensity errors upon reslicing.

Finally, in this context it is significant that MRI data are generally presented and stored in magnitude form although they are intrinsically complex, so that each pixel actually has both a signal magnitude and a phase associated with it. Use of magnitude reconstruction is expedient because it is both congruent with the properties of most image display methods in that only one scalar quality need be presented for each pixel, and because MRI phase varies for instrumental and other reasons and is difficult to keep under control. However, the nonlinear process of forming magnitude images generates aliased frequency components in the image data that again result in intensity errors upon reslicing. These errors occur on the dark side of bright edges and can be very intrusive in data from test objects. Such errors are frequently much less problematic with *in vivo* data. Another critical situation is with sign sensitive data, such as produced by inversion recovery[3] and some field echo sequences,[4] where signal cancellation, resulting in the so called rebound artifact, is produced at the boundary between tissues that present with opposed phases. In these cases the use of phase-corrected real data[3] solves the problem. However, in the most general situation, where the full complex nature of the data is essential, full complex data can be retained for the totality of the registration procedure. This may require modification of some of the widely available registration algorithms or, more pragmatically, the necessary coordinate transformations may be determined from magnitude data. Final reslicing and data comparison may then be performed with the underlying complex images.

A related property of image data is the point spread function (PSF),[5] which is the Fourier transform of the pass band of the imaging system if it has a linear response. In medical imaging, the PSF is generally well defined and well known, and it may be necessary to take it into account in subsequent processing steps such as image interpolation. The Gibbs fringes seen in MR images and in diffraction-limited optical images are a manifestation of the PSF and so are preserved when data are resliced with appropriate image interpolation algorithms. For images such as PET scans, where the intrinsic signal-to-noise ratio is low, it is the practice of some researchers to filter the data and trade off resolution for signal-to-noise ratio (see Chapter 5). The manner in which this is done clearly has a bearing on properties of the resulting data. In general, filtering of image data may be a necessary or desirable procedure which is only problematic if the changes induced in the data structure, such as alteration of the PSF, are not recognized and taken into account in subsequent analysis.

4.3   Image Format Conversion

Digital images are usually stored, displayed, and manipulated as streams of individual intensity values, with one intensity associated with each pixel. The details of how the information is stored are known as image formats. It is essential that any software used to read in such data is programmed to recognize and decode the appropriate format. In addition to the raw image information, image files generally also contain associated information such as patient details, how and when the data were acquired and, most importantly for image registration, the size of the matrix of pixels (number of rows and columns, numbers of slices), details of the spatial location, and length scales that relate the pixel grid to the physical world. This contextual and calibration information is usually stored as a single block of information known as an image header. The header may be part of the image file or stored as a separate file.

The minimum information required for image registration applications is the matrix size and dimensions (or, equivalently, field of view and slice thickness). Other voxel information may also be needed, such as the relationship of the image coordinates to the absolute coordinate frame of the scanner. This may be required to correct for image distortion or other hardware limitations (see Chapter 5).

In addition, the image or separate header file may contain patient-specific information. This can be convenient and can also be a useful check against mistakes that may be introduced by copying files and modifying file names. However, strict laws are now in place to protect the confidentiality of patients, so that unless the data is held in an appropriately secure location, it may be necessary to strip out any information that could be used to identify the subject directly.

Medical images are generally stored and may be archived in a proprietary format that may not be disclosed to the user by the system manufacturer. Subsequent processing requires the data to be exported from the scanner, and this again may be achieved using a variety of data formats. Although manufacturers are sometimes reluctant, or at least slow, to provide information on these file formats, much of this information is now in the public domain, as many groups have "reverse engineered" these formats. Details of the formats can be found on various locations on the Internet.* To deal with the requirement that images exported from equipment from one manufacturer may need to be imported to that of another manufacturer, a medical image standard known as DICOM3** has been devised and has now been widely adopted. This allows data to be freely exchanged between a wide variety of medical equipment including scanners and viewing consoles, as well as many proprietary processing software packages intended for use with medical images. A disadvantage of the DICOM3 standard is that the need to give it universal applicability makes it complex and unwieldy for many applications. Also, like many "standards," individual implementations of DICOM3 can vary in detail, so incompatibilities still occasionally occur. Another image format particularly widely used in the nuclear medicine environment is interfile.***

At the other extreme, there are very simple image formats consisting simply of pixel intensity values or pixel intensity values combined with rudimentary essential information such as the dimensions of the image pixel matrix. One popular format of this type is associated with the Analyse image

---

* Information about a wide range of formats used in medical imaging can be found at *http://www.cica.indiana.edu/graphics/image.formats.html*.
** DICOM is an acronym for Digital Information and Communications in Medicine and is a standard for image transfer developed and sponsored by National Electrical Manufacturers Association (NEMA). Information about DICOM standards can be found at *http://medical.nema.org/dicom.html*.
*** Information about Interfile can be found at *http://www.keston.com/Interfile/interfile.htm*.
For general information see *http://www.cica.indiana.edu/graphics/image.formats.html*.

analysis software,* which consists of a file containing only pixel values, usually stored in binary as short (2-byte) integers, and a separate header file, which contains a simple data structure of basic information.

In addition, there is a variety of widely used image formats not specifically designed for medical images. Common examples include tagged image file format (TIFF), graphics interchange format (GIF), Microsoft window bitmap (BMP), and a standard known as JPEG, developed by the Joint Photographic Experts Group. A specialist digital format developed by the Moving Picture Experts Group, known as MPEG, for storage of movie/video loops, is widely available and useful for displaying medical images of dynamic processes such as cardiac pulsations. Each of these image formats stores data in self-contained files that contain both the image data and header information detailing color maps, use of data compression, etc. In general, these formats do not have provision for integrated storage of patient, examination, or image acquisition details. As with other medical image-specific formats, information about file structures is widely available in the public domain.[†] Many proprietary software packages allow convenient import and export of images in the commonly used formats and also, frequently, conversion from one format to another.

A complicating factor in transferring data from one computer system to another arises from low level details of data storage. Key factors are the number of bytes used to store a given type of number format; for example, in most modern computers floating point numbers are stored as 4, 8, or 16 bytes, depending on the computer, operating system, and data precision. Even if the number of bytes per stored number matches or is corrected for, the order in which multiple bytes are stored has two standard variants. It may therefore be necessary to pass the data through a byte reversing program prior to use on another computer (see Figure 4.3). Some image analysis programs will do this automatically as required. An advantage of the GIF file format is that it only uses one byte per pixel intensity value and therefore does not suffer from this problem. A disadvantage is that this limits the dynamic range of the information that can be stored. In general, it is always prudent to check that the output of one system or package can actually be successfully imported to another.

A final issue associated with image transfer, particularly if images from different sources are combined, is the choice of coordinate system. The way that human images are displayed is a matter of convention; for example, the North American Radiological convention is to display transaxial images with right of the patient at the left of the image and the posterior side at the bottom regardless of how the subject was positioned in the scanner. An on-the-fly coordinate transformation is frequently performed in retrieving data from the hard disk, or other archive, and displaying it on a computer screen. That coordinate transformation may be user defined so that the same data may appear

---

* Analyse is a proprietry format developed at the Mayo Clinic (see *http://www.mayo.edu/bir*).
[†]See footnote on page 80.

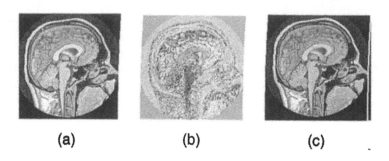

(a)   (b)   (c)

FIGURE 4.3
When data is transferred from one computer to another of a different make it is often
necessary to reverse the byte order of the numbers stored for each pixel value. (a) An image
of the brain stored and displayed on a Sun workstation as an array of short integers with
two bytes per pixel, (b) the same image copied to a Compaq Alpha workstation, and (c) the
image in (b) after byte reversal again displayed in the Compaq computer.

in different orientations depending on the current settings. On-screen labels
are generally provided to remove any ambiguity. However, image registration software may be required to align images originally stored with different
coordinate systems, so care is required to ensure consistency. Use of images
from test objects in which left-right, head-foot, and anterior-posterior orientations can be unambiguously determined provides a simple robust method
of ensuring that all data are presented to the registration algorithms and subsequent display system with appropriate consistency. An advantage of a
comprehensive format such as DICOM3 is that it retains image orientation
information that is likely to be lost in simpler formats.

4.4 Intensity, Size, and Skew Correction

Having achieved a consistent data format and a standardized convention
for the orientation of the data, it may still be necessary to manipulate the
images prior to image registration. Errors in scanner calibration or image
artifacts may need to be dealt with (see Chapter 5). Even with ideal performance, the acquisition techniques may have implications for subsequent
processing. Examples include changes in global intensity scaling during
segmented acquisition with radiotracers, or variation of intensity across
images produced by the use of surface coils in MRI. Algorithms designed to
register similar images such as those based on minimization of least-square-
intensity differences[6,7] may not work robustly if the images have differently
scaled intensity maps. This is easily corrected by manually or automatically
rescaling the images to matched intensity ranges. Most current registration
algorithms are not robust in the presence of large intensity variations across
the images, so it may be necessary to apply intensity correction schemes prior
to registration. MR scanners as well as post processing packages frequently

incorporate surface coil correction algorithms. These are typically based on low pass filtering of the data to suppress image structure and obtain an estimate of the underlying spatial intensity variations, which can then be used to normalize the intensity of the original images. The result is a much more homogeneous appearance, which is likely to avoid failures of registration algorithms but does not preserve intensity relationships between tissues. Recently, more sophisticated algorithms for image intensity corrections that appear to produce a more faithful final intensity distribution have been introduced.[8,9] (See also Figures 14.2 and 14.4 in Chapter 14).

Another discrepancy between images that may need correcting is differences in size, skew, or scaling between images or as a result of drift in scanner calibration with time. It is advisable to calibrate the scanners to be used for collection of images that will be registered both to check that the image dimensions and, in the case of CT, the gantry tilt, are correctly recorded in the header, and also to ensure that any file format conversion process correctly preserves this information. Tilting the gantry is common in CT acquisitions to reduce dose to the eyes or to generate a coronal slice orientation, but, since the direction that the bed moves is not also rotated, this results in the images being skewed (see Chapter 10, Figure 10.2). Correcting skew involves a slice-by-slice translation, which is normally carried out prior to registration. If this skew is not corrected, substantial errors can result. Spatial distortion of images may also need to be addressed. These factors are discussed in the next chapter and may be corrected as part of the registration process or as a preprocessing step.

4.5 Image Segmentation

Under some circumstances, it may be necessary or desirable to specifically exclude some regions of the images from the registration process. The process of dividing images into different regions is known as image segmentation. For example, in multimodality registration of PET and MR or CT images, the Woods algorithm[10] requires elimination of the skull and scalp from the anatomical MRI or CT images in order to produce reliable results. For rigid-body registration of single-subject, single-modality data to subvoxel precision, Hajnal et al.[11] found it helpful to exclude mobile tissue of the face and scalp in order to achieve the most precise results in the brain. This is because, although the brain is well approximated by a rigid body, other tissues may change their shape or other spatial relationships, and so the final global positional match achieved is influenced by both (see Figure 4.4). Other authors have found that, for the image data they considered, presegmentation was unnecessary.[12,13] In recent work on the spine, Little et al. used a composite model in which vertebrae were treated as rigid body surrounded by plastically deforming soft tissue (Figure 4.5).[14] This concept again requires image segmentation (of the vertebrae) as a preparation step.

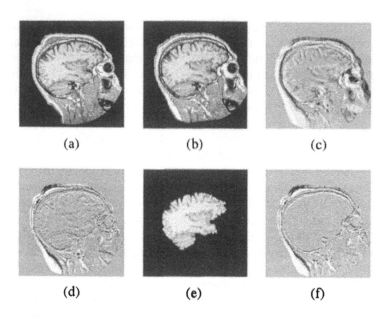

FIGURE 4.4
Serial MRI examination of a patient with a mild head injury: (a) baseline scan; (b) follow-up scan three days later; (c) difference image (b) minus (a); (d) difference image after registration of (b) to align it with (a); (e) segmented version of (a) used to exclude extra-cranial tissues; (f) subtraction image showing the result of registering (b) to (a) using only the segmented data in (e). Residual signals in the brain in (d) result from an inability of the registration algorithm to find a rigid-body transformation that accommodated both the brain and the changed hematoma. Excluding the soft tissue changes using the segmented image (e) allows the registration algorithm to determine a rigid-body transformation for the brain alone. The difference image (f) reveals that the brain is unchanged.

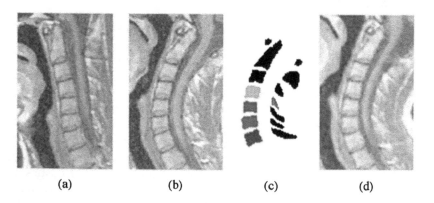

FIGURE 4.5
Example of spine registration showing two scans of the patient in different positions: (a) first position, (b) second position, (c) segmentation of vertebrae treated as rigid bodies by the algorithm, and (d) first image transformed to the coordinates of the second using a nonrigid registration algorithm.[14] Note that although the images shown are all 2D, the algorithm works on the 3D images.

Computer algorithms for image segmentation are widely available and range from simple intensity thresholding with or without manual intervention to complex automated procedures that include a wide range of image processing tools.[15] The segmented images may be stored as gray scale images with pixels in regions to be excluded reset to zero, or as coded masks used in conjunction with the gray scale images. Examples of coding schemes include labeling individual pixels or regions with a one for inclusion and a zero for exclusion, or with numerical values that are associated with designated tissue types.

4.6 Displaying Images

Many computer programs exist for displaying images in general and, in some cases, medical images in particular. When displaying medical images it is important that the images are correctly labeled. Confusion about the patient's identity or orientation (e.g., confusion over left and right in transverse sectional images) or incorrect information about details of data acquisition (e.g., which nuclear medicine tracer or MR sequence was used) could lead to incorrect diagnosis or treatment.

In addition to these usual concerns, a new set of display challenges arises when dealing with registered images. Once the images are in a single data space, it is natural to want to display them in a coherent way and explore spatial relations within the images. Many methods have been devised to achieve this, and the choice depends very much on the application. The following discussion is intended to introduce some frequently used methods and is not a comprehensive review of the topic. More detailed treatments can be found in numerous texts, for example, Bankman.[18]

A much used early technique was to display the images side by side on a workstation and employ a linked cursor so that the act of pointing to a location in one image automatically locates the corresponding location in the registered second image. This is useful for initial exploration and for locating a few localized features. For more global comparisons, image fusion has been used, where data from both images can be viewed as one. Simple methods for doing this include:

1. Color overlay, in which the data sets each contribute to each pixel, but in different colors, or one is coded in hue and the other in gray scale intensity. If features from one image are segmented they may be overlaid in isolation on another aligned image. For example, blood vessels extracted from an angiographic acquisition could simply be superimposed on an anatomical scan, so vessels can be related to anatomical landmarks, even though at the site of the vessels, none of the anatomic image can be seen (e.g., Chapter 10, Color Figure 10.5).

2. Interleaved pixel or checkerboard fusion, in which each pixel displays an intensity purely from one of the images being fused, with the represented image alternating in a regular interleaved pattern. This can be on a pixel-by-pixel basis, or in larger groups of pixels, forming a blocked appearance (e.g., Chapter 11, Color Figure 11.2). This method has the advantage of allowing extra colors to be displayed on older computers which only have eight bit frame buffers. It also provides a rapid means of manipulating color maps to fade one or another image in and out.

3. Dynamic alternating display, in which the computer switches rapidly from one image to the other either automatically or under user control.

4. Split view displays place two images in the same location on the screen with a movable dividing line, so that one image is seen on one side of the line and the other is seen on the other side.

5. Subtraction images is a simple method that is particularly useful in serial studies of the same subject. Subtraction of one registered image from another provides a direct display of change, which can then be related back to the source images. Subtraction images can be viewed separately (see Chapter 7) or overlaid on a source image, for example in color.

6. Displaying images in a standard space (e.g., an atlas such as that due to Talairach[16]) can help in comparison of images from different subjects. The data can be displayed directly, segmented features of interest can be positioned within the standard space, or features can be referred to simply by their coordinate locations within the standard space (see Chapter 14 for examples).

7. Segmenting a surface from one modality, and generating a rendered surface in which intensity is derived from the surface orientation but hue comes from a second set of registered images.

When nonrigid registration methods have been used, critical information may reside not just in the final images produced or difference images derived from them, but also in the deformations required to transform one image into the coordinates of the other. An example of this is a study of growth patterns in the brain during childhood, where brain images from subjects acquired serially over several years were aligned using transformations that included spatial distortions. The pattern of distortions required to make an early scan match a later one then reveals the pattern of growth in the intervening time.[17] Display of deformation fields is a major challenge because the deformations are generally spatial distributions of displacements that may vary in magnitude and direction from point to point in the image space. Such vector distributions, or in some cases tensor distributions (e.g., strain maps), are not easily displayed on flat screens designed to display variations in intensity and/or color. To achieve useful displays, researchers have used arrow pictures in which small variable length arrows are scattered over the display plane, with the direction of each showing the local direction of shift, and the length indicating the magnitude of the shift. Other methods include placement of a regular grid on the original image and displaying the distorted grid after registration is complete (see Chapter 13). Color coding of displacement has also been tried. Techniques for displaying deformation information are likely to develop further as applications for nonrigid registration are explored and precise requirements for the information to be extracted are defined.

4.7 Conclusion

Marshaling the data required to register images can entail a number of steps, ranging from file format conversion to image preparation by intensity correction, image segmentation, etc. Careful data preparation is essential to avoid errors that result in failed registration or data that are at risk of incorrect interpretation. However, the steps required are conceptually simple and, once established, can be made automatic or at least quick and efficient to operate. Such data preparation is likely to be required even when ideal scanner performance is assumed. In practice it is often necessary also to take account of imperfections in the data acquisition process itself. Such imperfections may cause errors that it is essential to correct or at least be aware of. The nature and consequences of these errors are the subject of Chapter 5.

Once image registration becomes a core part of a medical imaging application, it has consequences that have an impact on the whole imaging process, from the way examinations are performed to data acquisition methods, to image handling, image analysis, and, finally, on image presentation and interpretation. Some of the factors discussed in this chapter have implications for data acquisition efficiency, archiving, and processing strategies. It is the power of image registration to enhance and add value to medical imaging that makes these costs worth accommodating.

References

1. Noll, D.C., Boada, F.E., Eddy, W.F., A spectral approach to analysing slice selection in planar imaging: optimisation for through-plane interpolation. *Magn. Reson. Med.*, 38: pp. 151–160, 1997.
2. Stark, D.D. and Bradley, W.G. (eds.), *Magnetic Resonance Imaging* third ed., Mosby, St. Louis, 1999, Chapter 4.
3. Stark, D.D. and Bradley, W.G. (eds.), *Magnetic Resonance Imaging* third ed., Mosby, St. Louis, 1999, Chapter 5.

4. Stark, D.D. and Bradley, W.G. (eds.), *Magnetic Resonance Imaging* third ed., Mosby, St. Louis, 1999, Chapter 8.
5. Webb, S. (ed.), *The Physics of Medical Imaging*, IOP Publishing, Bristol, 1996.
6. Hajnal, J.V., Saeed, N., Soar, E.J., Oatridge, A., Young, I.R., and Bydder, G.M., A registration and interpolation procedure for subvoxel matching of serially acquired MR images, *J. Comput. Assist. Tomogr.* 19: pp. 289–96, 1995.
7. Friston, K.J., Ashburner, J., Poline, J.B., Frith, C.D., Heather, J.D., and Frackowiak, R.S.J., Spatial registration and normalisation of images, *Human Brain Mapping,* 2, pp. 165–189, 1995.
8. Vokurka, E.A., Thacker, N.A., and Jackson, A., A fast model independent method for automatic correction of intensity nonuniformity in MRI data. *J. Magn. Reson. Imaging.* 10: pp. 550–562. 1999.
9. Sled, J.G., Zijdenbos, A.P., and Evans, A.C. A nonparametric method for automatic correction of intensity nonuniformity in MRI data. *IEEE. Trans. Med. Imag.* 17: pp. 87–97. 1998.
10. Woods, R.P., Mazziotta J.C., and Cherry S.R., MRI-PET registration with automated algorithm, *J. Comput. Assist. Tomogr.*, 17, pp. 536–546, 1993.
11. Hajnal, J.V., Saeed, N., Oatridge, A., Williams, E.J., Young, I.R., and Bydder, G.M., Detection of subtle brain changes using subvoxel registration and subtraction of serial MR images, *J. Comput. Assist. Tomogr.*, 19, pp. 677–91, 1995.
12. Woods, R.P., Grafton, S.T., Holmes, C.J., Cherry, S.R., and Mazziotta, J.C., Automated image registration: I. General methods and intrasubject, intramodality validation, *J. Comput. Assist. Tomogr.*, 22, pp. 139–152, 1998.
13. Holden, M., Hill, D.L.G., Denton, E.R.E., Jarosz, J.M., Cox, T.C.S., Goody, J., Rohlfing, T., and Hawkes, D.J., Voxel similarity measures for 3D serial MR image registration, *IEEE Trans. Med. Imag.* 19:94–102, 2000.
14. Little, J.A., Hill, D.L.G., and Hawkes, D.J., Deformations incorporating rigid structures, *Comput. Vision Image Understanding,* 66: pp. 223–232, 1997.
15. Saeed, N., Magnetic resonance image segmentation using pattern recognition, and applied to image registration and quantitation, NMR in *Biomed* 11:157–67, 1998.
16. Talairach, J. and Tournoux, P., *Coplanar Stereotaxic Atlas of the Human Brain.* Thieme Medical Publisher, New York, 1988.
17. Thompson, P.M., Giedd, J.N., Woods, R.P., MacDonald, D., Evans, A.C., and Toga, A.W. Growth patterns in the developing brain detected by using continuum mechanical tensor maps, *Nature,* 404(6774): pp. 190–3, 2000.
18. Bankman, I. N. (Ed.) *Handbook of Medical Imaging Processing and Analysis.* Academic Press, San Diego, 2000, Section 5.

5

Correcting for Scanner Errors in CT, MRI, Spect, and 3D Ultrasound

Louis Lemieux, Dale L. Bailey, and David Bell

CONTENTS

0-8493-0064-9/01/$0.00+$.50
© 2001 by CRC Press LLC

5.1   Introduction

In this chapter we review image artifacts due to scanner errors relevant to image registration, and describe methods available for correction. Our discussion is restricted to the 3D imaging modalities: computed tomography (CT), magnetic resonance imaging (MRI), emission tomography (ET) (positron emission tomography [PET] and single-photon emission computed tomography [SPECT]), and ultrasound (US).

Three types of applications of medical imaging are particularly reliant on accurate images: image-guided surgery, multimodality image registration, and quantitative imaging. Generally, these are uses of images requiring calculation and application of mathematical mapping between image space and physical space or physical dimensions. Depending on the specific application, the registration mapping may be limited to determination of pixel dimensions or encompass position, orientation, and dimensional scaling of the image relative to real space. Applications in image-guided surgery are an example of the latter. Even if image registration can sometimes be limited to the relationship between respective image spaces alone, without reference to physical space, the degree of spatial integrity of each dataset used for registration taken individually is an important consideration in all cases. For example, in ET it is often desirable, even essential, to place the reconstructed functional data within an "anatomical framework." Although image distortion in ET is not a primary concern when registering with CT or MRI, a number of issues related to image quality can affect image registration and therefore require careful consideration. Another example is in longitudinal MRI studies, which can also be impaired by variations in image characteristics (such as voxel dimension), although mapping between image space and real space may not be sought. In the following sections, we begin by considering the nature and origin of artifacts in medical images, as this will allow us to define the scope of the problem. We then review specific relevant artifacts and describe the current state of the technology available to correct for these artifacts for each imaging modality.

5.1.1 Image Artifacts, Geometric Distortions, and Their Origins

The ideal image acquisition process results in a representation of the imaged object devoid of artifacts and noise. In other words, pixel intensities in the ideal image have a spatial distribution that matches exactly, to within a global dimensional scaling factor, that of the physical property(ies) of the object imaged. Artifacts can therefore be seen as occurrences of signal intensities that violate that correspondence. In the context of image registration, all artifacts are undesirable and can impair the registration process. However, the most relevant artifacts are image features that violate the requirement for an appropriately scaled, Cartesian mapping between image space and real space,* i.e., geometric distortions. Artifacts that appear as features superimposed onto the image, such as coherent noise or signal nonuniformity (e.g., due to radiofrequency inhomogeneity in MRI), must also be considered, as they may impede registration, although they do not represent geometric distortions. No further discussion of random image noise is necessary, as it is intrinsic to any data acquisition process, can originate in the imaged object or imaging device and, therefore, cannot be classified as scanner error. These considerations lead to discussion of the origin of image artifacts. Image artifacts can be categorized according to the location of their origin (either imaged object or imaging device) and the generating mechanism. The possible mechanisms of artifact generation are multiple, but can be categorized as either intrinsic or resulting from interactions between imaged object, environment, and imaging device. Mechanisms of artifact generation intrinsic to the imaged object include spontaneous movement and changes in its properties (e.g., temperature, mechanical properties, etc.). Mechanisms intrinsic

---

* For 3D imaging modalities. For projection methods, the mapping most often assumed is that of a point perspective.

to the imaging device* include physical or technical limitations of the imaging process and suboptimal or variable performance levels. Interactions between imaged object and imaging device, on the other hand, constitute an inherent part of the imaging process and also often lead to artifacts. For example, the imaging process may be optimized to capture accurately one specific component or aspect of the imaged object to the detriment of another, therefore leading to artifacts (e.g., chemical shift artifact in magnetic resonance imaging). Furthermore, artifacts resulting from the interaction between object and imaging device may also be unavoidable in certain circumstances (e.g., the streak artifact in CT; see Joseph[1]).

This chapter is concerned primarily with the issue of correcting image artifacts due to scanner errors, i.e., mechanisms intrinsic to the scanner or the imaging process itself and, to a lesser extent, consideration of artifacts intrinsic to the imaged object.

5.2   Geometric Distortion in Computed Tomography

CT is the oldest 3D medical imaging modality and has probably been the subject of the largest amount of technical development and refinements among all the modalities considered here. However, there is relatively little published work on the issue of CT geometric distortions, particularly in the context of image registration. This may be because CT is based on the absorption of radiation that traverses the body in a straight line, resulting in a very low degree of spatial distortion. Most artifacts in CT concern intensity, in particular the streak artifacts which have a variety of sources (see Joseph[1]). However, we will not discuss these in detail since most of these are either unavoidable, particularly and most importantly streaking due to the presence of metalic objects (e.g., stereotaxic frame) in the imaged volume, or do not constitute a significant problem for registration of images from modern scanners.

CT is closely linked to the development of frame-based stereotaxy for localization and co-registration; see Kelly and Kall.[2] Frame-based stereotaxy, by providing an external coordinate system in each slice, insures a high degree of robustness to images relative to scanner errors.[3] However, the advent of frameless stereotaxy, discussed in detail in Chapter 12, requires a reassessment of the sources of distortion and possible new methods to minimize these will need to be devised. Nonetheless, CT is generally assumed not to necessitate distortion correction in contrast to MRI.[4,5] Studies on the accuracy of localization in CT based on stereotactic frames have consistently reflected the low degree of geometric distortion in CT, with in-plane errors less than 1 mm and effectively limited by voxel dimensions, in particular slice thickness and separation.[6-9]

---

* We can also put into this category the factors related to the external environment (e.g., ambient conditions that fall outside the specified operational range of the device).

The main limitation to the spatial integrity of CT images lies in the mechanical elements of the imaging process, i.e., movement of the radiation source and detectors, as well as of the patient couch. Therefore, the following specific mechanisms can compromise the geometric integrity of images:

1. Error in the slice angle relative to the scanning axis due to uncertainty in the gantry angle and/or table bending due to the patient weight;

2. Error in the slice separation due to fluctuations in the couch speed relative to the prescribed value;

3. Error in the dimensions of the field of view due to imperfections and/or changes in the physical dimensions of the tube detector assembly.

Zylka and Wischmann devised a method to measure and compensate for all of the above sources of distortion in CT images.[10] By modeling the distortions as a second (or higher) degree polynomial and using an "N-shaped" localization device fixed to the table, the authors were able to observe distortions of the order of 2 mm, which depended on the gantry tilt angle. These will also vary depending on the mechanical properties of each scanner and the subject's body weight.

5.3 Spatial Inaccuracies in Magnetic Resonance Imaging

From the point of view of geometric distortions, MRI differs greatly from CT in at least three respects: first, the image acquisition process of MRI is fundamentally different, starting with the fact that it does not rely on any mechanical device. Second, the problem of geometric distortions is much more important in MRI, due to the fact that these are essentially unavoidable and can be quite large (5 mm or more).[6,11,12] Third, MR images obtained using different data acquisition schemes (conventional 2D and 3D Fourier transform imaging, echo-planar imaging, spiral imaging) and hardware (e.g., birdcage, surface coils) can be subject to substentially different image distortion effects. Therefore, the importance of the problem of image distortions was recognized in the early days of the application of MRI[11,13] and has been the subject of intense investigation over the past 20 years, resulting in a relatively large body of literature. There have been major advances in this field in the past decade, in particular improved main field homogeneity and the use of stronger readout gradients, which has significantly helped to reduce the magnitude of the problem in most standard applications. However, the problem of image distortion has not yet been resolved for all types of image acquisition sequences and applications.

MR image distortions can originate from limitations in the scanner or prop-erties of the imaged object.[14-16] The factors that are scanner-dependent, and therefore of greatest interest here, are

1. Gradient field nonlinearity;
2. Static field inhomogeneity;
3. Error in the field-of-view or slice thickness due to variations in the gradient field strengths;
4. Fields due to Eddy currents induced in scanner components by the switching gradients;
5. Imperfect slice or volume selection pulses.

In most standard imaging applications, the two most important sources of geometric distortion are gradient nonlinearity and field inhomogeneity,[14] although Schad et al.[12,17] seem to attribute a large part of the distortions to the effect of eddy currents. Gradient eddy currents have been much reduced in modern scanners by the widespread use of self-shielded gradient coils.

Although signal nonuniformity due to RF inhomogeneity is not a geomet-ric distortion, it can impede image registration in the most extreme cases (e.g., images acquired using surface coils, see Studholme et al.[18]) and there-fore merits discussion.

5.3.1   Magnitude of Geometric Distortions in MRI

The amount of geometric distortion can be measured using phantoms and/or phantoms combined with stereotactic frames.[6,8,12,14,19,20] The amounts of distor-tion observed vary widely and reflect the design and performance of different scanners (different manufacturers, levels of technological development, design, etc.), the slice orientation and imaging sequence used, and the design of the stereotactic frames. The magnitude of the distortion generally varies as a function of position, being larger in the peripheral region. Bakker et al. in a phantom study found localization errors of up to 7 mm and 4 mm in plane over a 40 cm field of view due to static field inhomogeneity and gradient nonlinear-ity, respectively.[14] Michiels et al. concluded that the degree of localization accu-racy achieved after optimization of the image acquisition and application of correction for both field inhomogenity and gradient nonlinearity is adequate for stereotactic neurosurgery.[21] However, Alexander et al. found discrepancies in stereotactic localization of the order of 4 mm between MRI and CT.[22] They did not attempt to correct the geometric distortions in MRI themselves, but rather proposed image fusion with CT as a means of assuring spatial accuracy while benefiting from the superior image contrast of MRI. In a frame-based localiza-tion study, Walton et al. found that 3D (volumetric) acquisitions give more accu-rate stereotactic localization.[23] Ramsey and Oliver, in a recent study on modern CT and MRI scanners, have found linear distortions in the range of 0 to 2 mm in

MR images with 3 mm and 5 mm slice thicknesses.[9] Although a direct comparison is difficult, it is fair to say that localization accuracy of MRI has tended to
improve since its advent.

Specific characteristics of each artifact generation mechanism and some correction methods available will now be discussed. Some correction schemes are
designed to correct for both gradient nonlinearity and field inhomogeneity;
these are discussed in each respective section.

5.3.2 Geometric Distortion Due to Gradient Field Nonlinearity

Gradient field nonlinearity is a consequence of limitations and imperfections in the design of the gradient coils.[24] Following the nomenclature proposed by Sumanaweera, the geometric distortions resulting from gradient
field nonlinearity are the *barrel* distortion (2D and 3D), the *potato chip* effect
(slice selection, 2D) and the *bow-tie* effect (2D). As gradient field nonlinearity
is solely dependent on geometry of gradient coils, its effects are constant in
time and independent of the imaging sequence used (for a given gradient).
Furthermore, the barrel effect is independent of gradient strength.[14] Walton[23]
et al. have more recently shown that geometric distortions due to gradient
nonlinearity are smaller in 3D acquisitions than 2D, as predicted by
Sumanaweera.[24] This is because a weak slice selection gradient is used to
excite the whole volume, therefore reducing considerably the magnitude of
the potato chip effect.

5.3.2.1 Correction

The distortions due to gradient nonlinearity, and in particular the barrel effect,
can be corrected by applying a theoretically or experimentally derived correction field.[12,14,17,22,25] In practice, many modern scanners incorporate such a
scheme in an automatic image reconstruction mechanism, e.g., General Elec-
tric's *Gradwarp*; see reference 8 in Sumanaweera.[15] In our experience with frame
based MRI stereotaxy, care must be taken as such correction schemes can fail
under specific circumstances; see Lemieux et al.[26] and Figure 5.1. The details of
these correction schemes are generally not published and, depending on the
manufacturer, it may be possible to switch off the correction temporarily. Furthermore, it is often impossible to determine when such correction schemes
were used in each specific study published. This would require, for example,
that the authors state the version of the scanner software used, which is rarely
the case (see also Sumanaweera et al.[24]).

5.3.3 Geometric Distortion Due to Field Inhomogeneity

Field inhomogeneity has three possible origins: imperfection of the field generated by the magnet, eddy currents induced in the conducting structures of
the scanner by the switching gradients, and spatial variations in the magnetic
susceptibility within the imaged volume.[4,15] Although the latter cannot be

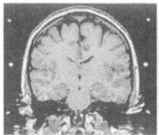 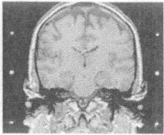

FIGURE 5.1

Illustration of geometric distortion due to gradient non linearity in MRI. On the left, the automatic correction scheme ("Gradwarp," see reference 8 in Moerland et al.[25]) has not worked properly following the selection of a rectangular field of view (24 cm × 18 cm). This is reflected in the apparent displacement of the middle fiducial markers of a stereotactic frame away from the imaginary lines joining the superior and inferior fiducials; the red lines have been superimposed to emphasize this point. The distortion was so severe as to render the surgical procedure unsafe. On the right, the distortion is significantly reduced following the selection of a square field of view (24 cm × 24 cm). See reference 26 for more details.

described as "scanner error," its effect is physically indistinguishable from the others and is present in virtually all images. Furthermore, the presence of metalic objects (stereotactic frame, surgical instruments, surgical implants, etc.) within the field of view will generally result in severe distortions. The geometric distortions due to susceptibility differences can be extremely complex due to field inhomogeneity dependency on both the material and shape of the imaged object, as well as its orientation relative to the static field. On the other hand, distortions resulting from magnet imperfections and eddy currents can often be modeled. Field inhomogeneity causes local variations in resonance frequency and therefore is sometimes referred to as an off-resonance effect. The consequence of this is that the resulting distortion is inversely proportional to gradient strength (bandwidth per pixel) and therefore can be minimized by proper selection of gradient strength and field of view. In standard spin warp imaging, the effect is limited to the frequency encode direction. In echo-planar imaging (EPI), the effect is present in both the read and phase encode ("blip") directions, the latter dominating because the bandwidth per pixel is lowest in the phase encode direction.[27] Geometric distortion in the phase encode direction in EPI can be very large and is still an important problem in many applications, such as diffusion-weighted imaging (DWI) and functional MRI; see Figure 5.2 for an illustration of the distortions in EPI. Another important source of distortions in EPI-DWI is eddy currents,[28] which are particularly problematic because the size of the distortion is a function of the amplitude of the diffusion-sensitizing gradients; therefore, it can vary during the acquisition process.

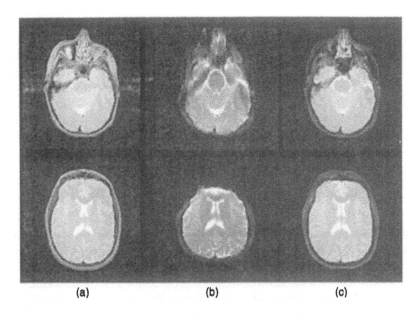

(a)   (b)   (c)

FIGURE 5.2
Illustration of image distortions in EPI: (a) conventional spin-echo; (b) single-shot EPI; (c) eight-shot EPI. TR = 2600 msec, TE = 80 msec. Both signal loss (dephasing) and geometric distortions can be seen in the EPI. The distortions are drastically reduced in multi-shot vs. single-shot EPI due to shorter echo train and resulting reduced accumulated phase error (images taken from *http://www.nmr.ion.ucl.ac.uk/~marks/epi/shots.html* with permission).

5.3.3.1   Correction

Correction schemes can be categorized into two groups: double acquisition with inverted gradients and phase unwarping based on field maps. Bakker et al.[14] and Chang and Fitzpatrick[29] described methods based on two acquisitions identical except for inverted gradients. This approach requires the identification of corresponding points in the two images. Using this approach, a reduction in the stereotactic localization error from 3.8 to 2 mm was obtained. Moerland et al. found a similar improvement using Bakker's method.[25] Maurer et al.[5] measured the effect of applying the method by Chang and Fitzpatrick[29] on the accuracy of CT-MRI registration and found an improvement in the range of 30 to 40%.

Sekihara et al. were the first to propose field mapping to correct for static field inhomogeneity.[13] Sumanaweera et al.'s approach is based on a field map (requiring two volume acquisitions) followed by the application of a phase unwarping algorithm to correct for positional errors throughout the imaged volume *in vivo*.[15] In a later development, Sumanaweera et al. extended their technique to remove the need for connectivity, which makes it applicable to images containing stereotactic frames.[19] This method results in an improvement of localization accuracy from 3.7 to 1.1 mm. The field mapping approach was used by Jezzard and Balaban to correct ("unwarp") EPI data.[27] Reber et al. use field maps obtained using high signal-to-noise ratio (SNR) EPI data for increased robustness.[30] Kadah and Hu propose an algebraic approach to the problem of identifying the optimal inhomogeneity distortion operator.[31] Ernst et al. propose coregistration with a reference (undistorted, non-EPI) image dataset as a correction method for EPI distortion.[32] The method is based on matching the brain surface to correct for global scaling and shearing errors in the EPI data. However, it cannot correct for distortion and signal loss due to local field inhomogeneity.

5.3.4 Error in Field of View (Voxel Dimensions) Due to Variations in Gradient Strength

Important fluctuations in imaging gradient amplitudes from prescribed values are common.[33] Furthermore, system calibration tolerances are typically much larger than stability effects. In frame-based stereotaxy, such fluctuations are largely irrelevant since the scaling factors can be derived from the frame. In the absence of a frame, the impact of uncertainty in the voxel dimensions is potentially important in certain applications of image registration, in particular longitudinal studies of morphological changes in the brain, image-guided neurosurgery combining CT and MRI, and radiotherapy planning.

5.3.4.1 Correction

Registration methods that incorporate linear scaling factors can compensate for such differences assuming that the dimensions of features used for matching have not varied in the interscan interval. To this effect the skull can be used as such an invariant structure and Freeborough and Fox have been able to observe very small changes in brain volumes by this means.[34] Alternatively a method based on the registration of a test object as part of a QA schedule has been proposed.[35] In particular, it has been observed that recalibration during normal servicing can introduce important variations in the scaling factors. The derived scaling factors can then be used as fixed factors in a rigid-body registration of head scans. Hill et al. proposed a method to measure the actual errors in the voxel dimensions based on scanning a purpose-built test object and registering the resulting images with a computerized version of the phantom.[36] The method was devised for application in image-guided neurosurgery using MRI and CT. A significant improvement in registration accuracy was obtained when using the scaling factors derived from the phantom when compared with the "free," nine-degrees-of-freedom registration.

5.3.5 Signal Nonuniformity Due to RF Inhomogeneity

Signal nonuniformity can be present in all MR images and in particular those acquired with smaller RF coils, such as surface coils.[37] Although RF inhomogeneity does not give rise to geometric distortions, the ensuing signal nonuniformity can be a significant problem for image registration.

In most modern volumetric images of the head acquired with a birdcage head coil, the level of nonuniformity is such that it does not affect rigid-body registration significantly, although it is still problematic for image segmentation.[38] However, images acquired with surface coils generally suffer from a high degree of signal nonuniformity, which can hamper registration severely.

5.3.5.1 Correction

In the context of image registration, this problem can be addressed in two possible ways: first, by correcting images prior to coregistration and, second, by using a registration method that is less sensitive to signal nonuniformity.[18] RF nonuniformity correction methods can be classified into two main categories: experimentally derived correction field maps and purely postprocessing. The first approach is based on the assumption that the nonuniformity field is solely dependent on geometry of the coil and therefore that a nonuniformity map obtained by scanning a uniform test object can be applied to all images acquired with the same coil.[37,39] This requires registration of the correction matrix with the image, which usually relies on the image position and orientation information supplied by the scanner (geometric prescription). This approach assumes that the effect is independent of the geometry and electrical properties of the imaged object, which is generally not the case.[40]

Postprocessing methods, on the other hand, usually rely on the assumption that signal nonuniformity due to RF inhomogeneity is restricted to low spatial frequencies.[41] A number of correction methods are available that require expert supervision.[42,43] Other methods have been proposed that form an integral part of segmentation algorithms.[44–46] This integrated approach is potentially extremely powerful, if complete segmentation of tissues within the region of interest is the desired outcome (otherwise the segmentation represents an unnecessary computational burden). Also, these methods currently either require expert supervision or are applicable to a single part of the anatomy. Sled et al. proposed a fully automated, nonparametric method that solely derives the intensity bias field and gives good results for whole-head data, providing input data of sufficient quality to allow subsequent precise segmentation of the brain.[47,48] Another nonparametric automatic postprocessing method has been applied successfully to standard brain images as well as images acquired using surface coils.[49]

5.4 Spatial Inaccuracies in Emission Tomography

Emission tomography (ET) is a technique for externally measuring radioactivity distributions *in vivo* in cross section. In contrast to the other modalities discussed in this chapter (apart from functional MRI), the data produced by emission tomography are *functional* images. These represent the biodistribution of a radioactively labeled pharmaceutical, which may have been introduced into the body by injection, inhalation, or ingestion. Emission tomography with radionuclide tracers is divided into two categories depending on the physics of the nuclear decay and detection process. In the first and most common form, SPECT (single photon emission computed tomography), photons emitted by the nucleus as a result of an energy transition or nuclear decay are detected by a gamma camera in a single event counting mode. The other form of emission tomography, PET (positron emission tomography), counts pairs of photons that arise from the annihilation of a positron with an electron. The feature that distinguishes PET from SPECT is that the radioactive nuclei decay by emitting a positron (a positively charged electron) rather than directly emitting a photon; the positron annihilates with an electron in the imaged body and produces two photons in exactly opposite directions.

SPECT systems have a lead collimator that defines lines of response, stored as projections on the crystal face for a given rotational angle. Gamma cameras commonly have one, two, or three detector heads. The heads rotate in a circular motion to acquire projection data at sufficient angles for reconstruction.

In PET detection, coincident events are recorded when two photons are detected on opposing sides of a circular array of detectors. A line of response is ascribed to the chord joining the locations where both photons were detected. The detector configurations common in PET vary.[50-55] In recent years many dual-head gamma cameras have become available with the ability to work in a coincidence mode, thereby permitting them to perform both PET and SPECT.[56]

An interesting recent development in "integrated imaging" has been to combine emission tomography and CT scanners into a single device.[57-59] SPECT/CT and PET/CT devices should be commercially available within the next few years. This approach obviously minimizes some of the problems of registration between modalities by using the same scanning couch and patient positioning, as well as making further use of anatomical data in attenuation, scatter, and partial volume correction of emission tomography data. Similar efforts have been made to combine PET and MRI or MRS.[60,61]

5.4.1 Sources of Spatial Inaccuracies and Measures to Prevent or Minimize Them

The data recorded by ET systems often require processing to compensate for a variety of effects before quantitatively accurate image reconstruction using methods such as conventional filtered backprojection can be employed. These include: photon attenuation *in vivo*; photon scattering *in vivo*; distortions intrinsic to the acquisition geometry; differences in performance within as well as between individual detector elements (uniformity); "gaps" in the projections, e.g., between the edges of flat detectors where the detectors meet. In addition, spatial distortions can arise at high counting rates ("pulse pileup").

Particularly problematic for image registration techniques are effects which lead to spatial and, to a lesser extent, intensity distortions. The main features which potentially limit the ability to coregister data from ET with anatomical modalities are due to the vastly different nature of the data: anatomy and high (~1 mm) resolution for MRI and CT compared with physiological function and intermediate resolution (4 to 15 mm) for emission tomography.

Registration of SPECT or PET data with anatomical data alone (i.e., without fiducial markers), often has the fundamental problem of trying to match dissimilar data. Functional data from emission tomography may contain insufficient anatomical detail for many algorithms. It is therefore imperative that systematic sources of error be minimized.

5.4.1.1 Geometric and Alignment Effects

5.4.1.1.1 Center of Rotation Errors

SPECT systems produce distortions in the reconstructed data if alignment of the detector heads and electronic alignment of the center of the data acquisition matrix are not carefully measured and corrected prior to reconstruction. The effect of this is to produce halo-like artifacts, which spatially distort the true distribution. Similarly, nonuniformities in detector response lead to "ring artifacts": circular intensity distortions in the reconstructed image. The reason for this is the use of a single (or very few) detector which is moved or rotated to various positions about the subject to acquire all of the data. Thus a nonuniform area will trace out a consistent, circular path at a set radius from the center of the acquisition matrix.

5.4.1.1.2 Nonuniform Sampling Effects

The sampling in emission tomography systems is usually greater towards the center of the field of view, and therefore any nonuniformity is greatly enhanced the closer it is to the center of the field of view. It has been calculated that a 2% nonuniformity at the center of the field of view can give an apparent 50% non-uniformity in the reconstructed image. This falls off rapidly with radius.[62] An example of nonuniformity "ring" artifacts is shown in Figure 5.3.

Full ring PET systems have a varying distance between adjacent parallel projections, decreasing towards the edge of the field of view, due to its circular geometry. This effect would cause spatial distortions if ignored; however, these are usually corrected prior to reconstruction. One effect that is not usually corrected by the reconstruction algorithm, though, is variation in the resolution of the system towards the edge of the field of view. The lines of response towards the edge of the field are measured at an increasing angle relative to the face of the crystals, thus decreasing the accuracy of localization. This leads to an ellipsoidal point response function as this degradation occurs preferentially for those lines of response at higher incidence angles to the detectors.

5.4.1.1.3 Voxel Dimensions

An important issue for accurate coregistration is the accurate measurement of the reconstructed voxel dimensions. In PET, for example, it is often assumed that the detector radius, which determines the dimensions of the coordinate

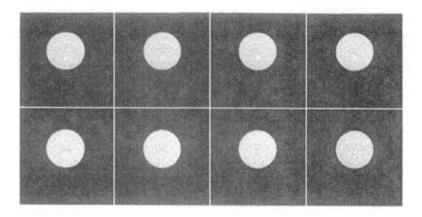

FIGURE 5.3
SPECT nonuniform artifacts resulting from poor uniformity correction are shown. The gamma camera was a dual-headed device with the heads opposed at 180° to each other. The reconstructed images show a 20 cm diameter cylinder which has been filled with water containing ^{99m}Tc and uniformly mixed. The nonuniformities exhibit as a "hot-spot" in the center of the image matrix (not the center of the object) seen in all images in the top row and the two right-most images in the bottom row, and a number of "cold" ring artifacts in the other images at varying radii. Note that the nonuniformities are centerd on the image matrix, not on the object. The object center is displaced above the image center.

system for the reconstruction algorithm, is simply the distance from the center of the tomograph to the crystal face. However, the mean free path (i.e., the average distance traveled) of the 0.511 MeV photons in the detector is around 1 cm for BGO scintillators (density(ρ) = 7.13 g $\cdot$ cm^{-3}). Therefore, the *effective radius* of the PET system is increased by this amount, and this affects the voxel spatial dimensions. In practice, a suitable method to avoid this effect is to measure the dimensions accurately with a calibrated test object. A circular disk of perspex which contains an array of fine holes drilled very accurately can be used. Into this tubing containing a radioactive solution is introduced. An example from a CT scan is shown in Figure 5.4. The same test object can be used in SPECT, PET, CT, and MRI with appropriate contrast (^{99m}Tc in SPECT, ^{18}F in PET, air in CT, and CuSO$_4$ for MRI) for the same purpose.

5.4.1.2   Physical Effects Causing Intensity Artifacts and Spatial Distortions

5.4.1.2.1   Attenuation Effects

Some physical effects cause changes in the spatial distribution of the reconstructed signal. Neglecting to correct for attenuation, for example, renders the projection data inconsistent at different radial angles, and this causes a number of distortions in the data. First, as the attenuation is greatest towards the center of the body, the reconstructed concentration in a homogenous structure

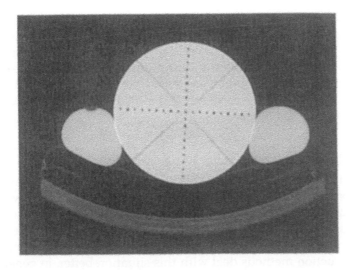

FIGURE 5.4
One slice from a CT scan of the test object used to measure voxel dimensions accurately is shown. The holes are precision drilled at 10 mm intervals in a solid cylinder of perspex ($\rho \sim 1.1 \mathrm{g} \cdot \mathrm{cm}^{-3}$). Fine tubing can be inserted into the holes and filled with radioactive or paramagnetic contrast.

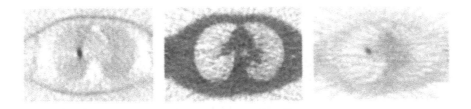

FIGURE 5.5
Distortion caused by not correcting the projection data for attenuation is shown. The image on the left is a PET reconstruction of an [^{18}F]-deoxyglucose (FDG) scan of the thorax. The patient has a single pulmonary nodule, seen in the right hilum, with high FDG uptake. The image in the center is the corresponding PET attenuation scan that is used for correcting the projections prior to reconstruction. It is, in effect, a low resolution CT scan. The image on the right shows the effect of applying attenuation correction to the emission data. The uptake in the nodule is now not distorted, especially in the anterior-posterior axis and the physiological distribution in the low-attenuation lungs is now more accurate. Both of these effects are errors caused by not applying attenuation correction to the projection data. (Image courtesy of Ms. Bernadette Cronin, Clinical PET Centre, Guy's & St Thomas' Hospital, London.)

will artifactually decrease towards the center of the object. Second, the inconsistency between projections will often cause "streaking" artifacts in areas of high contrast of radioactivity concentration (see Figure 5.5). This may cause difficulties for any registration algorithm that optimizes a voxel similarity measure. Attenuation may be corrected by multiplying the emission data with a correction factor file based on transmission measurements (for a review of transmission scanning in emission tomography, see Bailey[63]). The transmission data are similar to that measured in a CT scan, except that in emission tomography a gamma emitter is used for the source rather than an x-ray tube. Ideally, the data are acquired simultaneously with the emission data to reduce scanning duration and ensure accurate registration. The corrections are applied before reconstruction in PET and either before, during, or after reconstruction in SPECT.

5.4.1.2.2   Reconstruction Artifacts

The reconstruction algorithm may also produce artifacts, especially where there are extreme differences in the radioactive concentration between adjacent structures. An example often seen is when a radiotracer is excreted via the kidneys, and the bladder may contain high concentrations of urine compared with the concentration of the radiotracer in surrounding tissues. Iterative reconstruction methods deal with this situation better, in general, than analytical filtered back projection.

5.5   Spatial Inaccuracies in 3D Ultrasound Imaging

When performing an ultrasound scan, the transducer is moved so that a 3D image of the tissue structure is built up in the brain of the operator. However in order to analyze this information or for anybody else to visualize it, methods for the acquisition and display of 3D ultrasound (3D-US) images have been developed. An additional benefit of 3D-US is the display of image planes which are not accessible in 2D ultrasound; i.e., those corresponding to transducer positions and orientations which are physically unrealizable. This might include, for instance, looking down the neck of a patient as if the head had been chopped off!

A 3D ultrasound image is created by moving an ultrasound beam through a volume of tissue and acquiring a series of 2D images (slices) at a fixed time interval. For each slice, the position and orientation of the transducer is recorded. There are two principal acquisition methods used, which will be referred to as *freehand* and *fixed* geometry. In freehand scanning the transducer movement is controlled by the operator in the same way as for conventional 2D ultrasound. The position and orientation of the transducer is recorded by a position sensor attached to the transducer. In fixed geometry scanning the transducer movement is partially or completely controlled by the scanner or other device controlling the acquisition. In this case a position sensor is not used.

After acquisition has completed, the ultrasound data must be reconstructed so that a series of parallel slices is produced. The algorithm used for reconstruction depends on the acquisition method as well as a number of other factors. More information on acquisition and reconstruction methods is contained in Barry et al.[64]

The main interest here is in artifacts that give rise to position errors in the reconstructed data. Because of the way 3D-US data is acquired, a discussion of image inaccuracies in 3D-US must cover inaccuracies encountered in each of its constituents, namely: conventional 2D ultrasound scan acquisition, transducer position measurement, and the 3D acquisition process proper where 2D slice and position data are acquired dynamically.

5.5.1 Sources of Geometric Inaccuracies and Measures to Prevent or Minimize Them

5.5.1.1 *Conventional 2D Ultrasound Scanning*

The 2D ultrasound image acquisition process relies on the following two assumptions: 1) the ultrasound pulse travels in a straight line and 2) the speed of sound is constant. Departures from these assumptions will give rise to refraction and depth errors, both of which may have an impact on registration. A comprehensive description of 2D ultrasound artifacts is given in Cosgrove et al.[65]

5.5.1.1.1 *Refraction*

If an ultrasound pulse strikes a tissue interface at an oblique angle, the direction of travel will be changed if the speed of sound is different on either side of the interface. For most soft tissue interfaces the effect is small. However, if the propagation path includes fluid (such as in pelvic scans by the transabdominal route), the effect can be significant. The effect of refraction is to deviate the path of the ultrasound beam. Since the ultrasound image is built up by assuming that sound travels in straight lines, regions of tissue which are affected by refraction will be displayed incorrectly (see Figure 5.6).

It is very difficult to correct for refraction, since it is a fundamental property of ultrasound imaging. The effect can be reduced by avoiding large angles of incidence in regions of tissue where refraction is likely to be a problem.

5.5.1.1.2 *Depth Errors*

Depth is calculated by assuming a fixed speed of sound. Variations in the speed of sound will give rise to depth errors, which tend to be small for most soft tissue interfaces. However sound propagates in fat 10 to 15% more slowly than in most other soft tissues and prosthetic materials show a more marked deviation. The effect of this artifact can be reduced by avoiding regions in which it is significant.

5.5.1.1.3 *Spatial Resolution*

Refraction and depth errors will result in geometric distortion, i.e., image pixels will be displayed at incorrect locations. In contrast, variations in spatial resolution will change the volume of tissue that corresponds to each image pixel.

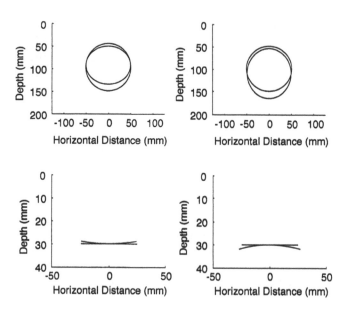

FIGURE 5.6

Geometric distortion resulting from ultrasound depth and refraction errors. In the upper figures, outlines of a circular reflector of radius 50 mm at a depth (to center) of 100 mm have been drawn. Superimposed on these are the new outlines due to propagation through a uniform low velocity layer (left) and high velocity layer (right) using a linear array transducer; i.e., parallel scan lines. In the lower figures, the horizontal lines represent a plane reflector of length 50 mm at a depth of 30 mm in a uniform medium. The curves represent the appearance of this plane reflector when the medium has two layers of different velocities separated by a horizontal interface when using a sector transducer. The ratio between the velocity of the upper layer and that of the lower layer is 0.9 (left) and 1.1 (right). The geometric distortion has been exaggerated for illustrative purposes—the maximum variation of the velocity of sound is only a few percent.

The tissue volume corresponding to an image pixel is determined by three components of spatial resolution, each of which is dependent on depth and, possibly, on the lateral position within the image. To a first approximation, the spatial resolution is determined by the width of the ultrasound beam in each of three directions: axial (along the beam), lateral (perpendicular to the beam and in the plane of the image), and slice (perpendicular to the image plane). Since the scan lines used to form an ultrasound image are not necessarily parallel, these three components may not correspond to conventional Cartesian axes. Each of these components can now be considered in turn:

1. Axial resolution is determined by the pulse width, which tends to broaden with depth due to frequency-dependent attenuation. However this is a small effect and in most cases the variation of axial resolution with distance along the beam can be neglected.

2. Lateral resolution is determined by the beamwidth within the scan plane, which will vary with distance along the beam according to the type of electronic focusing applied by the scanner. This results in good lateral resolution within a focal zone and poor lateral resolution elsewhere. There can be one or more focal zones applied to a given image. Multiple focal zones will give a more uniform lateral resolution over a greater distance along the beam than for a single focal zone. This is at the expense of frame rate.

3. Slice resolution is determined by the beamwidth perpendicular to the scan plane and this will be fixed by the transducer geometry. (It is possible to provide some control over slice focusing, but this requires 2D transducer arrays which are still at an early stage of development.) The transducer geometry will produce a point at which the slice beamwidth is a minimum; this point will not necessarily coincide with the minimum lateral beamwidth. The variation in slice beamwidth changes the slice component of the resolution cell.

The preceding description has looked at the variation of resolution with distance along the beam. This will not in general be the same as depth, so there will be lateral variations of resolution as a natural consequence of variation in beam angle. The only exception to this is for rectilinear scanning patterns. It is not generally possible to correct for variations in spatial resolution, although in recent years manufacturers have attempted to do so by using techniques such as dynamic focusing and aperture control.

5.5.1.2 Position Measurement

For freehand acquisition, a position sensor, which provides information on the position and orientation of the transducer, needs to be attached to it. Various technologies have been developed for position measurement: magnetic, optical, acoustic, and mechanical linkage being the main ones. Some error sources will apply to all sensor technologies and some will be specific to certain types. These are described in turn.

5.5.1.2.1 Sensor Design-Independent Errors

5.5.1.2.1.1 Latency This is the time delay between acquiring an ultrasound slice and making the position measurement. Since in freehand acquisition the transducer is moving fairly continuously, this latency means that the position measurement will never correspond exactly to the ultrasound slice.

The effect on the image is to cause an incorrect interpretation of the slice position, which will be manifested as spatial distortion (see Figure 5.7). The latency will be fairly constant for a particular position sensor and so this effect is systematic and spatial distortion will be in slice direction, i.e., along a line perpendicular to the image plane.

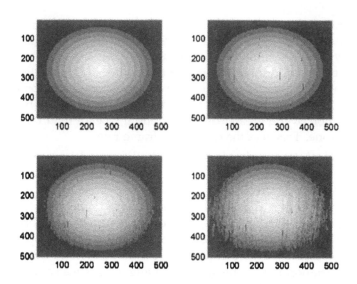

FIGURE 5.7
Reconstruction of a circular reflector for a simulated freehand ultrasound scan with increasing latency values. The upper images are a synthesized circular reflector (left) and a simulated freehand scan with zero latency (right). The lower figures show the effect of nonzero latency with the figure on the right having a larger latency than the left. The black streaks on the images are gaps in the data that are a consequence of using a simple nearest neighbor interpolation method. The highest latency value used was chosen in order to illustrate what could happen in an extreme situation. It is for illustrative purposes only and should not be regarded as a typical situation.

The effect of the artifact can be minimized by ensuring that the latency is significantly less than the interslice time interval. In most freehand scanning the slice acquisition rate will be equal to the scanner frame rate and most probably 20 to 40 Hz. In this case the interslice time interval will be 25 to 50 ms. Provided the latency is no more than a few milliseconds, the degree of spatial distortion is relatively small (a few percent of the interslice time interval). In principle, an approximate correction could be carried out for the effect of the latency if the transducer movement can be approximated by a simple function. However, given that the effect is likely to be relatively small, it is arguable whether it is worthwhile.

5.5.1.2.1.2 Uncertainty in Position Sensors   All position sensors will have a quoted accuracy for both position and orientation measurements. These place a fundamental limitation on the ultimate spatial resolution of the reconstructed data and cause nonlinear distortion and blurring. Orientation errors cause an increase in translation error with depth, since all pixels within a slice are subject to the same angle error, i.e., depth-dependent blurring/distortion. For a typical orientation error of 0.5°, the resulting translation error at a depth of 100 mm will be approximately 1 mm. This will be in addition to the sensor position error, which is typically 1 mm, so this effect can be significant.

5.5.1.2.1.3 Calibration of Sensor   In order to optimize sensor accuracy, a relationship must be established between the position of the sensor on the transducer and the ultrasound data. This is referred to as calibration and if done properly will mean that a given feature in the scanned volume will appear at the same position relative to a fixed reference point wherever the transducer is. The accuracy obtainable with the transducer-sensor system should equal that of the sensor alone. Any errors in the calibration process will degrade the sensor accuracy and therefore give rise to artifacts described above. A review of calibration methods is given in Prager et al.[66]

5.5.1.2.2   Sensor Design-Specific Errors

5.5.1.2.2.1 Electromagnetic Position Sensors   These devices function by measuring the strength of magnetic fields generated by sending current through three small wire coils which are mutually orthogonal. There are two distinct types using a.c. and d.c. fields.

Birkfellner et al.[67] investigated errors introduced by transducers and metal objects for both a.c. (Isotrak II, Polhemus Inc., Colchester, Vermont, U.S.) and dc (Flock of Birds, Ascension Inc., Burlington, Vermont, U.S.) sensors. They found that the Isotrak was affected by all metal placed within the useful range of the sensor and also by mounting it directly on the transducer casing. The Flock of Birds sensor was only affected by ferromagnetic metal and was relatively unaffected by directly mounting it on the transducer casing. However, the fundamental accuracy of the Isotrak was better than that of the Flock of Birds. In a clean environment, both devices performed according to the manufacturers' specifications. Errors can be minimized by removing all metal (Isotrak) or ferrous metal (Flock of Birds) from the sensor and mounting the sensor on an insulating rod attached to the transducer, rather than on the transducer casing itself (Isotrak). According to manufacturers' specifications, the fundamental accuracy of the Isotrak is about 0.75 mm and for the Flock of Birds is about 1.8 mm. The maximum measurement rate for the Isotrak is 120 measurements per second and for the Flock of Birds is 144 measurements per second. The average latency is approximately equal to half the minimum measurement interval. This equates to 4 ms for the Isotrak and 3.5 ms for the Flock of Birds.

Further information on errors produced by electromagnetic sensors may be found in references 68 through 71.

5.5.1.2.2.2 Optical Position Sensors   These devices function by tracking the position of a number of infrared markers on the transducer. The accuracy is greater than for electromagnetic systems and there are no errors introduced by electromagnetic interference, but the system tends to be more bulky. The main problem with optical systems is that line of sight must be maintained at all times, which places a restriction on the type of scanning with which they can be used. Sato et al. describe a system based around the OPTOTRAK optical sensor (NDI Inc., Waterloo, Ontario, Canada).[72] The latency of optical systems will increase with the number of markers that are tracked. When the OPTOTRAK system is used for tracking probe plus object, the latency will be 40 to 50 ms.

5.5.1.2.2.3 Acoustic Position Sensors   These are broadly the same as the optical devices with the infrared markers replaced by acoustic receivers. Since the speed of sound is very much less than that of light, the latency is much greater. King et al. describe a system based on the GP 8-3D acoustic sensor (Science Accessories Corporation, Stratford, Connecticut, U.S.) in which they evaluate accuracy of linear, angular, and volume measurements.[73] Hata et al. describe a system for US/CT registration based on a homemade acoustic sensor.[74]

5.5.1.2.2.4 Mechanical Arms   A system which uses a robot arm (Faro Medical Technologies, Lake Mary, Florida, U.S.) has recently been described.[75] They quote a "sub-mm" accuracy that yields a patient-image coordinate mapping accuracy of 2 to 3 mm. With such a mechanical system there are restrictions imposed in the scanning process due to the physical connection between the transducer and scanner. However no errors due to electromagnetic interference occur nor is line of sight required.

5.5.1.3   3D Acquisition Process

The 3D acquisition process consists of moving an ultrasound beam through a tissue volume which itself may be moving. Errors are therefore introduced by both the transducer and tissue motion. Also, freehand acquisition techniques introduce geometric distortions by collecting voxels in a spatially irregular fashion.

5.5.1.3.1   Transducer Motion

When a 3D ultrasound image is being acquired, the transducer is moving continuously. Therefore the position of the transducer when a pulse is transmitted is not the same as when the pulse is received. This causes the image plane to become distorted, since the transmitter positions (which are fired in sequence) will not lie on a straight line. If the slices are approximately parallel, the effect of these distortions is small, provided the interslice spacing is less than the slice beam width. However, for scanning geometries which have a rotational element, the effect may be more significant. Such scanning geometries could be a freehand acquisition where the transducer is "rocked" (i.e., rotated about a fixed point on the skin surface) or a transducer rotating under computer control. Rotating transducer systems have been described.[76,77] The magnitude of these errors can be calculated for particular scanning conditions and their effects can be determined.

Slices produced by the freehand scanning process will have a variable spacing and are unlikely to be parallel. This can cause a significant increase in the interslice distance with depth, especially if the acquisition involves "rocking" the transducer. One possible solution is to employ a technique called "spatial compounding," where tissue volume is repeatedly scanned from different directions. This reduces coherent noise (speckle) and increases the pixel density, thus reducing the interslice distance. Spatial compounding has been described in Rohling et al.[78]

5.5.1.3.2 Tissue Motion

Ultrasound is a contact scanning method and therefore a small amount of tissue compression will always occur, causing a greater degree of spatial distortion for more superficial scanning. Clearly the degree of compression can be minimized by using as little pressure as possible.

5.5.1.3.3 Nonuniform Sampling

In general, 3D ultrasound images which have been obtained by moving the ultrasound beam through a tissue volume will have nonuniform sampling. For images produced by moving the transducer under computer control (i.e., fixed geometry), the slices will be parallel and therefore the interslice sampling interval will be fixed. However different sampling intervals in the three directions are likely. For images that have been produced by a freehand sweep, the slices will not, in general, be parallel and the interslice sampling interval will not be fixed. Each of these types of nonuniform sampling will be considered in turn.

5.5.1.3.3.1 Fixed Geometry Here the sampling interval is constant, but has a different value in each of the three directions. This occurs frequently, since the interslice separation is often much larger than either of the in-plane sampling intervals. Provided the interslice separation is small enough to sample the tissue volume adequately, there are no special problems with this type of data. Precisely what constitutes "adequate sampling" will depend on the minimum size of the structure which needs to be resolved. For data display, it may be necessary to interpolate the data to give a cubic voxel.

5.5.1.3.3.2 Freehand Geometry There are two effects to consider here: the average interslice separation will vary and adjacent slices will not be parallel. The combination of these two effects produces a 3D dataset where the separation between data points varies in all three directions. Since the effect of a small change in transducer orientation increases with depth, large separations between data points will occur at large depths. Some degree of oversampling will therefore be necessary at smaller depths to compensate for this effect, in which case the acquisition method known as spatial compounding[78] can be used.

It is generally necessary to interpolate the data to a regular voxel array so that it can be displayed and/or compared with other imaging modalities; a number of different algorithms have been proposed.[79]

5.6   General Conclusions

We have described image distortions in CT, MRI, ET, and US that can influence image registration, both within and across modalities. The nature of each effect varies between modalities, reflecting the image generation mechanisms.

The problems of image distortion in CT are relatively minor when compared with MRI or 3D-US. This is why CT is often considered the spatial gold standard in multimodality registration and image-guided intervention studies. The problems of image distortion in MRI are multiple: geometric distortions due to imperfections in the scanner fields (static, gradients, and RF) and to interactions between the imaged object and the scanner fields. Scanner technology is constantly evolving, allowing the acquisition of images of increasing quality. However, new MR scanners, imaging sequences, and applications are constantly being developed, often giving rise to worse or even new artifacts, or to new demands on the accuracy of the images. Interventional MRI is a case in point; although the artifacts encountered generally belong to the categories described above, their importance is enhanced by the greater presence of instruments in the field of view and the need for a high degree of geometric accuracy. The constant expansion of MRI means that the issues of image artifacts in general and distortions in particular will remain an active area of research for many years to come. We also note that the use of postprocessing methods to correct for spatial inaccuracies in MRI is greater than in all other modalities. This may reflect both the magnitude of the problem and the desire to make MRI the superior modality to visualize and quantify structure. In ET, distortions generally result from fundamental physical or electronic limitations in the image formation process and often from a compromise between sensitivity and accuracy. In US, the great complexity of the interactions between the sound waves and the imaged tissue, resulting in the sometimes dramatic breakdown of the assumptions on which the method relies, imposes fundamental limitations on the achievable faithfulness of the reconstructed image. The amplitude of these geometric inaccuracies compared to other undesirable effects or limitations has resulted in a relative lack of interest in possible correction methods for US.

Using spatial resolution as a criterion, CT and MRI are generally superior to ET and US. On the other hand, distortions are the most important in MRI in relative terms, while CT and ET are often considered distortion free. Furthermore, one could argue that the magnitude of the distortions in US matches its spatial resolution. The implication of these observations is that the achievable quality of image registration will depend on the modalities involved and the aim of the registration. For maximum precision, relative differences in distortion can be modeled and integrated in the registration process. In general, such a model will be used to correct the most distorted modality. For applications involving an external coordinate system, the need to transform between image and world coordinates is likely to be a determining factor and may require distortion modeling for each modality.

References

1. Joseph, P.M., Artifacts in computed tomography. Newton, T.H. and Potts, D.G., Eds., *Radiology of the Skull and Brain: Technical Aspects of Computed Tomography*. C.V. Mosby, St. Louis, 1981.

2. Kelly, P.J. and Kall, B.A., *Computers in Stereotactic Neurosurgery*. Blackwell Scientific Publications, Boston, 1992.

3. Lemieux, L., Kitchen, N.D., Hughes, S.W., and Thomas, D.G.T., Voxel-based localization in frame-based and frameless stereotaxy and its accuracy. *Med. Phys.* 1994; 21(8):1301–1310.

4. Sumanaweera, T., Glover, G., Song, S., Adler, J., and Napel, S., Quantifying MRI geometric distortion in tissue. *Magn. Reson. Med.* 1994; 31:40–47.

5. Maurer, C.R., Aboutanos, G.B., Dawant, B.M., Gadamsetty, S., Margolin, R.A., Maciunas, R.J., and Fitzpatrick, J.M., Effect of geometrical distortion correction in MR on image registration accuracy. *J. Comput. Assist. Tomogr.* 1996; 20(4): 666–679.

6. Peters, T.M., Clark, J.A., Olivier, A., Marchand, E.P., Mawko, G., Dieumegarde, M., Muresan, L., and Ethier, R., Integrated stereotaxic imaging with CT, MR imaging, and digital subtraction angiography. *Radiology.* 1986; 161:821–826.

7. Maciunas, R.J., Galloway, Jr., R.L., Latimer, J., Cobb, C., Zaccharias, E., Moore, A., and Mandava, V.R., An independent application accuracy evaluation of stereotactic frame systems. *Stereotact. Funct. Neurosurg.* 1992; 58(1–4):103–7.

8. Walton, L., Hampshire, A., Forster, D.M.C., and Kemeny, A.A., A phantom study to assess the accuracy of stereotactic localization, using T1-weighted magnetic resonance imaging with the Leksell stereotactic system. *Neurosurg.* 1996; 38(1): 170–178.

9. Ramsey, C.R. and Oliver, A.L., Magnetic resonance imaging-based reconstructed radiographs, virtual simulation, and three-dimensional treatment planning for brain neoplasms. *Med. Phys.* 1998; 25(10):1928–1934.

10. Zylka, W. and Wischmann, H.A., On geometric distortions in CT images. *18th Conf. IEEE Eng. Med. Biol. Soc.* EMBS, Amsterdam, 1996.

11. Heilbrun, M.P., Sunderland, P.M., McDonald, P.R., Wells, T.H., Cosman, E., and Ganz, E., Brown-Roberts-Wells stereotactic frame modifications to accomplish magnetic resonance imaging guidance in three planes. *Appl. Neurophysiol.* 1987; 50:143–152.

12. Schad, L., Lott, S., Schmitt, F., Sturm, V., and Lorenz, W.J., Correction of spatial distortion in MR imaging: a prerequisite for accurate stereotaxy. *J. Comput. Assist. Tomogr.* 1987; 11(3):499–505.

13. Sekihara, K., Kuroda, M., and Kohno, H., Image restoration from non-uniform magnetic influence for direct Fourier NMR imaging. *Phys. Med. Biol.* 1984; 29(1):15–24.

14. Bakker, C.J.G., Moerland, M.A., Bhagwandien, R., and Beersma, R., Analysis of machine-dependent and object-induced geometric distortion in 2DFT MR imaging. *Magn. Reson. Imag.* 1992; 10:697–608.

15. Sumanaweera, T.S., Glover, G.H., Binford, T.O., and Adler, J.R., MR susceptibility misregistration correction. *IEEE. Trans. Med. Imag.* 1993; 12(2):251–259.

16. Reichenbach, J.R., Venkatesan, R., Yablonskiy, D.A., Thompson, M.R., Lai, S., and Haacke, E.M., Theory and application of static field inhomogeneity effects in gradient-echo imaging. *J. Magn. Reson. Imaging.* 1997; 7:266–279.

17. Schad, L., Ehricke, H.H., Wowra, B., Layer, G., Engenhart, R., Kauczor, H.U., Zabel, H.J., Brix, G., and Lorenz, W.J., Correction of spatial distortion in magnetic resonance angiography for radiosurgical treatment planning of cerebral arteriovenous malformations. *Magn. Reson. Imaging.* 1992; 10:609–621.

18. Studholme, C., Hill, D.G.H., Wong, J., Maisey, M.N., and Hawkes, D.J., Registration measures for automated 3D alignment of PET and intensity distorted MR images. *Proceedings in Image Fusion and Shape Variability,* Mardia, K.V., Gill, C.A., and Dryden, I.L., Eds., Leeds University Press, 1996.

19. Sumanaweera, T.S., Glover, G.H., Hemler, P.F., van den Elsen, P.A., Martin, D., Adler, J.R., and Napel, S., MR geometric distortion correction for improved frame-based stereotaxic target localization accuracy. *Magn. Reson. Med.* 1995; 34:106–113.

20. Mizowaki, T., Nagata, Y., Okajima, K., Murata, R., Yamamoto, M., Kokubo, M., Hiraoka, M., and Abe, M., Development of an MR simulator: experimental verification of geometric distortion and clinical application. *Radiology.* 1996; 199: 855–860.

21. Michiels, J., Bosmans, H., Pelgrims, P., Vandermeulen, D., Gybels, J., Marchal, G., and Suetens, P., On the problem of geometric distortion in magnetic resonance images for stereotactic neurosurgery. *Magn. Reson. Imaging.* 1994; 12(5): 749–765.

22. Alexander III, E., Kooy, H.M., van Herk, M., Schwartz, M., Barnes, P.D., Tarbell, N., Mulkern, R.V., Holupka, E.J., and Loeffler, J.S., Magnetic resonance image-directed stereotactic neurosurgery: use of image fusion with computerized tomography to enhance spatial accuracy. *J. Neurosurg.* 1995; 83:271–276.

23. Walton, L., Hampshire, A., Forster, D.M.C., and Kemeny, A.A., Stereotactic localization with magnetic resonance imaging: a phantom study to compare the accuracy obtained using two-dimensional and three-dimensional data acquisitions. *Neurosurg.* 1997; 41(1):131–139.

24. Sumanaweera, T., Adler, J.R., Napel, S., and Glover, G.H., Characterization of spatial distortion in magnetic resonance imaging and its implications for stereotaxic surgery. *Neurosurg.* 1994; 35(4):696–704.

25. Moerland, M.A., Beersma, R., Bhagwandien, R., Wijderman, H.K., and Bakker, C.J.G., Analysis and correction of geometric distortions in 1.5T magnetic resonance images for use in radiotherapy treatment planning. *Phys. Med. Biol.* 1995; 40:1651–1664.

26. Lemieux, L., Barker, G.J., and MacManus, D.G., Important geometric distortions in 3D gradient-echo images with rectangular field-of-view and implications for stereotaxy, in: *Proceed. Soc. Magn. Reson. 4th Scientific Meeting and Exhibition,* New York, 1996:600.

27. Jezzard, P. and Balaban, R.S., Correction for geometric distortion in echo-planar images from B0 field variations. *Magn. Reson. Med.* 1995; 34:65–73.

28. Moseley, M.E. and Butts, K., Diffusion and Perfusion, in Stark, D.D. and Bradley, Jr., W.G., Ed., *Magnetic Resonance Imaging.* C.V. Mosby; St. Louis: 1999.

29. Chang, H. and Fitzpatrick, J.M., A technique for accurate magnetic resonance imaging in the presence of field inhomogeneities. *IEEE. Trans. Med. Imaging.* 1992; 11(3):319–329.

30. Reber, P.J., Wong, E.C., Buxton, R.B., and Frank, L.R., Correction of off-resonance-related distortion in echo-planar imaging using EPI-based field maps. *Magn. Reson. Med.* 1998; 39:328–330.

31. Kadah, Y.M. and Hu, X., Algebraic reconstruction for magnetic resonance imaging under B_0 inhomogeneity. *IEEE. Trans. Med. Imag.* 1998; 17(3):362–370.

32. Ernst, T., Speck, O., Itti, L., and Chang, L., Simultaneous correction for interscan patient motion and geometric distortions in echoplanar imaging. *Magn. Reson. Med.* 1999; 42:201–205.

33. Hyde, R.J., Ellis, J.H., Gardner, E.A., Zhang, Y., and Carson, P.L., MRI scanner variability studies using a semi-automated analysis system. *Magn. Reson. Imaging.* 1994; 12(7):1089–1097.

34. Freeborough, P.A. and Fox, N.C., Modeling brain deformations in Alzheimer Disease by fluid registration of serial 3D MR images. *J. Comput. Assist. Tomogr.* 1998; 22(5):838–843.

35. Lemieux, L. and Barker, G.J., Measurement of small inter-scan fluctuations in voxel dimensions in magnetic resonance images using registration. *Med. Phys.* 1998; 25(6):1049–1054.

36. Hill, D.L.G., Maurer, C.R., Studholme, C., Fitzpatrick, J.M., and Hawkes, D.J., Correcting scaling errors in tomographic images using a nine degree of freedom registration algorithm. *J. Comput. Assist. Tomogr.* 1998; 22(2):317–323.

37. Wicks, D.A.G., Barker, G.J., and Tofts, P.S., Correction of intensity nonuniformity in MR images of any orientation. *Magn. Reson. Imaging.* 1993; 11:183–196.

38. Lemieux, L., Wieshmann, U.C., Moran, N.F., Fish, D.R., and Shorvon, S.D., The detection and significance of subtle changes in mixed-signal brain lesions by serial MRI scan matching and spatial normalization. *Med. Im. Anal.* 1998; 2(3):227–242.

39. Condon, B.R., Patterson, J., Wyper, D., Jenkins, A., and Hadley, D.M., Image non-uniformity in magnetic resonance imaging: its magnitude and methods for correction. *Br. J. Radiol.* 1987; 60:83–87.

40. Stollberger, R. and Wach, P., Imaging of the active B1 field *in vivo*. *Magn. Reson. Med.* 1996; 35:246–251.

41. Sled, J.G. and Pike, B., Quantitative experimental validation of an analytic model for intensity non-uniformity in MRI. *Proc. Intl. Soc. Magn. Reson. Med.* 1999; 7:2140.

42. Narayana, P.A. and Borthakur, A., Effect of radio frequency inhomogenity correction on the reproducibility of intracranial volumes using MR image data. *Magn. Reson. Med.* 1995; 33:396–400.

43. Meyer, C.R., Bland, P.H., and Pipe, J., Retrospective correction of intensity inhomogeneities in MRI. *IEEE. Trans. Med. Imag.* 1995; 14(1):36–41.

44. Wells III, W.M., Grimson, W.E.L., Kikinis, R., and Jolesz, F.A., Adaptive segmentation of MRI data. *IEEE. Trans. Med. Imag.* 1996; 15:429–442.

45. Held, K., Kops, E.R., Krause, B.J., Wells, III, W.M., Kikinis, R., and Muller-Gartner, H.W., Markov random field segmentation of brain MR images. *IEEE. Trans. Med. Imag.* 1997; 16(6):878–886.

46. Guillemaud, R. and Brady, M., Estimating the bias field of MR images. *IEEE. Trans. Med. Imag.* 1997; 16(3):238–251.

47. Sled, J.G., Zijdenbos, A.P., and Evans, A.C., A nonparametric method for automatic correction of intensity nonuniformity in MRI data. *IEEE. Trans. Med. Imag.* 1998; 17(1):87–97.

48. Lemieux, L., Hagemann, G., Krakow, K., and Woermann, F.G., Fast, accurate and reproducible automatic segmentation of the brain in T1-weighted volume magnetic resonance image data. *Magn. Reson. Med.* 1999; 42(1):127–135.

49. Vokurka, E.A., Thacker, N.A., and Jackson, A., A fast model independent method for automatic correction of intensity nonuniformity in MRI data. *J. Magn. Reson. Imaging.* 1999; 10(4):550–562.

50. Hoffman, E.J., Phelps, M.E., Huang, S.C., Mazziotta, J., Digby, W., and Dahlbom, M., A new PET system for high-resolution 3-dimensional brain imaging. *J. Nucl. Med.* 1987; 28(4):758–759.

51. Townsend, D.W., Wensveen, M., Byars, L.G., Geissbühler, A., Tochon-Danguy, H.J., Christin, A., et al., A rotating PET scanner using BGO block detectors: design, performance and applications. *J. Nucl. Med.* 1993; 34:1367–1376.

52. Bailey, D.L., Young, H.E., Bloomfield, P.M., Meikle, S.R., Glass, D.E., Myers, M.J., et al., ECAT ART—A continuously rotating PET camera: performance characteristics, comparison with a full ring system, initial clinical studies, and installation considerations in a nuclear medicine department. *Eur. J. Nucl. Med.* 1997; 24(1):6–15.

53. Karp, J.S., Muehllener, G., Mankoff, D.A., Ordonez, C.E., Ollinger, J.M., Daube-Witherspoon, M.E., et al., Continuous-slice PENN-PET: a positron tomograph with volume imaging capability. *J. Nucl. Med.* 1990; 31:617–627.

54. Townsend, D.W., Frey, P., Jeavons, A., Reich, G., Tochon-Danguy, H.J., Donath, A., et al., High density avalanche chamber (HIDAC) positron camera. *J. Nucl. Med.* 1987; 28:1554–1562.

55. Marsden, P.K., Ott, R.J., Bateman, J.E., Cherry, S.R., Flower, M.A., and Webb, S., The performance of a multiwire proportional chamber positron camera for clinical use. *Phys. Med. Biol.* 1989; 34:1043–1062.

56. Lewellen, T.K., Miyaoka, R.S., Kaplan, M.S., Kohlmyer, S.K., Costa, W., and Jansen, F., Preliminary investigation of coincidence imaging with a standard dual-headed SPECT system. *J. Nucl. Med.* 1995; 36(5):175P (Abstract).

57. Lang, T.F., Hasegawa, B.H., Liew, S.C., Brown, J.K., Blankespoor, S.C., and Reilly, S.M., et al., Description of a prototype emission-transmission computed tomography imaging system. *J. Nucl. Med.* 1992; 33(10):1881–1887.

58. Kalki, K., Blankespoor, S.C., Brown, J.K., Hasegawa, B.H., Dae, M.W., Chin, M., et al., Myocardial perfusion imaging with a combined x-ray CT and SPECT system. *J. Nucl. Med.* 1997; 38(10):1535–1540.

59. Beyer, T., Kinahan, P.E., Townsend, D.W., and Sashin, D., The use of X-ray CT for attenuation correction of PET data, in Trendler, R.C., Ed., *IEEE Nuclear Science Symposium and Medical Imaging Conference*; 1994; Institute of Electrical and Electronic Engineers; Norfolk, VA, 1994. 1573–1577.

60. Shao, Y., Cherry, S.R., Farahani, K., Meadors, K., Siegel, S., and Silverman, R.W., et al., Simultaneous PET and MR imaging. *Phys. Med. Biol.* 1997; 42:1965–1970.

61. Marsden, P.K., Shoa, Y., Cherry, S.R., Cave, A., Parkes, H.G., and Silverman, R.W., et al., Simultaneous acquisition of PET images and NMR spectra in a high field magnet. *J. Nucl. Med.* 1997; 38(5)Supplement: 45P.

62. Larsson, S.A., Gamma camera emission tomography. Development and properties of a multisectional emission computed tomography system. *Acta Radiologica* 1980; Suppl 363:30–32.

63. Bailey, D.L., Transmission scanning in emission tomography. *Eur. J. Nucl. Med.* 1998; 25(7):774–787.

64. Barry, C.D., Allott, C.P., John, N.W., Mellor, P.M., Arundel, P.A., Thomson, D.S., and Waterton, J.C., Three-dimensional freehand ultrasound: image reconstruction and volume analysis. *Ultra. Med. Biol.* 1997; 23(8):1209–24.

65. Cosgrove, D., Meire, H., and Dewbury K., *Abdominal and General Ultrasound* Vol. 1. Churchill Livingstone, Edinburgh, 1993.

66. Prager, R.W., Rohling, R.N., Gee, A.H., and Berman, L., Rapid calibration for 3-D freehand ultrasound. *Ultra. Med. Biol.* 1998; 24(6):855–869.

67. Birkfellner, W., Watzinger, F., Wanschitz, F., Enislidis, G., Kollmann, C., Rafolt, D., and Nowotny, R., Systematic distortions in magnetic position digitizers. *Med. Phys.* 1998; 25(11):2242–2248.

68. Rohling, R.N., Gee, A.H., and Berman, L., Automatic registration of 3D ultrasound images. *Ultra. Med. Biol.* 1998; 24(6):841–854.

69. Legget, M.E., Leotta, D.F., Bolson, E.L., McDonald, J.A., Martin, R.W., Li, X.N., Otto, C.M., and Sheehan, F.H., System for quantitative three-dimensional echocardiography of the left ventricle based on a magnetic-field position and orientation sensing system. *IEEE Trans. Biomed. Eng.* 1998; 45(4):494–504.

70. Hughes, S.W., D'Arcy, T.J., Maxwell, D.J., Chiu, W., Milner, A., Saunders, J.E., and Sheppard, R.J., Volume estimation from multiplanar 2D ultrasound images using a remote electromagnetic position and orientation sensor. *Ultra. Med. Biol.* 1996; 22(5):561–572.

71. Detmer, P.R., Bashein, G., Hodges, T., Beach, K.W., Filer, E.P., Burns, D.H., and Strandness, D.E., 3D ultrasonic image feature localization based on magnetic scanhead tracking—*in vitro* calibration and validation. *Ultra. Med. Biol.* 1994; 20(9):923–936.

72. Sato, Y., Nakamoto, M., Tamaki, Y., Sasama, T., Sakita, I., Nakajima, Y., Monden, M., and Tamura, S., Image guidance of breast cancer surgery using 3D ultrasound images and augmented reality visualization. *IEEE Trans. Med. Imag.* 1998; 17(5):681–693.

73. King, D.L., King, D.L., Jr., and Shao, M.Y., Evaluation of *in vitro* measurement accuracy of a three-dimensional ultrasound scanner. *J. Ultra. Med.* 1991; 10(2): 77–82.

74. Hata, N., Dohi, T., Iseki, H., and Takakura, K., Development of a frameless and armless stereotactic neuronavigation system with ultrasonographic registration. *Neurosurgery* 1997; 41(3):608–613.

75. Comeau, R.M., Fenster, A., and Peters, T.M., Intraoperative US in interactive image-guided neurosurgery. *Radiographics* 1998; 18(4) 1019–1027.

76. Tong, S., Cardinal, H.N., Downey, D.B., and Fenster, A., Analysis of linear, area and volume distortion in 3D ultrasound imaging. *Ultra. Med. Biol.* 1998; 24: 355–373.

77. Thrush, A.J., Bonnett, D.E., Elliott, M.R., Kutob, S.S., and Evans, D.H., An evaluation of the potential and limitations of three-dimensional reconstructions from intravascular ultrasound images. *Ultra. Med. Biol.* 1997; 23:437–445.

78. Rohling, R., Gee, A., and Berman, L., Three-dimensional spatial compounding of ultrasound images. *Med. Image Anal.* 1996/7; 1:177–193.

79. Rohling, R., Gee, A., and Berman, L., A comparison of freehand three-dimensional ultrasound reconstruction techniques. *Med. Image Anal.* 1999, 3(4):339–359.

6

Detecting Failure, Assessing Success

J. Michael Fitzpatrick

CONTENTS

6.1 Introduction

The goal of image registration is to find a geometrical transformation that aligns points in one view of an object with corresponding points in another view of an object. In medical applications one of these views will typically be a tomographic image such as CT, MR, SPECT, or PET, but may include x-ray or even video images. The other view may be chosen from one of these modalities or may be a physical view of the anatomy in space, a view which we treat here as merely another "imaging" modality. An object in medical applications is some portion of anatomy such as the brain, a limb, the chest, the liver, etc. Each view will always include approximately the same anatomical region. Typically the two views will be taken from the same patient, in which case the problem is that of intrapatient registration, but interpatient registration has application as well. Because most research on registration has focused on intrapatient three-dimensional images and rigid-body registration, this chapter likewise concentrates the most attention on this problem.

To be useful in any application, registration must be embedded in some larger system. The need for the embedding system arises because the transformation that the registration step produces as output is a mathematical mapping function, which is ill-suited for direct human use, particularly when three dimensions are involved. In rigid-body registration, the transformation itself is of little clinical relevance. In some nonrigid registration applications, however, the mapping can provide information about change in structures over time, or variability between individuals. In either case, the registration transformation serves as input to some other component of a larger system that leads ultimately to patient benefit. That next component may be an image viewer that presents resliced volumes or surface renderings to a physician during diagnosis or to a surgeon during image-guided treatment. It may be part of a robotically controlled treatment system, such as a bone drill in orthopedic surgery or a linear accelerator in radiotherapy, or it may be a segmentation algorithm that requires two or more modalities to distinguish among various tissue types. In every case, the job of the registration component is simply to deliver an aligning transformation. It is the job of the embedding system to make that transformation clinically useful.

Regardless of the combination of views, the next component in the embedding system, or the particular application, success or failure for the registration component of the system hinges on the quality of alignment of homologous points provided by the transformation that it produces. The alignment need not be perfect, but it must be adequate for the problem at hand. In order to determine whether a given registration system is indeed adequate for a given problem, or to determine whether it has performed adequately for a given pair of views, it is necessary to measure the degree of alignment. That measurement is the subject of this chapter.

6.2 Measures of Success

Our choice of the quality of alignment as the measure of success follows directly from our definition of registration, which is the determination of a transformation that aligns points in one view of an object with corresponding points in another view of an object. We note that other aspects of the performance of a registration system may also be considered in determining its success. Maintz and Viergever, for example, in a thorough annotated survey of papers on registration (through 1996) list precision, accuracy, robustness/stability, reliability, resource requirements, algorithm complexity, assumption verification, and clinical use as the items to consider as part of the assessment.[1] Our choice of the degree of alignment as the single measure of success simplifies assessment of registration methods and comparisons among them. A major benefit is that no patient outcomes are involved in this measure of success. Measuring registration success on the basis of patient outcomes necessarily convolves the quality of the alignment with the quality of the operation of each component of the embedding system through the chain from registration to diagnosis or treatment. In fact, such derived measures of success, in which improvement in registration accuracy is deduced from improved output of some subsystem further along the chain, may be all that is available when alignment cannot be measured directly. This derivative approach has been applied, for example, in the registration of bilateral mammograms by assessing the visual detection of abnormalities.[2] Such validations, which are capable of certifying a registration system as acceptable or of ranking systems, replace the problem of registration assessment with a different assessment problem. They are, however, to be avoided, if possible, in favor of the direct measure. The resulting simplification of the assessment report and sharper definition of registration quality are well worth the effort.

Most of the work and much of the literature on the subject of registration inevitably focuses on the quest for registration methods that produce a better alignment for some combination of modalities. The success of the registration, which we are relating monotonically to the quality of the alignment, has been estimated in published work by visual inspection, by comparison with a gold standard, or by means of some self-consistency measure. Although the great majority of studies of registration quality have been carried out for rigid-body registration algorithms, the same concepts are also applicable for nonrigid registration. The estimates of registration quality are employed in two distinct notions of success and, concomitantly, of failure. The first is success for a class of image pairs; the second is success for a given image pair. The former measure is useful when determining whether a method is applicable for a given clinical problem, while the second is useful as a safeguard against harmful errors for a given patient. In either case it is necessary to determine alignment error.

6.2.1 Alignment Errors

The measurement of registration success, whether for a class of images or for a given pair of images, will be some statistical estimate of some geometrical measure of alignment error. Many such measurements have been used to measure the quality of registration, but not all are of equal value. An understanding of their meanings is crucial to understanding and evaluating claims of registration accuracy.

6.2.1.1 Target Registration Error

A common geometrical measure, which we will call target registration error (TRE), is the displacement between two corresponding points after registration, i.e., after one of the points has been subjected to the registering transformation. The word "target" in the name of this error measure is meant to suggest that the error is being measured at an anatomical position that is the target of some intervention or diagnosis. Such errors would be expected to be more meaningful than errors measured at points with no intrinsic clinical significance. We let p represent a point in the first image of a pair to be registered, and q a point in the second image. A registration method applied to this pair leads to a transformation T that, without loss of generality, registers the first image to the second. The difference between the two vectors representing the transformed point and the corresponding point gives the target registration error. Thus,

$$\text{TRE} = T(p) - q. \tag{6.1}$$

If the direction of the error is important, the vector quantity must be reported; normally, however, only the magnitude TRE of the error is reported.

6.2.1.2 Fiducial Registration Error

An example of an error measure that lacks the intrinsic clinical meaning associated with TRE is fiducial registration error (FRE). This error is sometimes reported for systems that achieve registration by aligning pairs of points associated with specially selected "fiducial" features that are visible in both spaces. Both this error and TRE are illustrated in Figure 6.1. Fiducial features are selected not because of their clinical significance, but because of their locatability. They may be part of some easily visible anatomical features or they may be the centroids of specially designed fiducial markers that have been affixed to the anatomy before imaging. In either case the word "fiducial" is meant to suggest reliability. The reliability of anatomical points is enhanced by restricting their choice to clearly visible features; the reliability of the marker derives from its design, which typically insures that it is bright enough and large enough to render a consistent centroid in each image. The reliability of a point used in any point-based registration system is directly related to the consistency with which the identical geometrical location within the fiducial feature can be identified in each image space. An error in this localization step, which is commonly called the fiducial localization error (FLE) as illustrated in Figure 6.2, will propagate throughout the registration process, but if the magnitude of FLE is small, it can be expected that a transformation that aligns fiducial points will align less visible target points

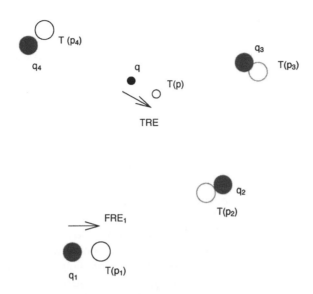

FIGURE 6.1

Schematic of point-based registration illustrating two measures of error. Black circles represent positions q_i in one space. The unfilled circles represent positions p_i in the other space after they have been mapped by the registering transformation **T**. The numbered positions are points used in the registration. Target registration error (TRE) is the registration error at a point not used to effect the registration fiducial registration error (FRE) is the alignment error between points used to effect the registration.

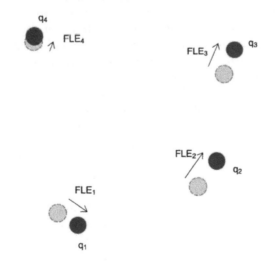

FIGURE 6.2

Schematic of point-based registration illustrating fiducial localization error (FLE). Black circles represent positions q_i at which points are localized in one of two spaces involved in the registration process. The dashed circles represent the actual positions. The black circles represent the position chosen by the localization process.

accurately as well. Fiducial registration error is typically reported as a mean, commonly in the root-mean-square (RMS) sense of the distance between corresponding fiducial points after a point-based registration has been effected. Thus,

$$\mathrm{FRE}^2 = \sum_i^N |\mathbf{T}(\mathbf{p}_i) - \mathbf{q}_i|^2, \qquad (6.2)$$

where N equals the number of fiducials used in the registration process and $\mathbf{p}_i$ and $\mathbf{q}_i$ are positions of fiducial i in the two image spaces.

TRE is more meaningful as a measure of registration success than FRE for two reasons. First, as pointed out above, TRE can be measured at clinically relevant points, whereas FRE is by definition limited to fiducial features whose positions are clinically relevant only by coincidence. Second, FRE may overestimate or underestimate registration error. The clinical relevance of TRE makes it dominant over FRE as a general measure of meaningful error, but if FRE were itself a good estimate of TRE, then it could serve as an easily measurable surrogate.

Unfortunately, it is not. The first problem is underestimation. Some components of registration error will not be reflected in FRE because the registration system uses these same fiducial point locations in its determination of the registering transformation. These hidden errors come about because the system does its best, within the limits of the set of transformations at its disposal, to align fiducial points pairs identified as corresponding, regardless of whether they do indeed correspond. For example, if the transformations being considered by the registration system are limited to rigid-body motion, then fiducial localization errors of the same magnitude and direction for every fiducial in a given image space will make no contribution to FRE. As a specific simple case, suppose FLE is exactly 3 mm in the x direction for all N fiducial points in the first image space and 4 mm in the z direction for all fiducials in the second. Because there exists a rigid transformation that will bring each of these purportedly corresponding pairs into perfect alignment, namely a translational motion of the first image of -3 mm in x and 4 mm in z, relative to the second, the resulting FRE for this case will be zero, while TRE will be displacement whose magnitude is 5 mm at all points. In general, for all rigid-body registration systems, to the extent that a given set of fiducial localization errors can be duplicated by means of a rigid-body motion, the registration error will be underestimated by FRE.

For nonrigid motion the situation may be worse. Any set of point pairs, however badly localized in either or both spaces, can be perfectly aligned, given a sufficiently versatile set of geometrical transformations. The FLE at each of the fiducial points will be interpolated exactly or approximately at all other points. Thus, by overfitting the fiducials in one space to their positions in the other space, the transformation may produce an FRE smaller than the true TRE. This problem is less insidious if the set of transformations is justified on physical grounds, meaning that the transformations include only those physically possible between the two spaces. For example, if two images of the same head are acquired, then for multimodality registration, where the desired accuracy is of the order of one mm, only a rigid transformation is justified (unless there is intervening surgical resection).* For nonrigid anatomy or intrapatient registration, the "registering" transformation may not reflect the physical transformation in regions where no points are available. It is helpful to view the problem of underestimation in terms of a null space. Regardless of the set of transformations, for sufficiently small errors FRE can be expected to be an approximately linear function of the N fiducial localization errors. The input space of FRE, as function of the FLEs, will always include a null subspace, which is the space of patterns of FLEs that can be completely compensated by one of the transformations in the set. If the localization error pattern has a component in that null space, then FRE will underestimate TRE.

The second problem is overestimation. This situation is common when random components to FLE are uncorrelated among the N fiducials used in the registration. In that case, the influence on the transformation by the localization error of some fiducials will tend to be cancelled by the influence of others. Here again rigid transformations provide a simple example. Suppose that in one image space FLE for half of the fiducials is 3 mm in the x direction, while for the other half it is 3 mm in the $-x$ direction. The optimal registration transformation will be the identity. For that transformation FRE will be 3 mm, while the resultant TRE will be zero at all points. In more realistic situations the cancellation is less complete.

The relationship between the expected FLE and the expected TRE depends on both the number and placement of the fiducial points. For uncorrelated FLEs, the relationship for rigid-body registration has been subject to conjecture for many years but is now well understood in the RMS sense for isotropic error patterns.[4,5] The relationship between FRE and FLE, which is due to Sibson,[6] is surprisingly simple,

$$RMS(FRE) = (1 - 2/N)^{1/2}RMS(FLE), \qquad (6.3)$$

where N is again the number of fiducial points used in the registration. This equation is of great importance because it provides a means to bridge the gap from self-consistency to accuracy. (See also Section 6.3.2 for another means.) Here FRE represents self-consistency, and TRE, whose statistics can be determined from those of FLE, represents accuracy. Equation 6.3 makes it possible to validate the accuracy of the system without resorting to comparison with any other system. This method for "bootstrapping" its accuracy gives the point-based, rigid-body system a special place in the arena of validation.

A caveat should be given here regarding the problem of the null space of FRE mentioned above. To the extent that there is a consistent, rigid displacement of

---

* The brain does pulsate within the closed skull by about 0.5 mm with the cardiac cycle.[3]

the fiducial markers in a given space relative to the object to be registered, the use of Equation 6.3 will underestimate FLE, and hence TRE.* Such consistency will be negligible for displacements caused by the effects of noise or voxelization on the marker localization algorithm. There may be a consistent effect from spatially nonuniform brightness, such as that caused in MR by radiofrequency (RF) inhomogeneity, but such an effect will be negligible because of the small extent of the typical fiducial feature. It may well be appreciable, however, for geometrical distortion resulting from static field inhomogeneity in MR scanners. Such distortion patterns may, for example, produce a consistent translation of a marker's image relative to the head image when it is located just external to the head. Scaling and skewing errors in the image, which, for example, may be caused by errors in MR gradient strength or CT gantry angle, will invalidate the relationship in Equation 6.3, with both over- and underestimation of FLE possible. Image distortion is discussed at greater length in Chapter 5.

6.2.1.3   Other Error Measures

Other measures of alignment error may be used as well. Distances between lines and, more commonly, between surfaces may be clinically relevant in some cases, but they reveal only part of the displacement error. Distances between lines are insensitive to displacements in either space parallel to the line in the respective space; distances between surfaces are similarly insensitive to displacements parallel to the surfaces. Distances between surfaces, used in some systems as cues for registration, are known to be poorly related to TRE for such systems[7] but are still used for validation when no other means is available.[8,9] Combinations may be used also with distances measured between points and lines, points and surfaces, or lines and surfaces.

For rigid-body registration, error reports may include angular displacement. Angular displacements specified relative to the directions of the coordinate axes are independent of the positions of those axes and the origin of the coordinate system. (The translational components of the error do, however, depend on the origin when there are nonzero rotational components.) It is also possible to identify for any rigid motion a single axis of rotation such that rigid motion is completely specified by a single angular displacement about that axis along with a single translational component in the direction of that axis. Since the inverse of a rigid transformation is rigid and the composition of any two rigid transformations is likewise rigid, any error in the determination of a rigid transformation has itself the form of a rigid transformation. Thus, an angular displacement would appear to be a simple, convenient method for specifying alignment error. Unfortunately, its meaning is severely limited by two factors: it is a global measure that cannot be focused on a clinically important region, and the magnitude of local displacement that results from rotation depends on the distance from an axis of rotation that has no

---

* To be precise, the problem only occurs if the rigid displacement relative to the object is different in the two spaces to be registered.

clinical meaning. Thus, the significance of angular motion is typically difficult to interpret clinically.

6.2.2 Statistics

As mentioned earlier, registration success may be determined for a class of image pairs or a given image pair. The former measure is useful when determining whether a registration system is appropriate for a given clinical problem, while the latter is useful as a safeguard against harmful errors during subsequent routine clinical use. Once a measure of alignment error is chosen, it can be measured and reported, but because of the complex variation among images, it will be necessary to perform many registrations and make many measurements before a clear picture of system accuracy can emerge. The accuracy report is therefore necessarily statistical. Common, meaningful statistics include the mean and standard deviation, the root-mean-square, which is often used for Euclidean distance measures, the median, which may be more meaningful than either of the former measures in the face of outliers, and other order statistics, such as 90 or 95% thresholds. Such statistics, gathered in experiments on a well-defined class of images, can be used in predictions of clinical performance on future data sets of the same class. Indeed, the primary purpose of gathering statistics on experimentally measured image registration accuracy is the prediction of clinical success or failure. For example, statistics gathered from experimental measurements of TRE on a system for registering CT or MR with specified imaging parameters (e.g., slice thicknesses, field-of-view, pulse sequence, contrast administration, etc.) for a given anatomy (e.g., head, liver, etc.) and given pathology (e.g., tumor, diffuse white matter lesions, etc., or normals), can be used to predict the expected value of TRE, or preferably its distribution, in a similar clinical situation. If the distribution is available, then the probability of success can be stated as the probability that TRE will fall below the acceptable threshold.

Except in rare cases, TRE will vary with position. Thus, the location, or locations, at which TRE is measured is a critical part of the description of the experimental situation as well. For example, if the clinical target is near the optic nerve, then the value of TRE at the center of the cerebellum is not a reliable predictor of clinical success or failure. The mean TRE throughout the brain is a valuable statistic but is still inferior to a point-by-point accounting, even when it is supplemented by the variance. A maximum value provides more protection against disaster, but such a conservative measure may preclude the use of a system that would in fact benefit the patient for a particular target point. It should perhaps be emphasized that experimental error statistics are meaningful predictors of clinical error only when the clinical situation is sufficiently similar to the experimental situation. We discuss this notion of similarity further below.

A second, and equally important, purpose of gathering registration statistics is detection of clinical failure. A successful registration need not mean that the alignment is perfect, but it does mean that the alignment error is below some threshold. While registration accuracy cannot be determined directly for a given clinical case (otherwise, there must be a superior registration method available), there may be some measurement that can be made for a given case to indicate whether the accuracy is likely to be acceptable. The relationship between that measurement and a clinically meaningful measure of accuracy, such as TRE, will be statistical and must be verified experimentally. The function that is optimized during the registration process can serve this purpose, but its statistics must be carefully established to give it predictive power. The primary example is FRE for a point-based rigid-body system. Experimental measurements of FRE can be used to determine the distribution of FRE values for a properly working point-based system.[6] During a clinical registration, FRE can be reported and compared with that distribution. If the value is very large, at or above the 95% level observed experimentally, for example, the system may not be working properly.

6.3   Methods for Estimating Error

The most straightforward method for estimating registration error is to compare a given registration transformation with a "ground truth" transformation, one whose accuracy is high. Ground truth may be obtained from some *gold standard* registration system, which we define as any registration system whose accuracy is known to be high. We devote most of this section to these gold standard methods.

6.3.1   Gold Standards

Gold standards may be based on computer simulations, phantoms or cadavers, or patients, where the latter category is understood to include normals as well. Phantoms may range from rectangular blocks of plastic to realistic anthropomorphic models[10] and are second only to computer simulations in providing known transformations. They are inferior, however, to patient images and computer simulations in image fidelity. For this reason they cannot be considered seriously in registration validation except for development work or as applied to the stereotactic frame, whose accuracy can be expected to be largely unaffected by differences between the phantom and a patient. For that reason we will discuss only this single application of phantom validation (see Section 6.3.1.2). Similarly, because of physiological changes at death, cadaver studies have limited use but are also appropriate for validating stereotactic frames and, to a certain extent, any systems based on bone-implanted marker systems. Gold standards based on patients are the most difficult to establish. They may be based on target features, fiducial marker systems, visual inspection, or other methods.

6.3.1.1 Computer Simulations

Computer simulations are image pairs generated by computer. While it is possible to model the anatomy and imaging process to produce both images to be registered, computer simulations are typically produced by modifying one acquired image to produce a second simulated image that has been modified by a known geometrical transformation. The second image may be of the same or different modality. Simulations have the primary advantage that the transformation is known exactly, and the secondary advantage that any transformation is readily available. They are especially apt for development work, but they lack the realism arising from the sometimes subtle anatomical changes that accompany respiration, the cardiac cycle, and involuntary or voluntary motion during image acquisition. Such motion can cause warping in CT, in which slices are acquired serially, and blurring and other reconstruction artifacts in MRI, PET, or SPECT, in which information is gathered from multiple slices in parallel. Motion can cause other artifacts such as changes in magnetic susceptibility patterns in MR or scatter patterns in the other modalities, each of which is difficult to predict and varies with patient position and orientation. Validations based on simulations can, however, provide an upper bound on success, which can be of great value when a registration system is under development.

The simplest application of computer simulation is intramodality registration. If the second image is to be of the same modality as the first, the modification that produces it is purely one of geometrical transformation. Because a transformed voxel position will rarely fall on an integral voxel position, interpolation is necessary (see Chapter 3). If the resolution in the first image is strongly nonisotropic, the simulated image interpolation artifacts may be unacceptable in the generated image. For this reason, computer simulation for registration validation is typically based on MR volume acquisitions, whose resolution can be made virtually isotropic.[11-13] For intermodality registration it is necessary to identify tissue types and generate new gray level values (in addition to the new values resulting from interpolation) according to the physical processes of the second imaging modality. Collins et al.[13] have produced one high-resolution image of the head segmented into four tissue types and background expressly for this purpose.*

For intrapatient registration, it is most common to determine rigid-body transformations which, as stated above, are appropriate in most cases for the brain. In other intrapatient applications, nonrigid transformations may be more appropriate than model changes in soft tissue due to natural motion, resection, growth, atrophy, or other physical changes (see Chapters 13 and 15). For interpatient registration the transformation is either affine or a nonrigid transformation with additional degrees of freedom, and must model human variation. Such transformations are discussed in Chapters 13 and 14. Simulated images for validation in the nonrigid regime must be approached with

---

* This image and simulated images generated from it are available at http://www.bic.mni. mcgill.ca/brainweb/.

great care. Simulation of intrapatient motion should be based on tissue mechanics or growth models, and simulation of interpatient variation must be anatomically sound. Models based on splines and other convenient mathematical formulations will tend to favor registration systems that employ transformations with similar formulations, and therefore are highly suspect as standards for nonrigid validation. The overriding problem is that, unless constraints of some kind are placed on the motion, the number of parameters necessary to specify the physical transformation of a continuous, nonrigid object, or between two such objects, is large. In fact, absent such constraints, the number is infinite. When the constraints of rigidity are inappropriate, then the choice of constraints becomes the overriding issue in the registration.

6.3.1.2   *Target Features*

Rigorous attempts to use experimental statistics to predict clinical registration accuracy were first applied to the stereotactic frame.[14] The frame, which is rigidly attached to bone, usually the skull, is used to effect a registration between the physical patient and an image of that patient, typically for guiding biopsy needles or radiation beams to lesions within the head. In these applications the head is held motionless in the scanner and (optimally) in the same orientation relative to gravity as during treatment. Furthermore, major resection is not involved. Thus the relationship between skull and brain remains rigid. The frame is in fact appropriate only for rigid anatomy because all positioning is measured relative to the frame, a (removable) part of which is visible in the image. The rigid combination of frame and anatomy makes the registration problem much easier than the general one and potentially more accurate, because registration cues can be taken from a device that is built expressly to provide such cues.

Use of the frame for registration also makes the job of validating accuracy easier and potentially more reliable. Because neither the anatomy nor the pathology are involved in frame-based registration, its accuracy is largely unaffected by them and can be determined by means of carefully controlled experiments on phantoms. In 1992, Maciunas et al. carried out a large scale experiment of this kind on several frames.[14] They employed a phantom to which, in addition to the frame, imageable markers were attached. These markers served as *target features*, meaning that they played the role of the targets of therapy. By localizing a given target both in image space and physical space, applying the transformation determined by the frame to the localized point, and then measuring the disparity between the registered point and the physical point, TRE can be estimated. It can thus be seen that the target feature is in effect a gold standard that provides a transformation at only one point. Using this gold standard, the study found that a mean TRE of 2 mm was possible.

Maurer et al. in 1997[15] also used the target-feature approach to estimating TRE for a registration system based on specially designed, skull-implanted fiducial markers. The accuracy of any marker-based system can be expected to share some of the stereotactic frame's independence of anatomy and pathology. Maurer et al. demonstrated this independence by showing that the differences between measurements of TRE on 100 patients and measurements on a phantom were statistically insignificant.[15] The target feature was a marker identical in design to the fiducial marker and implanted in the skull, but it was not used in the registration process. The mean measured TRE was found to be 1.0 mm for registrations of CT (3 mm slices) to physical space, and 1.4 mm for registrations between MR (3 mm slices) and either of these modalities.

To achieve this accuracy, a considerable effort was expended both in the design of the markers and the design of algorithms to localize them. The resulting FLE for this system is about 0.3 to 0.4 mm in CT images with 3 mm slices, in MR images with 1 to 5 mm slices, and in physical space.[15–17] A similar study, also based on a skull-attached marker as target feature, has been carried out for a similar skull marker system. The mean TRE for registrations of CT (2 mm slices) to physical space was measured for 20 neurosurgical patients and found to be 1.7 mm.[18] The theoretical dependence of TRE on position suggests that attachment to the skull in each of these studies should provide an upper bound on RMS (TRE) (see Chapter 3), but the possibility of brain motion, which is not reflected in these measures, limits the reliability of these systems for validation to nonsurgical applications and skull base surgery.[19, 20]

Target features are also appropriate for validation in nonrigid registration for both intrapatient and interpatient applications. Miga et al., for example, used an array of implanted target markers in a porcine model,[21] and Edwards et al. used implanted electrodes[22] to validate their respective models of brain deformation during surgery. Naturally occurring features may be used as targets for validation as well. Woods et al., for example, employed cortical landmarks comprising prominent gyri and sulci to validate a method for inter-subject registration of PET and MR images.[23] Because these latter target features are not point objects, their measure of error was the smallest distance between voxels in the features. A similar method has been used in a cadaveric study to validate rigid systems.[24] It is difficult to translate such measures into TRE.

6.3.1.3 Fiducial Marker Systems

A fiducial marker system can provide an excellent gold standard for both intramodality and intermodality rigid registration. The transformations some of these systems produce can provide submillimetric accuracy, and actual patient images can be used. The primary disadvantage is that high accuracy comes at the price of high invasiveness. Thus, the availability of such images may be rare, and the set of available transformations is typically limited.

The stereotactic frame provides such a system and has been used, for example, to validate retrospective algorithms for PET-to-MR[25,26] and a point-based system for neurosurgery based on skull-implanted markers.[18] Point-based fiducial systems have the advantage over the frame in that they do not rely on maintaining a prescribed shape among the fiducials. Thus, errors caused by subtle bending of the N-bars or head ring of a frame are not a problem for fiducial systems. Fiducial systems are, however, like the frame, subject to errors caused by relative motion of the marker and anatomy between image acquisitions, or between image acquisition and physical localization. Such problems may be severe for skin-attached markers. The use of large numbers of skin markers enhances their accuracy only marginally because of correlated FLEs as they ride together on moving skin. Bone-implanted fiducial marker systems are far less prone to consistent motion and therefore gain the advantage of the bootstrapping feature, explained above, in which accuracy can be inferred without independent validation. Thus, point-based validation systems based on bone-implanted markers provide self validation as well. This benefit derives from the known statistical relationships among FLE, FRE, and TRE, as described above, which follow from the independence of FLE among the markers. Thus, while FRE is untrustworthy as a direct measure of registration accuracy, it can be exploited as an indirect measure if the theoretical chain is followed correctly from its experimental measurement via the estimate of the distribution of FLE to the prediction of the distribution of TRE (see Chapter 3). With this theory in hand, it is possible to provide statistical error bounds on the estimate of accuracy provided by point-based validation. The point-based standard is superior to the target-marker approach because it provides a dense set of TRE estimates, one at every point in space, whereas the target-feature approach provides an estimate at only the points occupied by features. Thus, for rigid-body registration in M dimensions, if there are M or more features available, it makes sense to use the point-based registration approach. This approach also typically interpolates feature localization errors by incorporating a single-least-squares fit for all of them.

6.3.1.4   Other Standards

Because a gold standard is simply a system whose accuracy is known to be high, any registration system with a known error may in principle be used as a gold standard. Wong et al., for example, used a mutual information method as a gold standard for validating accuracy of the human visual system in the detection of PET-to-MR misregistration.[27] The visual system has been used in countless reports as a gold standard for evaluating automatic registration methods.[23,28–33] It can play an important role during the development stages of any automatic registration system as a means to assess its potential and guide its refinements. It is also clearly applicable whenever the goal of the system is to produce automatic registrations that are on par with those that could be done manually. The purpose of the automatic registration in that case is to substitute inexpensive computer time for expensive expert time.

Visual inspection for validation can perhaps serve best by providing quality assurance in clinical use as a safeguard against harmful errors for a given patient. Because visual inspection has the last word on accuracy when used in quality control, it may appear that automatic registration followed by visual inspection is no better than direct, interactive registration. A useful advantage, however, in this division of duties is that the human visual system appears to be good at recognizing a very bad registration, but not so good at finding a very good one.[34] Many registration systems rely on optimization procedures that will perform properly for the large majority of patients but will occasionally fall into a nonglobal optimum that produces a bad result. The distribution of this latter mode is typically far wider than that of the properly working system, thus greatly increasing the overall variance in TRE. Visual inspection can detect very bad registrations, effectively truncating the distribution at some detection level. By catching these large outliers, visual inspection can return a system nearly to its correctly working state. As a result of efforts to quantify the accuracy of visual inspection as a means of failure detection in intermodality registration, it appears that when suitable interactive image viewing software is available, the human visual system can be relied on to detect a TRE greater than 4 mm for MR-to-PET[27,35] and 2 mm for MR-to-CT.[34] Thus, for automatic systems that tend to remain below these levels when working properly, the benefit of visual inspection should be well worth the effort.

6.3.2 Registration Circuits

A simple consistency measure has recently been proposed when at least three images of the same modality, A, B, and C, are to be registered.[36-38] By independently registering A to B, B to C, and C to A in what might be called a registration "circuit," it is possible to follow a target point from A to B to C, and back to A. If the TREs for the three registration processes are uncorrelated, then the RMS (TRE) for a single registration will be equal to RMS (TRE)/$\sqrt{3}$ for the circuit. For an n-image circuit the ratio is $\sqrt{n}$. Here, in analogy to Equation 6.3, the relationship between the circuit error and the error for a single registration provides a bridge between consistency (circuit TRE) and accuracy (single-registration TRE) when registration errors are uncorrelated. This approach has been proposed for serial MR registration problems, where it may be important to measure TRE values as small as 0.2 mm[38] or even 0.05 mm.[12] The circuit may be the only approach available for such applications in view of the difficulty of producing a gold standard with this extreme accuracy. The same approach can be used for intermodality registration if two images of each modality are available. One needs only to arrange the images so that modalities alternate around the circuit.

While this approach is reasonable when no gold standard is available, a potentially serious weakness lies in its assumption that the errors between registrations are uncorrelated. The assumption will inevitably be violated because of the fact that successive registrations, A to B and B to C, say, share a common image. Noise or imaging artifacts in B will tend to cause B to be shifted in the same direction relative to A in the A-B registration as it is relative to C in the B–C registration. These two displacements, while they contribute to each of the two single-registration TREs, will tend to cancel in the circuit, erroneously reducing their contribution to the TRE of the circuit. Thus, dividing the TRE of the circuit by $\sqrt{n}$ can be expected to underestimate TRE for a single registration. To compute RMS values, many sets of n registrations would need to be made, but these correlated errors will not be reduced in the mean. The problem does not occur for the point-based, rigid-body problem when data are gathered for Equation 6.3 because no image contributes to more than one registration.

6.4   Accounting for Error in the Standard

Comparison with a standard introduces the error of the standard into the validation. The target feature, for example, even when it is based on a marker designed to be accurately localizable, will not provide a perfect estimate of TRE. The effect of its localization error can be seen in Figure 6.3. Here the white and gray circles with dashed borders represent positions in space two. $T(\mathbf{p})$ is the transformed position arising from $\mathbf{p}$ in space one. The black circle with solid border represents the erroneously localized position $\mathbf{q} + TLE_q$ in space two as determined by the localization process, and the white circle with solid border represents the transformed position in space two of the

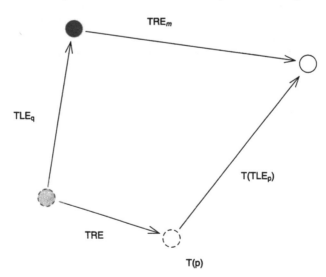

FIGURE 6.3
Schematic of registration error measurement based on a target feature. Because of target localization error (TLE), the measured target registration error (TRE_m) differs from the true target registration error (TRE). $\mathbf{p}$ and $\mathbf{q}$ represent the true positions of the marker in the two spaces; T is the registering transformation.

erroneously localized position in space one. For rigid-body transformations, this latter transformed position is $T(p) + T(TLE_p)$.

The true TRE will, in general, be different from the measured value, TRE_m, because of the error in localization, which we will call target localization error (TLE) in analogy with fiducial localization error. In a given measurement, either TRE or TRE_m may be larger in magnitude, but we should expect the true error TRE to be smaller in the RMS sense than the measured error TRE_m. This expectation is based on the assumption that the localizations of the target are uncorrelated with the registration error, a reasonable assumption because the target feature is not used in the registration process. If we make the further common assumption that there is no bias in the errors (i.e., the mean of each Cartesian component is zero), then the RMS errors are related in this simple way,

$$RMS(TRE) = \sqrt{RMS(TRE_m)^2 - RMS(TLE_p)^2 - RMS(TLE_q)^2}. \quad (6.4)$$

If the target localization error can be estimated, then Equation 6.4 should be used in estimating RMS (TRE); otherwise RMS (TRE_m) serves as an upper bound.

A similar situation holds when TRE is determined by comparison with another registration system used as a gold standard. Since the errors of the two systems are likely to be uncorrelated, the relationship between actual TRE and the measured value TRE_m is similar,

$$RMS(TRE) = \sqrt{RMS(TRE_m)^2 - RMS(TRE_g)}, \quad (6.5)$$

where TRE_g is the target registration error for the gold standard.

6.5   Independent Validation

System developers have used point-based methods to validate their own registration systems,[30,39] but there has been only one large-scale effort to carry out independent validations of many methods. An international effort to validate retrospective registrations of the head by using a set of patient images with a point-based method as a gold standard was undertaken in 1995 by 12 institutions in the U.S., Belgium, England, France, and The Netherlands.[40] In this project, coordinated by researchers in the U.S. at Vanderbilt University, a set of CT, MR, and PET images of patients was acquired at Vanderbilt and made available via the Internet to researchers at the other institutions. The patients were part of a separate, independent study in which skull-implanted markers were being used for image-guided surgery—the same markers as those used in the marker-based validation documented by Maurer et al.[15] A subset of the patients was also outfitted with stereotactic frames. All traces of the markers and the frame N-bar were erased from the images before their posting on the Internet, and the experimental situation was carefully documented with regard to image acquisition. The anatomy included an approximately consistent region of the heads of tumor patients. The frame, when present, was used as a calibration device to correct for scaling errors in MR and, for some patients, corrections were made for distortion arising from static field inhomogeneity.[41] Retrospective systems were then applied to the images by researchers at the institutions outside Vanderbilt and the resulting transformations were communicated, again via the Internet, back to Vanderbilt for comparison with the gold standard transformations, which were sequestered throughout the evaluations.

Erasure of the markers and sequestering of the standard transformations blinds the user of the retrospective method to the correct transformations. This feature is an important aspect of the study. It produces an assessment more likely to predict clinical performance, because the system assessed cannot be given inadvertent "hints" by the operator based on known answers. The results of the study revealed that a median TRE below one millimeter is possible for MR-to-CT rigid registration of head images, and a median of 3 mm is possible for MR-to-PET. The study also showed that large errors sometimes occur without warning, suggesting that some standard of quality assurance, such as visual inspection, should be employed in clinical use.

These are important results, but they must be applied with care because of limitations in the data set. The images came from a limited patient population (patients with tumors that were about to be surgically resected) and include only a limited variety of image acquisition protocols and scanners. Nevertheless, the study has been of value in establishing with some certainty a benchmark for retrospective registration accuracy, and the data set has been, and continues to be, of value as a tool for developers. The evaluation service has been in continual use since the original posting of the data set on the Internet in early 1996, both to support the work of developers[42] and to provide a means of independent validation in published accounts of new methods.[43–46]* New patient data sets including other regions of the anatomy, with new and better gold standards, would doubtless be welcomed by the image registration community.

6.6   Conclusions

Validation is an essential part of the registration process. It infers agreement on the goal of registration, which we have taken to be the alignment of points in one view of an object with corresponding points in a second view of an object. The objects in these views are typically the same, usually a patient or

---

* Available at *http://cswww.vuse.vanderbilt.edu/~image/registration/*.

some part of a patient's anatomy. We have focused on three-dimensional views and adopted a generalized notion of a "view" which includes not only images acquired with imaging systems (for example, CT, MR, PET, or SPECT), but also the physical view of the anatomy (for example, the view during surgery). This notion of views accommodates both intramodality and intermodality registration, and intrapatient and interpatient registration as well. We define several measures of error including *target registration error*, or TRE, which is the disparity in the positions of two corresponding points after registration. Regardless of the views, our definition of registration leads to a recommendation of TRE as the quantity of choice to be reported in the validation process.

TRE can be expected to vary with the registration situation, which comprises the imaging modalities, anatomy, and pathology. Also, for a given registration situation TRE can be expected to vary with position within a view. Experimental validation of a registration system should thus be extended to a clinical situation only to the extent that the clinical situation matches the experimental one. The degree of the required match will vary with the registration system, but the same modality pair should always be used.

The most commonly accepted strategy for validation is to compare the system to be validated against a *gold standard*, which we define as any system whose accuracy is known to be high. Gold standards may be based on computer simulations (typically by acquiring one image and generating a second with a known geometrical transformation, phantom images), cadavers, or patient images. Computer simulations provide arbitrarily accurate geometrical transformations but, like phantoms, are less realistic than cadaver or patient images. Simulations should also be approached with great care in nonrigid validations because of the bias of such validations in favor of registration methods that employ similar nonrigid transformations, whether or not they are physically meaningful. Validations based on pairs of acquired patient images represent the most desirable class of standards because of the inclusion of all the physical effects of the patient on image acquisition, but suffer from the difficulty of establishing the true transformation between acquired (as opposed to simulated) images.

The simplest method for establishing the transformation between acquired images, effective both for phantoms and patients, is based on the *target feature*, which is any object that can be localized independently in each view. The root-mean-square (RMS) disparity in the two localizations of the target feature after registration provides an upper bound on the RMS of TRE at the location of the feature. A more desirable method for rigid-body registration is based on a registration system that employs several fiducial features as registration cues. The major advantage of this type of system as a validation standard is that its accuracy can be determined without reference to other standards. This is accomplished by exploiting theoretically established statistical relationships among fiducial localization error (FLE), fiducial registration error (FRE), and TRE to translate self-consistency into accuracy. FRE plays an important role in this translation, but is a poor measure of registration error.

Visual assessment has often been used as a standard and has recently been subjected to validation. A self-consistency method is considered based on the registration circuit, in which a set of three or more images are registered in pairs. One major effort at validation is described. It involves intrapatient, intermodality, rigid-body registration of the head for CT, MR, and PET images and is based on a gold standard that employs bone-implanted fiducial markers.

Most validation efforts have been concentrated primarily in rigid registration. While not all the problems in this field are solved, progress has been substantial, and considerably more is known about rigid registration than nonrigid registration. Improved validation for rigid systems is still of vital importance, but the greatest challenges in assessing the success of registration systems will lie in the nonrigid regime.

Improving registration accuracy is an important goal, but without a means of validation no registration method can be accepted as a clinical tool. It is hoped that this discussion of accuracy assessment will lead others to work to improve available methods and to find new methods for assessing accuracy. Such methods will accelerate progress towards improved registration systems and will make existing methods accessible to physicians and surgeons and, ultimately, to their patients.

Acknowledgments

The author wishes to acknowledge the support of the Engineering and Physical Sciences Research Council of the U.K. and the Vanderbilt University Research Council, Nashville, Tennessee for their monetary support of this work. He also wishes to thank Professor David Hawkes, Dr. Derek Hill, and the other members of the Computational Imaging Science Group in the Division of Radiological Sciences and Medical Engineering at Guy's, Kings', and St. Thomas' Schools of Medicine and Dentistry, King's College, London, for their hospitality and stimulating discussion while this work was undertaken.

References

1. J.B.A. Maintz and M.A. Viergever. A survey of medical image registration. *Med. Image Anal.*, 2:1–36, 1998.
2. M.Y. Sallam and K.W. Bowyer. Registration and difference analysis of corresponding mammogram images. *Med. Image Anal.*, 3:103–118, 1999.
3. B.P. Poncelet, V.J. Wedeen, R.M. Weisskoff, and M.S. Cohen. Brain parenchyma motion: measurement with cine echoplanar MR imaging. *Radiology*, 185:645–651, 1992.

4. J.M. Fitzpatrick, J. West, and C.R. Maurer, Jr. Predicting error in rigid-body, point-based registration. *IEEE Trans. Med. Imaging*, 17:694–702, 1998.
5. J.B. West and J.M. Fitzpatrick. The distribution of target registration error in rigid-body, point-based registration. *Proc. Information Processing in Medical Imaging*, Springer Lecture Notes in Computer Sciences, 1613:450–465, 1999.
6. R. Sibson. Studies in the robustness of multidimensional scaling: perturbational analysis of classical scaling. *J.R. Statist. Soc. B*, 41:217–229, 1979.
7. C.R. Maurer, Jr., G.B. Aboutanos, B.M. Dawant, R.J. Maciunas, and J.M. Fitzpatrick. Registration of 3-D images using weighted geometrical features. *IEEE Trans. Med. Imaging*, 15:836–849, 1996.
8. S.J. Nelson, M.R. Day, P.J. Buffone, L.L. Wald, T.F. Budinger, R. Hawkins, W.P. Dillon, S. Huhn, M.D. Prados, S. Chang, and D.B. Vigneron. Alignment of volume MRI images and high resolution [^{18}F]fluorodeoxyglucose PET images for the evaluation of patients with brain tumors. *J. Comput. Assist. Tomogr.*, 21:183–191, 1997.
9. E.I. Parsai, K.M. Ayyangar, R.R. Dobelbowwer, and J.A. Siegel. Clinical fusion of three-dimensional images using bremsstrahlung SPECT and CT. *J. Nucl. Med.*, 38:319–324, 1997.
10. R.P. Woods, S.R. Cherry, and J.C. Mazziotta. Rapid automated algorithm for aligning and reslicing PET images. *J. Comput. Assist. Tomogr.*, 16:620–633, 1992.
11. J.V. Hajnal, N. Saeed, A. Oatridge, E.J. Williams, I.R. Young, and G.M. Bydder. Detection of subtle brain changes using subvoxel registration and subtraction of serial MR images. *J. Comput. Assist. Tomogr.*, 19:677–691, 1995.
12. L. Lemieux, U.C. Wieshmann, N.F. Moran, D.R. Fish, and S.D. Shorvon. The detection and significance of subtle changes in mixed-signal brain lesions by serial MRI scan matching and spatial normalization. *Med. Image Anal.*, 2:227–242, 1998.
13. D.L. Collins, A.P. Zijdenbos, V. Killokian, J.G. Sled, N.J. Kabani, C.J. Holmes, and A.C. Evans. Design and construction of a realistic digital brain phantom. *IEEE Trans. Med. Imaging*, 17:463–468, 1998.
14. R.J. Maciunas, R.L. Galloway, Jr., J. Latimer, C. Cobb, E. Zaccharias, A. Moore, and V.R. Mandava. An independent application accuracy evaluation of stereotactic frame systems. *Stereotact. Funct. Neurosurg.*, 58:103–107, 1992.
15. C.R. Maurer, Jr., J.M. Fitzpatrick, M.Y. Wang, R.L. Galloway, Jr., R.J. Maciunas, and G.S. Allen. Registration of head volume images using implantable fiducial markers. *IEEE Trans. Med. Imaging*, 16:447–462, 1997.
16. C.R. Maurer, Jr., R.J. Maciunas, and J.M. Fitzpatrick. Registration of head CT images to physical space using a weighted combination of points and surfaces. *IEEE Trans. Med. Imaging*, 17:753–761, 1998.
17. D.L.G. Hill, C.R. Maurer, Jr., C. Studholme, J.M. Fitzpatrick, and D.J. Hawkes. Correcting scaling errors in tomographic images using a nine degree of freedom registration algorithm. *J. Comput. Assist. Tomogr.*, 22:317–323, 1998.
18. F.C. Vinas, L. Zamorano, R. Buciuc, Q.H. Li, F. Shamsa, Z. Jiang, and F.G. Diaz. Application accuracy study of a semipermanent fiducial system for frameless stereotaxis. *Comput. Aided Surg.*, 2:257–263, 1997.
19. D.L.G. Hill, C.R. Maurer, Jr., R.J. Maciunas, J.A. Barwise, J.M. Fitzpatrick, and M.Y. Wang. Measurement of intraoperative brain surface deformation under a craniotomy. *Neurosurgery*, 43:514–528, 1998.

20. C.R. Maurer, Jr., D.L.G. Hill, A.J. Martin, H. Liu, M. McCue, D. Rueckert, D. Lloret, W.A. Hall, R.E. Maxwell, D.J. Hawkes, and C.L. Truwit. Investigation of intra-operative brain deformation using a 1.5 Tesla interventional MR system: preliminary results. *IEEE Trans. Med. Imaging,* 17:817–825, 1998.

21. M.I. Miga, K.D. Paulsen, F.E. Kennedy, P.J. Hoopes, A. Hartov, and D.W. Roberts. Modeling surgical loads to account for subsurface tissue deformation during stereotactic neurosurgery. *IEEE SPIE Proc. Laser Tissue Interaction IX, Part B: Soft Tissue Modeling,* 3254, 501–511, 1998.

22. P.J. Edwards, D.L.G. Hill, J.A. Little, and D.J. Hawkes. A three-component deformation model for image-guided surgery. *Med. Image Anal.,* 2:355–367, 1998.

23. R.P. Woods, S.T. Grafton, J.D.G. Watson, N.L. Sicotte, and J.C. Mazziotta. Automated image registration: II. Intersubject validation of linear and nonlinear models. *J. Comput. Assist. Tomogr.,* 22:153–165, 1998.

24. P.F. Hemler, S. Napel, T.S. Sumanaweera, R. Pichumani, P.A. van den Elsen, D. Martin, J. Drace, and J.R. Adler. Registration error quantification of a surface-based multimodality image fusion system. *Med. Phys.,* 22:1049–1056, 1995.

25. R.P. Woods, J.C. Mazziotta, and S.R. Cherry. MRI-PET registration with automated algorithm. *J. Comput. Assist. Tomogr.,* 17:536–546, 1993.

26. Y. Ge, J.M. Fitzpatrick, J.R. Votaw, S. Gadamsetty, R.J. Maciunas, R.M. Kessler, and R.A. Margolin. Retrospective registration of PET and MR brain images: an algorithm and its stereotactic validation. *J. Comput. Assist. Tomogr.,* 18:800–810, 1994.

27. J.C.H. Wong, C. Studholme, D.J. Hawkes, and M.N. Maisey. Evaluation of the limits of visual detection of image misregistration in a brain fluorine-18 fluoro-deoxyglucose PET-MRI study. *Eur. J. Nucl. Med.,* 24:642–650, 1997.

28. D.L. Collins, P. Neelin, T.M. Peters, and A.C. Evans. Automatic 3D intersubject registration of MR volumetric data in standardized Talairach space. *J. Comput. Assist. Tomogr.,* 18:192–205, 1994.

29. H.M. Kooy, M. Van Herk, P.D. Barnes, E. Alexander, III, S.F. Dunbar, N.J. Tarbell, R.V. Mulkern, E.J. Holupka, and J.S. Loeffler. Image fusion for stereotactic radiotherapy and radiosurgery treatment planning. *Int. J. Radiat. Oncol. Biol. Phys.,* 28:1229–1234, 1994.

30. P.A. van den Elsen, J.B.A. Maintz, E.-J.D. Pol, and M.A. Viergever. Automatic registration of CT and MR brain images using correlation of geometrical features. *IEEE Trans. Med. Imaging,* 14:384–396, 1995.

31. J.B.A. Maintz, P.A. van den Elsen, and M.A. Viergever. Evaluation of ridge-seeking operators for multimodality medical image matching. *IEEE Trans. Pattern Anal. Mach. Intell.,* 18:353–365, 1996.

32. P. Thompson and A.W. Toga. A surface-based technique for warping three-dimensional images of the brain. *IEEE Trans. Med. Imaging,* 15:402–417, 1996.

33. C. Studholme, D.L.G. Hill, and D.J. Hawkes. Automated 3D registration of MR and PET brain images by multi-resolution optimisation of voxel similarity measures. *Med. Phys.,* 24:25–35, 1997.

34. J.M. Fitzpatrick, D.L.G. Hill, Y. Shyr, J.B. West, C. Studholme, and C.R. Maurer, Jr. Visual assessment of the accuracy of retrospective registration of MR and CT images of the brain. *IEEE Trans. Med. Imaging,* 17:571–585, 1998.

35. U. Pietrzyk, K. Herholz, and W.-D. Heiss. Three-dimensional alignment of functional and morphological tomograms. *J. Comput. Assist. Tomogr.,* 14:51–59, 1990.

36. P.A. Freeborough, R.P. Woods, and N.C. Fox. Accurate registration of serial 3D MR brain images and its application to visualizing change in neurodegenerative disorders. *J. Comput. Assist. Tomogr.*, 20:1012–1022, 1996.

37. R.P. Woods, S.T. Grafton, C.J. Holmes, S.R. Cherry, and J.C. Mazziotta. Automated image registration: I. General methods and intrasubject, intramodality validation. *J. Comput. Assist. Tomogr.*, 22:139–152, 1998.

38. M. Holden, D.L.G. Hill, E.R.E. Denton, J.M. Jarosz, T.C.S. Cox, J. Goodey, T. Rohlfing, and D.J. Hawkes. Voxel similarity measures for 3D serial MR image registration. *IEEE Trans. Med. Imaging*, 19:94–102, 2000.

39. M.J. Clarkson, D. Rueckert, D.L.G. Hill, and D.J. Hawkes. Registration of multiple video images to pre-operative CT for image guided surgery. *Medical Imaging 1999: Image Processing*, Proc. SPIE 3661-01:14–23, 1999.

40. J.B. West, J.M. Fitzpatrick, M.Y. Wang, B.M. Dawant, C.R. Maurer, Jr., R.M. Kessler, R.J. Maciunas, C. Barillot, D. Lemoine, A. Collignon, F. Maes, P. Suetens, D. Vandermeulen, P.A. van den Elsen, S. Napel, T.S. Sumanaweera, B. Harkness, P.F. Hemler, D.L.G. Hill, D.J. Hawkes, C. Studholme, J.B.A. Maintz, M.A. Viergever, G. Malandain, X. Pennec, M.E. Noz, G.Q. Maguire, Jr., M. Pollack, C.A. Pelizzari, R.A. Robb, D. Hanson, and R.P. Woods. Comparison and evaluation of retrospective intermodality brain image registration techniques. *J. Comput. Assist. Tomogr.*, 21:554–566, 1997.

41. H. Chang and J.M. Fitzpatrick. A technique for accurate magnetic resonance imaging in the presence of field inhomogeneities. *IEEE Trans. Med. Imaging*, 11:319–329, 1992.

42. W.M. Wells, III, P. Viola, H. Atsumi, S. Nakajima, and R. Kikinis. Multi-modal volume registration by maximization of mutual information. *Med. Image Anal.*, 1:35–51, 1996.

43. F. Maes, A. Collignon, D. Vandermeulen, G. Marchal, and P. Suetens. Multimodality image registration by maximization of mutual information. *IEEE Trans. Med. Imaging*, 16:187–198, 1997.

44. J. Ashburner and K. Friston. Multimodal image coregistration and partitioning—a unified framework. *Neuroimage*, 6:209–217, 1997.

45. Thévanaz P. and Unser M. An efficient mutual information optimizer for multiresolution image registration. *Proc. IEEE SPIE Conf. Image Processing, Vol I*, 833–837, 1998.

46. C. Studholme, D.L.G. Hill, and D.J. Hawkes. An overlap invariant entropy measure of 3D medical image alignment. *Pattern Recogn.*, 32:71–86, 1999.

Section II

Applications of Rigid-Body Registration

7

Registration and Subtraction of Serial Magnetic Resonance Images of the Brain: Image Interpretation and Clinical Applications

Angela Oatridge, Joseph V. Hajnal, and Graeme M. Bydder

CONTENTS

7.1 Introduction

Various methods of aligning MR images with images from other medical imaging modalities or other MR images have been described in previous chapters. Clinical applications of registration of MR images to other MR images are currently almost exclusively directed at detecting change in the brain and allied structures. Even with this restriction, relatively few examples in which clinical applications dominate over technical or methodological issues can be found. In this chapter, we will discuss our experience in applying image registration methods to clinical problems. With the increasing availability of MR scanners, more and more patients have repeat examinations, and radiologists are frequently asked to report on changes that reflect the subject's progression or regression and may require a change in existing treatment or the start of new treatment. We have employed a rigid-body registration technique to monitor change in the brain in individual subjects who underwent serial MRI examinations. This approach allows disease progression and response to treatment to be monitored with great sensitivity. It fits naturally with the noninvasive nature of MRI.

A feature of serial studies of individual subjects is that the images obtained at each examination are likely to show the same anatomic regions with the same or similar contrast properties. This makes the problem of determining the transformation (T; see Chapter 3) that maps one image to the next in the series much easier to solve. However, similarity of images and the requirement to detect change with maximum sensitivity means that the spatial match can and must be to subvoxel precision, and the voxel intensity values in the final registered images must have minimal interpolation errors. A closely related topic is image registration as applied to fMRI (see Chapter 8), in which a sequence of similar images is generally acquired at intervals of a few seconds, and changes in subject position with time are corrected by retrospective image alignment. In clinical applications, a wider range of sequence types may be required and images may be acquired weeks or months apart, rather than seconds or minutes.

The similarity of the images and the requirement of subvoxel precision favors registration algorithms based on voxel similarity measures rather than landmark or fiducial systems. Virtually all currently available registration algorithms using voxel similarity measures have been successfully applied to single subject serial studies (see Chapter 3 for technical details). Methods by Woods[1] and Friston[2] have found wide application in fMRI. Those by Hajnal,[3] Lemieux,[4] Freeborough and Fox,[5] and Studholme et al.[6] have also been used for more medically oriented studies.

A critical issue in serial MRI studies is the threshold for detection of change, which is the level of change that must occur for it to be detected against background noise and artifacts. In our experience, artifacts are usually the limiting factor in MRI. In addition to the full range of MRI acquisition artifacts, artifacts associated directly with the registration process are important. To control the latter it is necessary to match the data processing involved with registration to the properties of the original MRI data and vice versa. Serial MRI studies typically employ either (a) three-dimensional (3D) data sets or (b) two-dimensional (2D) multislice data sets. Since the subjects occupy three spatial dimensions, the data and registration algorithms must also reflect this. Data requirements for 3D coverage have been discussed in Chapter 4. While the necessary conditions are satisfied for true 3D sequences, this is frequently not achieved with 2D slice methods.[7]

Comparing precisely registered images acquired at different times is greatly facilitated by generating subtraction images derived from positionally registered scans. On these images, signals from unchanged structures cancel out, producing a neutral background against which real differences can be identified more clearly. These registered subtraction images require a different approach to interpretation than conventional images.[3,8-10] This chapter describes a formalism for analyzing them and shows examples of the application of image registration and subtraction, as well as how quantification can be applied to various problems.

7.2 Methods

Three-dimensional images were acquired with true 3D radiofrequency (RF) spoiled T1-weighted pulse sequences on a 1.0T Marconi HPQ plus scanner (Marconi Medical Systems, Cleveland, Ohio). For whole head studies, a nonselective RF excitation pulse was employed (TR 21 msec, TE 6 msec, flip angle 35°) and images were acquired in the sagittal plane with frequency-encoding

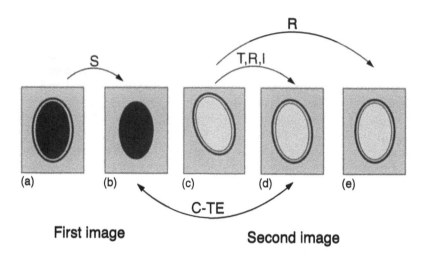

FIGURE 7.1

Implementation of registration (STRICTER). The first image obtained is shown on the left
and is shaded black (a). The second image (shaded gray) is obtained at a different position
in the same coordinate system (c). Segmentation (S) removes the skull and scalp from the
first image (a) to give (b). Translation (T) Rotation (R) and sinc Interpolation (I) of voxel
values are used to produce image (d) which is matched with the segmented version of the
first images (b). A Chi-squared (C) Test (TE) is used to asses the accuracy of this match.
Following this first attempt as a match, more accurate values for the translation and rotation
are chosen in order to reduce the value of χ^2 and the process is repeated. When the optimal
match has been found in this way the second image is Reformatted (R) into the same position
as the first image. The original, unsegmented first image (a) can now be compared with the
reformatted second image (e) which is precisely aligned.

direction head to foot to avoid aliasing. Data matrices of $152 \times 256 \times 114$ with
two NEX or $192 \times 256 \times 140$ and one NEX were acquired in a volume of 25×25
$\times$ 18 cm to produce nominally isotropic phase-encoded resolution of 1.6 mm^3 or
1.3 mm^3, respectively.

Two-dimensional multislice images were acquired with a Gaussian slice
profile at a TR of 6140 msec and a TE of 80 msec for 64 slices. Slice thickness
(full width at half maximum) was 4.4 mm with a 50% overlap, yielding a slice
separation of 2.2 mm. A 25 cm field of view with a 125×125 matrix was used
to provide approximately isotropic sampling.[8,11,12]

Registration proceeded in the order segmentation, translation, rotation
and interpolation, chi-squared test, and reformatting (STRICTER). The stages
are illustrated in Figure 7.1.

This procedure produces an optimal global match for brain tissues. The
inclusion of a segmentation step, by which the skull and all extracranial tissues are excluded from the process of determining the spatial transformation
from one image to another (the transformation T in Chapter 3), ensures that
the correct global transformation for the brain is found. This is a precautionary
measure ensureing that extraneous tissue changes, which can be substantial
with some disease processes or over long periods of time, do not influence the

registration process. Thus the brain is precisely aligned, irrespective of other changes. Provided the rigid-body approximation is valid, accuracy of the spatial match for an unchanged brain determined using a voxel similarity measure is limited by the signal-to-noise ratio (SNR) of the images. For the sum of squared differences (Chapter 3), labeled Chi squared, this is conceptually straightforward and easily demonstrated[3] (see also Chapter 6). Typical matching accuracies of less than 0.01 mm in each axis and less than 0.01 of a degree in each rotation angle were routinely achieved and validated with phantoms.

If the brain has changed, the definition of a position of spatial match becomes less certain. The concept of a null hypothesis is adopted to deal with this situation. In this case our null hypothesis is that the brain is an unchanged rigid body that has simply been imaged in slightly different poses. Under these conditions, after image registration, voxel intensity values in regions of the images that represent brain must differ only by noise (see Figures 4.2 and 4.4 in Chapter 4). This can be achieved to any desired degree of precision, provided the properties of the data and the data processing are appropriately matched.[3] Neglecting image artifacts for a moment, residual voxel intensity differences can now be unambiguously viewed as evidence of brain change (in shape, size, signal intensity, etc). The registration process used minimizes these differences in a least-squares sense. The pattern of changes detected after image registration is an unbiased measure of brain change as referenced to the null hypothesis.

To visualize the pattern of change, difference images were produced by subtracting baseline images from registered follow-up images or by subtracting an earlier registered follow-up image set from a later one. Although the registered images and difference images were acquired in the sagittal planes, reformatting images into the transverse and coronal planes, or any plane when required was possible.

The process of reformatting the images to achieve the fully registered data from which subtraction images are formed requires image interpolation (see Chapter 3). In order to ensure that, after realignment, voxel intensities in the reformatted images were what they would have been if the scan had been acquired in the final position, sinc interpolation was employed.[3] This allowed the null hypothesis condition, in which voxels in regions of unchanged brain subtract to leave only noise, to be achieved.

An example of two 3D T1-weighted images acquired a month apart and the subtraction image derived from them is shown in Figure 7.2.

7.3   Image Interpretation—General

The information provided by subvoxel registration was utilized at three different levels. First, accurate alignment of images alone made detection of differences easier, since change in precisely corresponding anatomical areas could be properly attributed to genuine differences in the tissues or

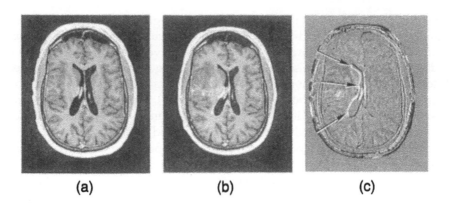

(a)   (b)   (c)

FIGURE 7.2
Astrocytoma grade III: Registered contrast-enhanced T1-weighted RF spoiled images
before (a) and four weeks after (b) treatment with Temozolamide. The difference image
[(b) − (a)] is shown (c). The white line around the right lateral ventricle (large arrow) is
largely due to an interplateau shift (c) of the ventricles towards the midline. There are
also increases in signal intensity in (c) due to increased contrast enhancement (arrowed).
Border zone shifts are also seen in the right hemisphere where the tumor is present (small
arrows) (c).

fluids being studied. Second, it was possible to use the precisely registered
images to produce subtraction images for direct visualization of change,
and, third, precise registration provided a basis for accurate serial measurements either directly from the images or through the use of computerized
algorithms.

The overall approach was to examine baseline, registered follow-up, and
subtraction images simultaneously. Collateral information was obtained
from regions apart from those of immediate interest, including tissues
other than the brain. This provided a means of recognizing artifacts and
checking the fidelity of the registration. On each image, validation of the
registration process was assessed by examining regions where there were
boundaries between tissues that produced steep changes in signal intensity and checking that these were reduced to the noise level of the difference image. The large amount of data acquired and the ability to review
the images in different planes ensured that this could be performed at
many different locations.

Interpretation of accurately aligned baseline and follow-up images follows
established principles. In this study, the sequences used were mainly sensitive to tissue mobile proton density, T1 and T2. Disease processes which
increased mobile proton density T1 and T2 included inflammation, demyelination, edema, and most tumors. Diseases that tend to decrease proton density T1 and T2 included late scar formation, calcification, and subacute
hemorrhage. The effect that these changes produce on image signal intensity
can be determined using simple models.[13–15]

7.4 Interpretation and Registered Subtraction Images

Interpretation of precisely registered difference images involves additional considerations. Once residual changes due to artifacts and misregistration of deformed or displaced extracerebral tissues have been discounted, changes on the difference images can be attributed to (a) change in the intrinsic signal intensity of one or more tissues or fluids; (b) change in site, shape, or size of one or more tissues or fluids; or (c) a combination of (a) and (b). These changes can generate either positive or negative signals on difference images. In order to understand the type of change present and to locate the anatomical context in which the change has occurred, one must refer to the source image from which the difference image has been generated.

7.4.1 Interpretation of Pure Changes in Signal Intensity

When changes in signal intensity of a tissue or tissues occur, individual or groups of voxels will have different intensity values, which can be detected provided the change dominates over the level of artifact and noise in the images. The detection of changes in signal intensity is usually simpler on difference images than on source images because signals from unchanged tissues and fluids are reduced to a common background level (shown schematically in Figure 7.3). This can be particularly useful for detecting

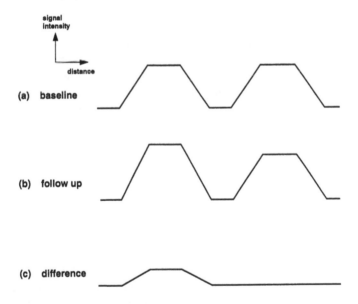

FIGURE 7.3
Profiles of the signal intensities of tissue and/or fluid with distance demonstrates the effect of a local change in signal intensity on the difference image. The follow-up scan (b) shows a small change in one region. The difference in this region is more clearly shown by subtracting (a) from (b) to give (c). This shows the local increase in signal intensity.

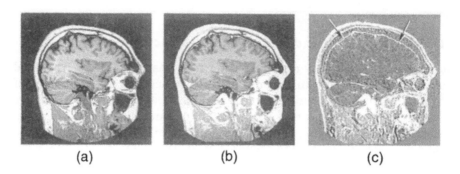

(a)   (b)   (c)

FIGURE 7.4
Contrast enhancement: Normal volunteer aged 63 years. Registered T1-weighted RF spoiled images before (a) and after (b) intravenous gadolinium DTPA with difference image [(b) − (a)] shown in (c). Enhancement is seen in the meninges (arrows), vascular layer of the scalp, skin, veins, sinuses, and nasal mucosa in (c).

changes in regions where the anatomy is complex and where there are variable partial volume effects (such as in boundary regions). Difference images are also useful for recognizing signal changes in tissues with intensities at the extremities of the image intensity range. Whereas on source images these are at the top or bottom of the gray scale, on difference images they are referred to the neutral (zero change) level. Global changes in signal intensity may only become obvious on difference images where the brain has a nonzero signal in relation to the noise on the image outside the scalp.

Image registration can be useful in ensuring that pre- and postcontrast images are precisely matched. In most circumstances it is unlikely that any structure in the brain will significantly change in site, shape, or size in the time between the pre- and postscans, so differences on registered images are almost always due to pure changes in signal intensity (Figure 7.4).

Normal enhancement occurs in tissues such as the meninges or cortical veins. These areas are subject to considerable partial volume effect from adjacent tissues, such as brain and CSF, producing variable baseline intensity values. By performing accurate registration it is possible to ensure the same set of partial volume effects on pre- and postcontrast images. As a result, more uniform enhancement of meninges, cortical veins, and ependyma is seen on difference images than on conventional images. It is possible to perform double subtractions (i.e., the difference between the contrast enhancement with time from one examination to the next).

On T1-weighted images, the facts that the contrast agent normally only gives positive enhancement and that there should be no change in brain site, shape, or size, provide an additional check on the fidelity of the registration procedure. Under these circumstances, immediate post- minus pre-enhancement difference images should only show positive changes, whereas a misregistration artifact typically shows both positive and negative effects. In some cases we have found that the image differences introduced by the contrast agent appear to be partially offset by a very slight positional mismatch when χ^2 is minimized. This results in weak negative signals that tend to follow high contrast boundaries. This can be avoided by modifying the definition of χ^2 to include only those voxels for which the postcontrast scan has lower intensity than the precontrast scan. This ensures that the pattern of enhancement does not influence the spatial match. Algorithms that employ mutual information as a voxel similarity measure are also likely to achieve correct alignment when there is signal change due to contrast enhancement.

7.4.2 Interpretation of Pure Changes in Site, Shape, or Size

Changes in site, shape, or size are manifest as a local shift in position of at least some part of the brain and its surrounding tissues or fluids. The size and distribution of these local shifts provide information about the nature of the overall change (i.e., whether it has been one of site, shape, size, or a combination of these).

7.4.2.1 Model for Analyzing Shifts

The effects of shifts can be analyzed using a simple model of two tissues (and/or fluids), one with a higher plateau of signal intensity, the other with a lower plateau, and a border zone (region of partial volume effects) between them (Figure 7.5a). (Although Figure 7.5a is shown in one spatial dimension, the model is used in three dimensions). At the ventricular margin with a typical T1-weighted pulse sequence, white matter or central gray matter forms a higher plateau, and CSF a lower one. Likewise, within the brain, white matter forms a higher plateau and gray matter a lower one. With a heavily T2-weighted pulse sequence, the central white matter has a low signal intensity (lower signal plateau) and the CSF has a high signal intensity (higher signal plateau). The principles outlined later are the same, but because of the reversal in sign of the gray and white matter and CSF, the polarity of changes for the same shift is reversed.

It is sometimes useful to regard the cortex as part of a composite (or double) border zone between central white matter and CSF. Shifts can be thought of as larger, in which one plateau crosses the border zone so that it overlays the other plateau, and smaller, in which the displacement is less than the width of the border zone.

Larger (interplateau) shifts produce a high and constant (full scale) central signal change on difference images (Figures 7.5b, 7.5c). The full scale signal change on the difference image is locally monophasic. It is positive when the high signal plateau has shifted into the region of the low signal plateau (e.g., Figure 7.2, lateral margin of right lateral ventricle), and vice versa. The intermediate regions on either side of the full scale change correspond to the two border zones on the source images. The origin of interplateau shifts is usually clear from the source images. The size of the shift in the direction of the

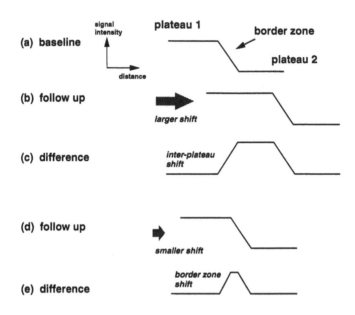

FIGURE 7.5
Plateaus and border zones showing interplateau and border zone shifts. A tissue or fluid with a higher signal intensity in shown in plateau 1 and one with a lower signal intensity is shown in plateau 2 (a). This is appropriate for central white matter (plateau 1) and CSF (plateau 2) using a T1-weighted pulse sequence. There is a border zone (region of partial volume effects) between them, in which signal intensity changes with distance. A larger, interplateau shift of the image is shown in (b) and subtraction of (a) from (b) is shown in the difference profile (c). This has a central full scale change (plateau 1 minus plateau 2) with two intermediate zones on either side. A smaller border zone shift, which is less than the border zone in width is shown in (d). This results in a difference profile (e) which is smaller than (c) in both amplitude and width.

maximum signal intensity gradient is equal to the width of the full scale region plus a fraction of the width of the border zone region (see later).

Smaller shifts (where higher and lower plateaus do not overlap) primarily involve border zones. On difference images they produce smaller changes in signal intensity than the full scale changes seen with interplateau shifts (Figures 7.5d, 7.5e and Figure 7.2, right hemisphere). The precise effect depends on the size and direction of the local signal intensity gradient and the shift.

7.4.2.2 Effect of Signal Intensity Gradient Size

In the limit of a vertical slope (idealized maximum signal intensity gradient) there is a step function change in signal intensity on the difference image over the width of the shift. (It is really an interplateau shift; see Figure 7.6.) With smaller signal intensity gradients (less than vertical slopes) the same shift results in a rise that is more gradual and to a lower height, but over a wider area. The area under the difference curve is the same in each case (i.e., the

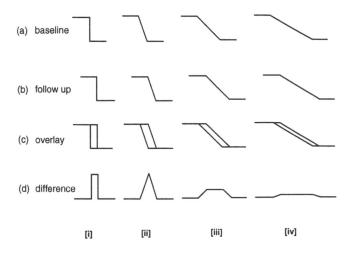

FIGURE 7.6
Profiles of two plateaus and a border zone showing the effect of change in signal intensity gradient size for a constant border zone shift. Initial image profile (a), shifted image profile (b), overlay (c) of (b) on (a), and subtraction of (a) from (b) is shown in (d) for vertical signal change (infinite slope) [i] and decreasing slopes [ii], [iii], and [iv]. As the slope is decreased, the width of the difference profile is increased and the height decreases after image [ii]. This makes the change less easy to detect against background noise (not shown). The area under the curves (d) is the same in each case for the constant shift which is illustrated.

area of a parallelogram, base × height). The steep gradient produces the highest contrast to noise value; eventually as the slope decreases, the change on the difference image becomes so slight that it merges into the noise of the image and is not detectable.

7.4.2.3 Effects of Signal Intensity Gradient Direction

At the junction between the higher signal tissue plateau (e.g., white matter) and the border zone, it is possible to draw an iso-intensity contour (a line of constant signal intensity and hence zero signal intensity gradient). The local direction of maximum signal intensity gradient is perpendicular to this (Figure 7.7). The same applies to the junction between the border zone and the lower signal intensity plateau. The size of the gradient generally decreases as the width of the border zone increases, since the two plateaus have a constant signal intensity difference. An iso-intensity contour divides the image into voxels of higher signal intensity on one side and lower signal intensity on the other. It is convenient to indicate the signal intensity gradient direction with an arrow showing the direction of *decreasing* signal intensity across a contour because then, if the shift has a component parallel to the direction shown, there will be an *increase* in signal on the difference image. If the shift has a parallel component, but in the opposite direction, there will be a decrease in signal on the difference image. A high signal intensity gradient inplane generally corresponds to a low signal intensity gradient throughplane and vice versa.

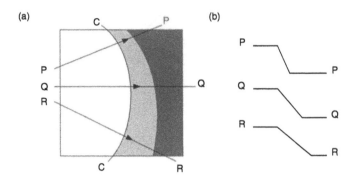

FIGURE 7.7
Plan (a) and profiles (b) of two plateaus and a border zone showing signal intensity gradients in different directions. The profiles (PP, QQ, and RR) show the signal intensity changes in passing from one plateau across the border zone to the other plateau. The contour (CC) marks the edge of the high signal plateau. At each point on CC the maximum signal intensity gradient is perpendicular to the contour. The direction of the gradient defined as being from high to lower signal intensity is indicated by the arrows. An estimate of the slope of the signal intensity gradient through PP, QQ, and RR can be obtained by noting that the slope is inversely related to the distance between the two plateaus.

7.4.2.4   Effects of Size of Shift

As shown in Figure 7.8 the initial effect of a shift is to show a small change on the difference image (i.e., a border zone shift). If the shift is increased, a peak is reached when one plateau just crosses the boundary zone to reach the other plateau. This peak is maintained in intensity and widens as the shift is increased further (i.e., an interplateau shift). The area under the curve on the difference image increases in direct proportion to the size of the shift (i.e., area of a parallelogram) and is independent of the magnitude of the signal intensity gradient. Using the plateau model, the size of the component of a shift parallel to the local gradient direction will be the width shown on the difference image multiplied by the mean difference signal as a fraction of the full scale signal intensity.

7.4.2.5   Effects of Shift Direction

Shifts are usually both inplane and throughplane, but may be thought of as predominantly one or the other. With inplane shifts it is possible to visualize on the same image the tissue or fluid which has shifted (or will shift; e.g., Figure 7.2), whereas with throughplane shifts the tissue or fluid moving into the slice comes from adjacent slices. In order to visualize plateaus and border zones in three dimensions it is therefore necessary to consider adjacent slices (which are one voxel apart with 3D acquisitions).

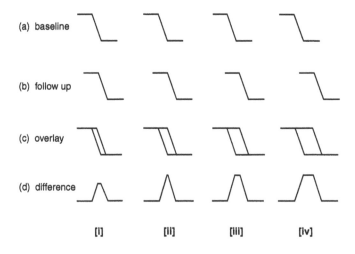

FIGURE 7.8
Effect of shift size. Baseline image profiles (a), successively displaced image profiles (b), overlays (c) of (b) on (a), and differences (d) for increasing shifts [i]-[iv]. As the shift is increased, the height of the difference increases to a maximum and the width of this maximum then increases. The area under the difference curve is directly proportional to the shift difference.

The effect of inplane shifts is shown in Figure 7.9. There is an increase in signal intensity on the side to which the high signal tissue or fluid has shifted on the difference image. The difference is maximal at the point of the maximum signal intensity gradient in the direction of the shift. When the displacement is perpendicular to the local intensity gradient, no signal intensity change is seen. This effect is seen in the right lateral ventricle in Figure 7.2c, where a positive change is seen at the lateral margin and a negative change at the medial margin.

The effect of rotation is to produce differential shifts. These produce changes on the difference images where there is a radial edge, since this has a circumferential intensity gradient component that is parallel to the local shift direction. The displacement increases with radial distance from the center of rotation.

The mechanism for signal change produced by throughplane shifts is the same as for inplane shifts, i.e., changes are produced on difference images whenever the shift has a component parallel to the local signal intensity gradient. However, the visual appearance of difference signals produced by throughplane shifts is more heterogeneous than that produced by inplane shifts (Figure 7.10).

The practical effects of both inplane and throughplane shifts for a transverse and a coronal slice taken from the same 3D data set are shown in Figures 7.11 and 7.12. The images were produced by shifting the volume data by a single voxel (approximately 0.97 mm) in each of the principal matrix directions in turn and then subtracting the original images from the displaced images.

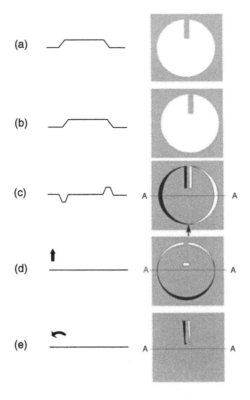

FIGURE 7.9
Effect of the shift direction (inplane). Profiles (left) and plans (right) of an object are shown in the initial position (a) with shift to the right (b) and on the corresponding difference image (c). Difference image profiles along the lines AA and plans are shown for an upward inplane displacement (d) and counter-clockwise rotation (e). The changes in signal on the difference images can be directly related to the signal intensity gradients and shifts. A shift that is perpendicular to the local signal intensity gradient produces no change on the difference image (e.g., c, arrow).

Figure 7.11a shows a transverse slice taken from the volume set, and Figure 7.11b shows the adjacent slice. The difference images in Figures 7.11c–7.11e show the effect of left-right, postero-anterior, and head-foot shifts, respectively, of just one voxel. The inplane shifts in Figures 7.11c and 7.11d produce predictable results in which edges (border zones) in Figure 7.11a are accentuated as high or low signal according to the pattern of the local signal intensity gradients.

The result of the throughplane displacement (Figure 7.11e) is more complex. The origin of individual regions of positive or negative signal difference can be determined by careful comparison of Figures 7.11a and 7.11b, since Figure 7.11e is simply Figure 7.11b minus Figure 7.11a. However, while some regions contain curvilinear changes of the same type seen with inplane shifts, in many areas the overall effect does not correspond overtly to the anatomic structures visible in Figure 7.11a or 7.11b. This is because the regions on the

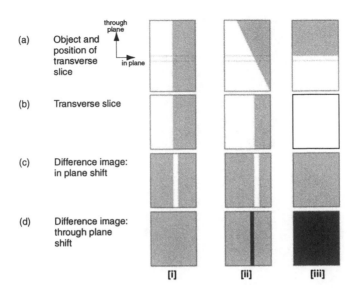

FIGURE 7.10
Effects of inplane and throughplane shifts. Three objects with differently oriented boundaries between regions of high and low signal are shown (a[i]-[iii]). The position of a transverse slice through each object is also shown (a, dotted lines). The corresponding images are shown (b[i]-[iii]). For an inplane shift to the right the difference image shows a linear change in both (c[i]) and (c[ii]) but no change in c(iii). For a throughplane shift a variety of patterns are seen. There is no change in (d[i]), change along a line in (d[ii]) and a change within the whole plane in (d[iii]). In the last case there is a steep gradient throughplane which is not apparent from the image (b[iii]). Inplane shifts produce predictable difference signals where there are inplane edges (c[i]) and c[ii]). However, throughplane shifts, which reveal the presence of throughplane intensity gradients, can produce either linear or regional difference patterns (d[ii-iii]). In this diagram white indicates positive signal, gray is zero, and black is a negative signal.

difference image where the largest signal intensity changes occur are those with the maximum **throughplane** signal intensity gradient. These are just the places which tend to have the smallest **inplane** signal intensity gradients because they arise where tissue boundaries are parallel or nearly parallel to the slice plane (cf. Figure 7.10[iii]). Small inplane gradients imply a relatively uniform appearance in the source image with little hint of the throughplane differences.

A similar effect is seen in Figure 7.12, but this time it is the postero-anterior shift (Figure 7.12d) which produces throughplane differences from the slice in Figure 7.12a to that in Figure 7.12b. Note that simply by reformatting to the coronal plane, the head-foot displacement that was difficult to interpret in Figure 7.11e is transformed to the anatomically linked pattern in Figure 7.12e.

A throughplane shift in a case of cerebral atrophy is shown in Figure 7.13. The movement of the upper surface of the corpus callosum upwards into the region of the pericallosal sulcus and gray matter produces an increase in signal on the transverse difference image (Figure 7.13c).

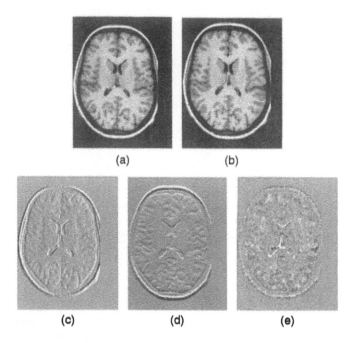

FIGURE 7.11
Simulated effects of inplane and throughplane shifts on anatomic images: a volume data set with cubic voxels (0.97 mm on each side) was copied, displaced by one voxel in each of three orthogonal directions, and then the original data was subtracted from it. A transverse slice from the volume set (a), the adjacent slice (b), and difference images for left-right (c), postero-anterior (d), and head-foot (e) displacements are shown. Image (e) results from subtracting (a) from (b). The differences produced by inplane shifts (c, d) show monophasic and multiphasic curvilinear changes that can easily be related to the anatomy in (a). Intense signals with a simple geometry can be seen around the skull and scalp (c, d). The pattern of throughplane changes (e) is less clearly related to the anatomy shown in (a). The ventricular system produces curvilinear features as expected from Figures 7.9a[ii]-7.9d[ii]. However, there are more widespread changes that are patchy or mottled rather than curvilinear. These arise from throughplane differences between (a) and (b) that have little or no inplane component. Close inspection is necessary to relate the differences in (e) to the source images (a) and (b).

7.4.2.6   Effects of Change in Shape (without Change in Signal Intensity)

Change in shape involves change in site of at least some of the tissue or fluid, but it does not necessarily produce a change in size. A change in shape will in general be accompanied by corresponding shifts elsewhere in the image. Recognition of these may be straightforward for simple structures and larger changes, but difficult for complex structures and smaller changes. It requires an overview of the site and direction of the shifts at different locations in the brain.

7.4.2.7   Effect of Change in Size (without Change in Signal Intensity)

This will also involve change in site and possibly shape. The associated shifts may be focal or general. The focal changes may be centered on a particular region while general changes are centered on the structure itself.

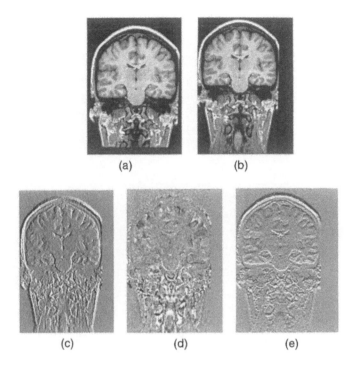

(a)　　　　　　　(b)

(c)　　　　　(d)　　　　　(e)

FIGURE 7.12
The same image data as in Figure 7.11 are shown, but reformatted into the coronal plane. Anatomic image (a), adjacent slice (b), and differences produced by a one voxel shift in the left-right (c), postero-anterior (d), and head-foot (e) directions are displayed. Note that the throughplane direction is now postero-anterior (d) and this image shows nonspecific changes in signal intensity as well as monophasic and multiphasic curvilinear changes.

Change in size is typically not associated with compensatory (i.e., equal and opposite) changes in the corresponding regions. Recognition of change in size also requires an overall assessment of the site, size, and direction of shifts.

7.4.2.8　*Etiology*

Changes in site (as well as shape and size) are typically due to mass effects. The latter term includes displacement of otherwise normal tissue by a disease process. Mass effects are typically associated with tumors but may be seen with many other diseases such as abscesses, hematomas, trauma, edema, and demyelination. The effects may be local or general. Reduction in size may take the form of localized or generalized atrophy. This occurs typically in degenerative conditions but also in cerebral infarction, trauma, etc.

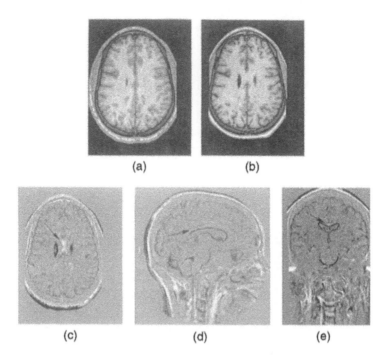

(a)   (b)

(c)   (d)   (e)

FIGURE 7.13
Throughplane shift: Registered transverse T1-weighted RF spoiled images prior to bone marrow transplantation (a) and eight months later (b). The difference image is shown in (c). The corresponding registered difference images in the sagittal (d) and coronal (e) plane are also shown. With the cerebral atrophy the corpus callosum has shifted superiorly and its superior surface encroaches on the region previously occupied by the pericallosal sulcus and gray matter giving the high signal in (c) (arrow). The small size of shift is apparent in (d) and (e) (arrows). Cerebral atrophy has developed and this produces low signal margins around the ventricular system and the external surface of the brain.

7.4.3 Interpretation of Changes in Signal Intensity Combined with Changes in Site, Shape, or Size on Difference Images

Changes in signal intensity and shifts frequently occur together. In many pathologies, the areas of abnormal tissue have increased T1 and T2 and may also produce mass effects. The increase or decrease in signal intensity may take it beyond the plateau levels in the model used to describe shifts. As a result, shifts may produce signal differences which are beyond the "full scale" of the model. Using the T1-weighted 3D volume sequences described here, this occurred with very short T1 lesions due either to subacute hemorrhage or contrast enhancement. A lesion involving the higher plateau (e.g., white matter) that lengthens its T1 decreases the size of the difference between the two plateaus so the interplateau difference is less than full scale.

When the changes in signal intensity and shifts are at different sites, they can be treated independently (as with displaced but otherwise normal tissue around a space-occupying lesion). When they occur together, some further consideration is necessary. The key concept is that a difference in signal intensity of a tissue or fluid in the boundary zone not only produces a change in its own right, but also changes the signal intensity gradient so that the effect of a shift may be increased or decreased. The detailed change depends on the pulse sequence being employed. For example, with a T1-weighted sequence, a lesion with increased T1 would decrease its signal intensity and also decrease the gradient at its interface with CSF. The decreased signal intensity would produce a negative signal on the difference image and the effect of any shift in producing a change on the difference image would be reduced.

When a lesion is characterized only by an increase or decrease in its signal intensity relative to the surrounding normal tissue (and has no mass effect) it may be difficult or impossible to distinguish a change in its signal intensity from a change in its size. The change in signal intensity usually changes the signal intensity gradient in the border zone, and this determines the threshold for detecting the border of the lesion in relation to the image noise and artifact level. In this situation, a decrease in signal intensity difference between the lesion and its surroundings usually appears to be accompanied by a decrease in size, but if the signal intensity gradient in the border zone is maintained the lesion size may appear unchanged. A "pure" change in signal intensity may thus be inextricably linked to a change in size of the lesion.

7.5 Regional and Tissue-Specific Appearances on Difference Images

In this section, specific anatomical regions are considered in more detail and a wider range of tissues and fluids is discussed.

7.5.1 The Ventricular System

The boundaries of the ventricles are smooth, continuous, and regular; their signal intensity gradients are predictable both inplane and over adjacent slices (Figures 7.12 and 7.13). The border zone for shifts in certain directions is quite narrow. In this situation, full scale changes due to relatively small interplateau shifts are readily seen when the shift is parallel to the maximum signal intensity gradient. Locally monophasic curvilinear changes are typically seen with smaller border zone shifts.

Changes within the ventricles may be complicated by the presence of the choroid plexus and other structures which may produce multiphasic effects. Large shifts may lead to complete overlap of the ventricular system with the brain, and there may be changes in the shape of the ventricles as well as size.

7.5.2   The Brainstem and Cerebellum

The brainstem also presents continuous and predictable boundaries, although the cerebellar folia show a more complex, but still regular, pattern. The signal intensity gradients associated with the cerebellar folia sensitize them to shifts in the superior-inferior and postero-anterior directions.

7.5.3   The Cerebral Cortex

In contrast to the ventricular system and brainstem, the cerebral cortex is convoluted and the signal intensity gradients are highly variable in both magnitude and direction. The sulci are generally wider in the frontal lobes than in the occipital lobes. The major fissures (central and lateral) are wider again. Because of the many different gradient directions, the cortex is sensitive to shifts in many directions. It can be divided into (a) a superficial part representing the external surface and including the tips of the gyri and (b) a deeper part consisting of infolded cortex below the external surface. The superficial gyri form part of the general external shape of the brain and have a reasonable degree of regularity about their position. Their signal intensity gradients reflect this, and it is possible to recognize shifts of the superficial cortex using the simple plateau model, although the plateaus are not so well defined as with the ventricular system.

The deeper infolded cortex is notable for the fact that there are frequently two border zones in close proximity, with signal intensity gradients that are opposed ("reverse slopes") or obliqued. The cortex is subject to shifts which may move both of these border zones in the same direction producing biphasic changes (i.e., Figure 7.2, right hemisphere). There are also other processes which move the sulcal border zones in opposite directions, either towards one another (as in generalized brain swelling) or apart (as in cortical atrophy, i.e., Figure 7.13). Combinations of the different signal intensity gradients and different inplane shifts in both border zones within sulci (and fissures) of different widths result in a variety of appearances, some of which are illustrated in Figure 7.14.

Adjacent to the cortex are blood vessels as well as meninges; shifts which involve these may result in more complex multiphasic changes.

7.5.4   Global Change in Brain Size

When there is a global change in brain size, the matching process effectively aligns the central portion of the two volume images of the brain. As a result, the more peripheral regions are progressively displaced from their original positions. If slices are imaged perpendicular to a radius from the center out to the periphery, there will be a progressive throughplane shift which reaches a maximum at the outer surface. This effect will generally be greatest for transverse slices at the superior aspect of the brain and at the inferior aspect of the cerebellum. For parasagittal slices, the largest changes are at the lateral extremities of the hemisphere, since these are furthest from the center of the brain. The effect is reversed for generalized reduction in size. To obtain more

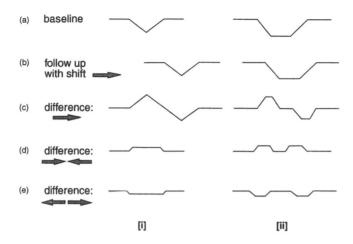

FIGURE 7.14
Intensity profiles showing effects of shifts on sulci and fissures. Wedge [i] and trough [ii] profiles are shown in (a). A displacement is shown in (b) and the corresponding differences in (c). Effects of sulci moving together (d) and apart (e) are also shown.

accurate images of local changes, the matching process can be restricted to smaller volumes around the area of interest.

7.5.5 Blood Vessels and Venous Sinuses

With the T1-weighted sequence used in most of this study, only minimal inflow effects were seen in proximal arteries, but changes in signal intensity were more obvious with angiographic sequences. The signal intensity in many vessels reflected the T1 of blood which is intermediate between brain and CSF. The blood vessels may be circular, elliptical, or triangular in cross section, and subtraction of these following an increase or decrease in size may produce different effects that can be predicted from the plateau model (Figure 7.15). There may also be positional shifts of blood vessels.

7.5.6 Meninges

Because the images are matched to the brain, shift of the brain within the cranial cavity may appear as a shift of the dura and skull into the subarachnoid space surrounding the brain. This shift then shows up along the smooth outline of the dura and adjacent skull rather than the convolutions of the cortex.

7.5.7 Other Extracerebral Tissues and Fluids

The process of registering the brain also aligns tissues and fluids surrounding it, as long as these are in fixed relation to the brain. If they are not in fixed relation, differences will be seen on the subtraction images. Such tissues may undergo changes in their own right, and these need to be interpreted with

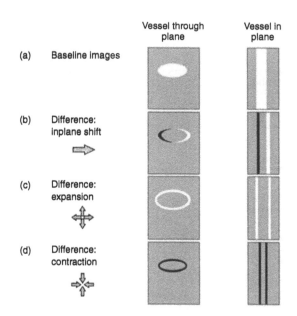

FIGURE 7.15
Views of blood vessels (inplane and throughplane) and surrounded by CSF for a T1-weighted image are shown in (a). The difference for an inplane shift is shown in (b) and the effects of expansion (c) and contraction (d) on difference images are also shown.

reference to the brain. Susceptibility effects from air in the nasal sinuses may impact on brain signal with T2-weighted sequences. The scalp shows changes in most subtraction images consistent with differences in blood distribution within it. Changes are seen in the neck due to changes in the relative position of the head and neck at the craniovertebral junction. Marked contrast enhancement is seen in blood vessels, the nasal mucosa, scalp, and the skin.

7.6   Artifacts and Failed Registration

Difference images are subject to all of the artifacts present on the source images, and subtraction usually makes these more obvious. Artifacts may be produced by global motion of the subject as well as more localized motion of structures such as the eyes and the pharynx. The use of phase encoding in two directions as required by the 3D acquisition increases the vulnerability of the sequence-to-motion artifact in different directions. In addition, phase wrap artifacts, in which signals from outside the defined field of view or at the edges of the excited slab get aliased to appear within the images, can be intrusive but are usually easily recognized. For the 2D multislice acquisitions fully interleaved single sequences were used, with all slices being excited within each TR. This ensured a coherent data set, even if artifacts were present.

However, it is not uncommon to use serially interleaved methods, in which, for example, every second slice is obtained in one complete acquisition, followed by a separate, repeat run to acquire the omitted slices. With this latter approach, subject motion can result in spatially inconsistent data, so that the two scans cannot be treated as one, but neither component scan has full enough spatial coverage to be reformatted without error.

Susceptibility artifacts may be very largely replicated if the patient is in virtually the same position on both examinations. However they are inherently anisotropic with respect to B_0 and may not therefore be correctable by rigid body translation and rotation. The problem is likely to be greater with T2-weighted sequences than the T1-weighted sequences and the T2-weighted spin echo sequences used in this study.

The difference images provide an inbuilt check of the fidelity of registration. If the program fails to obtain a satisfactory match, monophasic or multiphasic changes will be seen in border zones. Interplateau shifts may also be seen. The changes may be widespread and generally will have the character of a whole brain shift superimposed on any underlying changes. Unregistered images provide a useful guide in this context.

Difference images tend to reveal artifacts more strongly than the original anatomical images. This is because subtraction of registered images cancels out the signal from unchanged anatomy, whereas the artifacts present in the source images are likely to be different for each acquisition and so do not cancel. A notable feature of many difference images is biphasic changes along strong edges that run perpendicular to the primary or secondary phase encode directions. These are often caused by patient motion at a level that is insufficient to produce overt artifacts on the source images, but which has the effect of slightly reducing the image resolution by making the extreme edges of the raw k-space data inconsistent.[10]

Changes in scanner calibration can also often readily be detected on difference images. For example, changes in gradient scaling, which alter the apparent size of imaged objects, are manifest as progressively increasing difference signals from edges perpendicular to the scaled axis. Methods for correcting calibration errors are discussed in Chapter 5.

7.7 Approach to Diagnosis of Changes to the Brain on Difference Images

It is necessary to relate the causes of changes on difference images (i.e., pure changes in signal intensity, throughplane and inplane border zone shifts, and interplateau shifts) to the appearances they produce, i.e., (a) nonspecific changes in signal intensity; (b) monophasic curvilinear changes; (c) multiphasic curvilinear changes, and (d) interplateau changes. Changes of different types may be present on the same image. Their relation to underlying causes is summarized in Table 7.1. A formal approach to image interpretation is described in Table 7.2.

TABLE 7.1

Typical Appearances of Changes on Difference Images

Cause	Pure Change in Signal Intensity	Throughplane Border Zone Shift	Inplane Border Zone Shift	Interplateau Shift
Overall appearance	Nonspecific change in signal intensity	Monophasic curvilinear change	Multiphasic curvilinear change	Interplateau change
Signal intensity	Often monophasic (locally) Variable	Monophasic (locally) Less than full scale	Multiphasic (locally) Less than full scale	Monophasic (locally) Full scale
Site	Anatomic Physiologic Pathologic Distribution / Inplane plateau but throughplane border zone	Ventricular margin Brainstem margin etc.	Cerebral cortex Cerebellar hemisphere etc.	Brain margins, i.e., around ventricles and subarachnoid space (for brain/CSF)
Shape	Variable	Curvilinear	Curvilinear	Follows brain margins (for brain/CSF)
Size	Variable	Local size of border zone	Local size of border zone	Often extensive, but may be local with or without reversed phase
Segments	Depends on anatomy, physiology, pathology / Mottled, patchy, or circumscribed area	Narrower curvilinear directional dependence	Broader curvilinear etched, bas relief, directional shadowing	Uniform central region

Notes:

(i) Shifts are shown from smallest (pure change in signal intensity) to largest (interplateau).

(ii) The specificity of appearances also increases from left to right across the page.

(iii) Interplateau shifts may be throughplane and/or inplane and are accompanied by smaller changes due to throughplane and inplane border zone shifts.

(iv) Throughplane border zone shifts produce a heterogeneous range of appearances, i.e., nonspecific change in signal intensity as well as monophasic and multiphasic curvilinear changes.

(v) Inplane border zone shifts produce monophasic and multiphasic curvilinear changes.

(vi) Monophasic curvilinear changes typically occur at ventricular margins, brainstem margins, etc. where interplateau shifts first appear with larger shifts.

(vii) Reformatting into a perpendicular plane may convert a nonspecific throughplane shift to a more specific inplane plane shift.

TABLE 7.2

Approach to Image Interpretation

---

1) *Review source images*
   Define any signal intensity changes and shifts.
2) *Review difference images*
   Define significant abnormalities (i.e., non artifactual areas of increased or decreased signal intensity). These should fit into one or more of the four categories described in Table 7.1, i.e., nonspecific change in signal intensity, monophasic curvilinear change, multiphasic curvilinear change, or interplateau change.
3) *Assess interplateau shifts*
   For interplateau changes determine the shift direction (inplane or throughplane) by direct reference to the source images including different slices. The shift size is equal to the width of the full scale region on the difference image plus a fraction of the width of the associated border zone region (see later).
4) *Assess signal intensity gradients*
   In the regions of other changes on the difference images, use the source images to define the inplane contours and signal intensity gradients (which are perpendicular to the contours), noting the direction of decreasing signal. Define the throughplane signal intensity gradients in the slice of interest (these tend to be reciprocally related to the inplane gradients). Define the throughplane signal intensity gradients between slices by comparison of adjacent source images in the relevant areas.
5) *Assess border zone shifts*
   Determine shifts in the border zones by noting
   (a) signal on the difference image is produced by a shift with a component parallel to the maximum signal intensity gradient;
   (b) the difference image signal is positive when the shift is in the direction of decreasing gradient and vice versa;
   (c) the size of the shift in the direction of the maximum gradient is equal to the width of the change on the difference image multiplied by the average fraction of the full scale signal intensity;
   (d) local changes in signal intensity may exaggerate or minimize the signal difference produced by a shift;
   (e) profiles from source and difference may help resolve shift direction and size; and
   (f) reformatting the images into a perpendicular plane may transform a nonspecific change in signal intensity due to a throughplane shift to the curvilinear change of an inplane shift.
6) *Assess overall pattern of shifts*
   Review the overall pattern of shifts for changes in brain site, shape, or size on a focal or general basis.
7) *Assess pure changes in signal intensity*
   Note that with a pure change in signal intensity no shift is detectable. (A pure change in signal intensity may, however, be accompanied by an inseparable change in lesion size).

7.8 Clinical Applications—General

There are many potential uses for this technique and the applications described merely constitute a starting point that reflects local interest. The monitoring of physiological changes of the brain was necessary to establish a baseline for recognition of changes in disease. The importance of radiographic positioning and its effects on changes to the shape of the brain were studied. Also the appearance of growth and development in children needed to be identified.

Another unexpected finding was a reduction in brain size (atrophy rather than edema) during the third trimester in patients with pre-eclampsia. Also observed were atrophic change and swelling in first episode schizophrenia over a 6 to 12 month period. Many other applications of this technique are possible and results are awaited with considerable interest.

7.9   Physiological Changes

7.9.1   Effect of Head Position

Figure 7.16 shows interplateau and border zone shifts produced by changing head orientation from right-side down to left-side down. The image shows shift of the ventricular system and changes in many gyri. These changes may provide a basis for measuring brain compliance in health and disease, including quantification of the elastic properties of the brain.

7.9.2   Menstrual Cycle

In the four females studied, registration of repeated examinations showed very small changes. The most consistent finding on the difference images was a border zone shift related to the lateral ventricles consistent with an increase in their size at the end of the second half of the menstrual cycle. This change

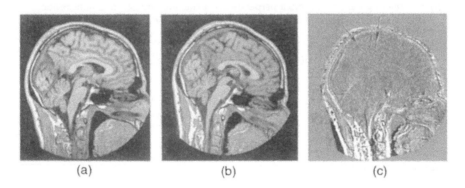

(a)   (b)   (c)

FIGURE 7.16
Change in the superior sagittal and straight sinuses with head flexion: Sagittal T1-weighted images in upright position (a) and with head flexion (b). The registered difference image [(b) − (a)] is shown in (c). The signal from the inferior sagittal sinus has increased, probably as a result of an increase in size. The superior sagittal sinus shows a more complex change posteriorly (c). Border zone shifts are noted in the region of the superior cerebral sulci (c) (arrows).

is consistent in sign, but may be smaller in size than the previously reported finding of increase in CSF volume later in the menstrual cycle detected with a volume measurement technique.

7.9.3 Pregnancy

During normal pregnancy, the brain decreases in size, reaching a maximum reduction at term. After delivery it regains its original size over a period of four to six months (Figure 7.17). [16,17]

7.10 Contrast Enhancement

Normal enhancement in the meninges, diplocic veins, scalp, skin, and other structures was more clearly demonstrated than with conventional unregistered images.[18] In addition, abnormal enhancement was more clearly demonstrated in patients with meningeal disease and other conditions (Figure 7.18).

Registration and subtraction were of particular value in the following situations:

(a) *Recognition of small degrees of enhancement*: When the level of change was small, differences may be much less than those produced by misregistration, particularly when the changes are at boundaries. Diffuse generalized enhancement may also be more readily recognized on subtraction images in relation to the noise level of the surrounding images. This type of change may be missed with conventional display strategies.

(b) *Enhancement in tissues of fluids with very high or very low baseline signals*: The usual window level and width settings may place the changes due to enhancement off the top or the bottom of the display gray scale, and so render changes difficult to recognize. Subtraction reduces all tissues and fluids to a common baseline and makes changes of this type easier to visualize.

(c) *Enhancement at interfaces, boundaries, and other regions of complex anatomy*: In these situations there are frequently partial volume effects, and even a small displacement of the brain between pre- and postcontrast images produces a difference in these effects, resulting in spurious changes in signal intensity. Precise registration provides the same partial volume effects on the before and after images, so that enhancement can be readily recognized.

(d) *Assessment of enhancement when thin slices are used*: While use of thin slices reduces partial volume effects, it may increase problems due

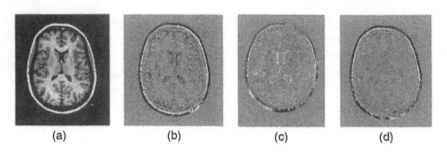

(a)   (b)   (c)   (d)

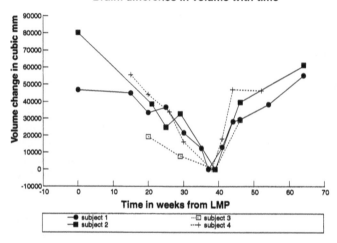

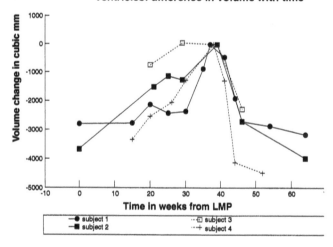

FIGURE 7.17
Pregnancy: T1-weighted baseline images taken prior to pregnancy (a). Subtraction images from prior to delivery minus baseline (b), six weeks after delivery minus prior to delivery (c), and six months after delivery minus baseline (d). The brain decreases in size before delivery and increases after delivery back to its normal size. Figure (e) shows change in brain volume, and Figure (f) shows change in ventricular volume with time.

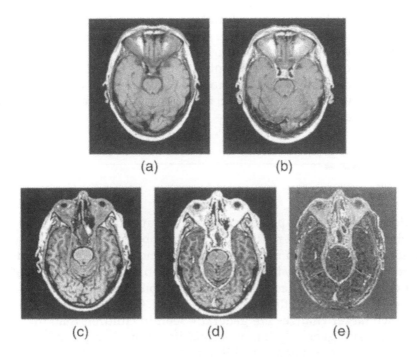

FIGURE 7.18

Contrast enhancement Wegener's disease: T1-weighted spin echo images (SE 720/20) before (a) and after (b) contrast enhancement; T1-weighted volume images before (c) and after (d) contrast enhancement, with subtraction image, (d) − (c), shown in (e). The tentorial enhancement is best seen on the registered volume and subtraction images (e) (arrows).

to overt misregistration. The same absolute displacement may appear as only a slight difference in position of a thick slice, and so permit valid image interpretation, but when a narrow slice thickness is used, the same displacement may take the region of interest into a completely different slice and create uncertainty in interpretation. Precise registration enables the patient position to be maintained, and allows the advantage to thin slices to be utilized.

(e) *Follow-up studies.* Assessing changes in the degree of enhancement between examinations may be rendered difficult by misregistration between examinations. This problem can be overcome by accurate alignment of images on serial examinations.

The technique may also be used to provide angiography.

In a number of conditions, such as detection of metastases and demonstration of enhancement in multiple sclerosis (MS) plaques, scans delayed by one or two hours may be more useful than immediate postinjection scans. Misregistration problems are usually increased in this situation, since the patient is taken out of the scanner and positioned back again later. Results from this technique may be improved by registration. It may also be possible to reduce the dosage of contrast enhancement if subtraction is used routinely. The need for triple dose enhancement may also be reduced.

A limitation of the technique in contrast studies is that of increased acquisition times because of the need to produce isotropic volume data sets. Even slab imaging takes 2–30 s. As a result, the technique is not particularly suited to the timescale of dynamic studies.

7.11 Pediatrics

In children physiological, pathological, and therapeutic changes of the type described above may be present.[19] These may be complicated by growth and development, which may be normal or abnormal. Growth and development includes not only increase in size of the brain, but also cortical folding, myelination, and decrease in brain proton density, T1 and T2. The surrounding tissues and fluids may also change. Growth of the skull means that much larger changes are generally seen in children than in adults, where the skull generally imposes rigid limits on changes in brain size. Because of the large changes in children, it is often useful to match examinations in successive pairs so that the differences between any two image sets are minimized (Figure 7.19). The small subarachnoid space over the cortex also makes segmentation more difficult than in adults.

Changes in children may be quite complex, with, for example, the ventricular system showing changes due to expansion and contraction at different phases of growth (Figure 7.20).

In the late phase of neonatal infarction (one to nine months) increased growth can be seen atthe margins of the lesion (Figure 7.20). The rapidly proliferating tissue seen in the late phase of infarction did not have the features

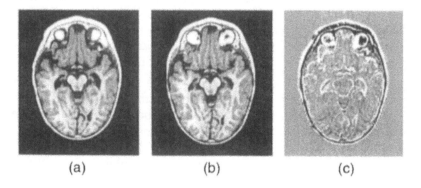

(a)   (b)   (c)

FIGURE 7.19
Growth and development in a child aged 10 months (a) and 14 months (b) on registered T1-weighted images with subtraction images (c) = (b) − (a). The white line around the gyral tips of the brain in (c) indicates growth of the brain.

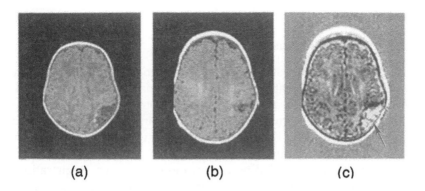

FIGURE 7.20
Neonatal infarction: T1-weighted scan at 4 weeks (a) and at 14 weeks (b), with registered difference image (c). The highlighted area in (c) (arrow) shows that growth in the brain adjacent to the infarction has been more rapid than elsewhere.

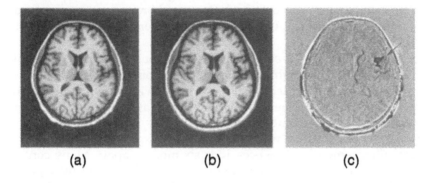

FIGURE 7.21
Adult infarction: T1-weighted scans 1 week after infarction (a) and 12 months after (b). The registered difference image (c) shows the infarct (arrow) as a low signal area and dilatation of the adjacent lateral ventricles.

of gliosis (long T1 and T2), and followed the configuration of the brain. It may provide an anatomical substrate for neurological plasticity.

7.12   Adult Infarction

Registration can be used to detect subclinical infarction[20] and show atrophic changes associated with the lesion. The development of an infarct with adjacent ventricular dilatation is shown in Figure 7.21. The technique may also be of value in distinguishing infarction from low-grade glioma and in serial studies.[21]

7.13 Multiple Sclerosis

There is considerable interest in monitoring the progress of multiple sclerosis (MS) with and without treatment; some cohorts have now been studied for several years. The expected annual change in lesion burden is about 5 to 10%. This is of the same order as misregistration errors inherent with conventional techniques, thus assessing the effectiveness of new therapies such as interferon may be difficult in short term studies.

Twelve patients were studied on two or more occasions. Registration not only allowed changes to be identified in specific lesions, but also separation of differences in contrast enhancement from other changes using "difference of difference" images (i.e., difference of post-minus precontrast enhancement scans at two different times). Changes in unenhanced lesion T1 were much more readily recognized with the subtraction images, including effects due to both increased and decreased T1. Obvious changes were seen in the T1 of areas where no enhancement was observed. Decreased brain size was observed in patients who had treatment with steroids and others who did not have this treatment.

Subvoxel registration revealed that many lesions are more complicated than they appear at first sight, with some undergoing remission and others in very close proximity undergoing exacerbation with both parallel and discordant contrast enhancement. Also observed was shortening (as well as lengthening) of T1 in the acute phase.

For example, a 31-year-old woman with MS was examined with and without contrast enhancement on two occasions six months apart. Many contrast-enhancing lesions were either much better seen or only seen on the registered images. There were changes in lesion signal intensity and the degree of enhancement, as well as evidence of decreased brain size on the follow-up scans (Figure 7.22). This may have been due to brain swelling at the time of the initial examination that had been partly or completely resolved when the follow-up study was performed. It may also have been due to progressive atrophy. The patient did not receive steroids. Registration and quantification may also be used to detect and monitor atrophic change in MS.[21]

7.14 Tumors

On the registered difference images, increased tumor size was manifest as encroachment on the ventricular system and subarachnoid space.[22,23] Figure 7.23 (a) shows an astrocytoma grade III before treatment. After one month, the registered difference image (Figure 7.23 (c)) shows tumor expansion in

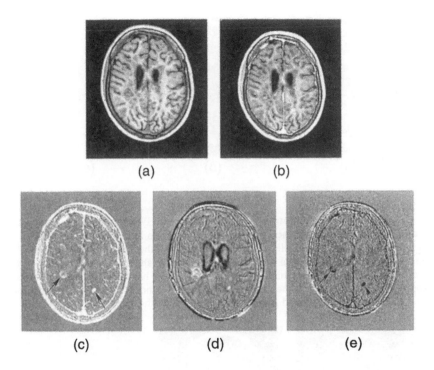

(a) (b)

(c) (d) (e)

FIGURE 7.22
Multiple Sclerosis: A 31-year-old female with MS: initial unenhanced (a), enhanced (b), and registered subtraction (c) images. A repeat pre- and postenhancement scan was performed six months later. The difference image on the unenhanced scans six months apart is shown in (d), and the difference between the earlier "post minus pre" scans and the later "post minus pre" scans is shown in (e). The enhancing lesions are see better in (c) (arrows). The ventricular system has increased in size in (d), and there is evidence of decreased brain size. Some lesions appear bright because they have shortened their T1 time (d). Lesions that were enhancing in (b) now appear dark on (e); they no longer enhance (arrows).

spite of treatment. Differences in contrast enhancement were also demonstrated by comparison of the subtracted (post-minus precontrast) images on each examination.

In tumor regression following treatment, T1 may be decreased. This produces an increased signal on the difference image. Decreased mass effect can also be demonstrated (Figure 7.24).

Registration may allow earlier recognition of tumor growth and response to therapy than conventional techniques. A cohort of inoperable and partially resected meningiomas has been studied to assess their rate of growth (Figure 7.25).

T2-weighted images may also be used for registration.[11] Figure 7.26 shows a mixed pattern of response to progression.

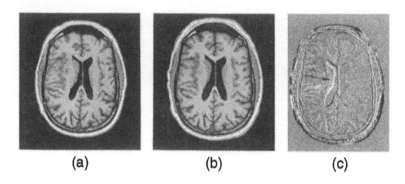

(a)   (b)   (c)

FIGURE 7.23
Astrocytoma grade III in a 42-year-old male examined with IV Gadodiamide (a) and again one month later (b), with subtraction of (a) from (b) shown in image (c). The increase in image size can be seen on the aligned source images, but the extent of the mass effect is better seen in (c) (arrow). Positive and negative interplateau shifts are seen around the right lateral ventricle. Border zone shifts are seen on the right hemisphere. Smaller negative interplateau shifts are seen at the ventricular margins on the left, as well as more subtle border zone shifts anteriorly and posteriorly within the left hemisphere.

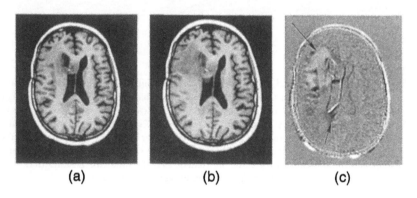

(a)   (b)   (c)

FIGURE 7.24
Astrocytoma: T1-weighted scans before (a) and six weeks after (b) treatment with Temozolamide; (c) difference image. Most of the tumor has decreased in size and shortened its T1 following treatment (long arrow) but some has progressed (short arrow).

7.15 Schizophrenia

The first study with CT showing ventricular enlargement in schizophrenia was published 20 years ago. It was a cross-sectional study. Longitudinal studies without registration have shown no change in the brain with CT, and increase in size of the caudate nucleus in patients treated with antipsychotics. Using registration, atrophic changes were demonstrated in the five first-episode schizophrenics who were studied six months apart (Figure 7.27).

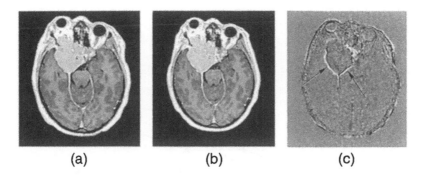

(a) (b) (c)

FIGURE 7.25
Meningioma: Contrast-enhanced T1-weighted images from volume acquisition obtained initially (a) and 13 months later (b). Subtraction of (a) from (b) in image (c) shows by the white and dark lines (arrows) that the tumor has grown between the scans.

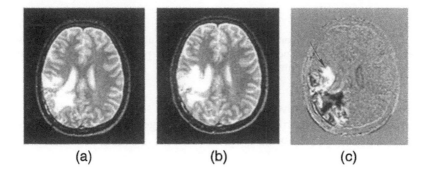

(a) (b) (c)

FIGURE 7.26
Astrocytoma: T2-weighted images before (a) and after (b) treatment. Subtraction of (a) from (b) is shown in (c). The responding areas appear dark in (c) but the more anterior white area has progressed (arrow).

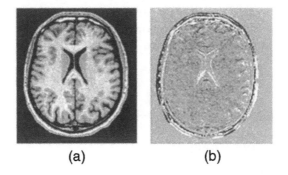

(a) (b)

FIGURE 7.27
Schizophrenia: Registered subtraction image, showing differences that developed over six months after first admission. The ventricles have increased in size, and abnormalities (biphasic changes) are seen in the left temporal lobe.

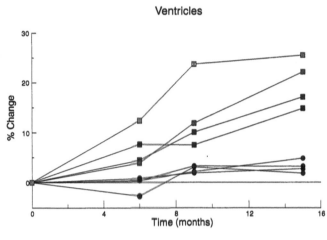

FIGURE 7.28
Alzheimer's disease: Plot of percentage change in ventricular size for patients with Alzheimer's Disease (squares) and normal controls (circles). The patients show a greater increase
in ventricular volume than controls.

Another three patients showed evidence of brain swelling, two studies were
equivocal, and one was negative. These changes may reflect difference
phases of the first episode of this illness.[24,25]

7.16 Alzheimer's Disease

Fox, Freeborough, and Rosser[5,26,27] have used registration, subtraction,
and quantification to demonstrate atrophic changes in Alzheimer's disease. They found marked changes compared with controls (Figure 7.28).
Some pre-symptomatic patients also had early changes detectable with
registration and quantification.

7.17 Postoperative Changes

Although three published serial studies of the brain following coronary
artery bypass surgery (CABS) have been negative except in patients who had
clinical evidence of strokes, registration of serial scans has shown abnormalities in most patients studied to date.[28]

In monitoring the effect of treatment, effects of drugs on brain size need to be recognized. In particular, steroids and ACTH may produce a change in brain size due to treatment, not the primary pathologic process. Likewise, alcohol and states of hydration may affect brain size.

7.18 Bone Marrow Transplantation

In order to determine the nature and frequency of changes to the brain in patients undergoing chemoradiotherapy and BMT, we performed registered serial MRI studies in 15 patients with CML (13 allografts and 2 autografts).[29]

Repeated studies performed 4 to 339 days after transplantation showed ventricular enlargement and cortical atrophy in all of the 13 patients who had allografts. The changes were evident at 4 to 6 days, and became more obvious in later follow-up cases. Similar changes were seen in one patient with an autograft, but no significant change was seen in other autografted patients or in the normal controls.

Cerebral atrophy has been described following long term administration of steroids, and reversibility of the findings may follow decrease or cessation of steroid use. The appearances are typically described with long term use (six months to five years) and cumulative doses of 4000 to 58,000 mg of prednisone. Assessing the potential effect of steroids is complex. All 15 patients in this study had steroids at some stage in their illness. The total dosage for allograft patients varied from the equivalent of 100 to 20,250 mg of prednisolone. There was no evidence of reversibility of ventricular size in any patients. This might have been expected in patients having a reduction in their dosage or stopping treatment with steroids. The onset of brain changes occurred at the same time as treatment with steroids, cyclophosphamide, and TBI, but there did not appear to be a particular association with steroids given in the previous 48 hours.

7.19 Quantitation of Brain Change

Quantified measurement of the size of various brain structures and pathologies can readily be achieved from MR images. A number of examples have been cited in this chapter and many computerized tools are now available for such measurements including some designed specifically for use in conjunction with registered images.[25,30,31] Although there may be technical problems in achieving reliable quantitation for some structures, for example, due to complexity of shape or ambiguity in the precise location of a boundary, in many scientific and clinical serial studies a key prerequisite to measurement is identification of the nature or pattern of change to be quantified. An illustrative example is provided by Figure 7.26, which shows a case of an astrocytoma that was monitored before and after treatment. An intuitively natural measurement to make might be the total tumor volume, which might then be correlated with outcome. However, as shown in the subtraction image, Figure 7.26c, although the tumor responds to the treatment, that response is heterogeneous. Thus measurement of a global volume decrease would fail to capture a critical factor of localized lack of response, which then acts as a locus for future tumor growth and can result in poor final outcome. The registered subtraction technique allows the pattern of change to be identified and can be used to guide measurement as required. This is a powerful feature of the registration methodology.

7.20 Conclusion

Use of image registration allows changes to be detected on serial examination in many diseases when conventional approaches produce equivocal or negative results. This is likely to increase the sensitivity of MRI for many neurological applications. Effects due to treatment may also be monitored with this technique. Pediatrics is notable for the fact that there are also changes due to growth and development, and these may be affected by disease and treatment. The technique appears likely to have many applications.

The work described in this chapter has exclusively employed rigid-body registration for serial studies of the brain. Rigid-body registration may also have clinical applications in other organs or body parts, most notably for normally rigid structures such as bones. In addition to monitoring disease progression or regression, other emerging applications are perfusion imaging and dynamic contrast-enhanced angiography. In both these methods, images are acquired in quick succession following contrast administration, and uncorrected changes in subject position during the examination can cause problems. Finally, recent developments in nonrigid registration methods are likely to have clinical applications when combined with serial MRI examinations. These are outside the scope of this chapter, but various examples of early work are discussed in Section III.

References

1. Woods, R.P., Mazziotta, J.C., and Cherry, S.R., MRI-PET registration with automated algorithm, *J. Comput. Assist. Tomogr*, 17, 536, 1993.
2. Friston, K.J., Ashburner, J., Poline, J.B., Frith, C.D., Heather, J.D., and Frackowiak, R.S., Spatial registration and normalisation of images, *Human Brain Mapping*, 2, 16, 1995.

3. Hajnal, J.V., Saeed, N., Oatridge, A., Soar, E.J., Young, I.R., and Bydder, G.M., A registration and interpolation procedure for subvoxel matching of serially acquired MR images, *J. Comput. Assist. Tomogr.*, 19:289, 1995.
4. Lemieux, L., Wieshmann, U.C., Moran, N.F., Fish, D.R., and Shorvon, S.D., The detection and significance of subtle changes in mixed-signal brain lesions by serial MRI scan matching and spatial normalization, *Med. Image Anal.*, 2(3): 227–242, 1998.
5. Freeborough, P.A., Woods, R.P., and Fox, N.C., Accurate registration of serial 3D MR brain images and its application to visualizing change in neurodegenerative disorders, *J. Comput. Assist. Tomogr.*, 20, 1012, 1996.
6. Studholme, C., Hill, D.L.G., and Hawkes, D.J., An overlap invariant entropy measure of 3D medical image alignment, *Pattern Recognition*, 32, 71–86, 1999.
7. Noll, D.C., Badda, F.E., and Eddy, W.F., A spectral approach to analysing slice selection in planar imaging: optimization for through-plane interpolation, *Magn. Reson. Med.*, 38, 151, 1997.
8. Hajnal, J.V., Saeed, N., Soar, E. J., Oatridge, A., Young, I.R., and Bydder, G.M., Detection of subtle brain changes using subvoxel registration and subtraction of serial MR images, *J. Comput. Assist. Tomogr.*, 19, 289, 1995.
9. Bydder, G.M., Detection of small changes to the brain with serial magnetic resonance imaging, *Br. J. Radiol.*, 68, 1271, 1995.
10. Oatridge, A., The Use of Subvoxel Registration and Subtraction of Serial Magnetic Resonance Imaging for Detecting Small Changes to the Brain. Ph.D. thesis, Leeds Metropolitan University, 1999.
11. Hajnal, J.V., Oatridge, A., Murdoch, J., Saeed, N., and Bydder, G.M., Multislice data acquisitions for multiplanar reformatting and image registration, *Proc. Intl. Soc. Magn. Reson. Med.*, 6, 560, 1998.
12. Oatridge, A., Saeed, N., Hajnal, J.V., and Bydder, G.M., Subvoxel registration and subtraction of 2D multislice magnetic resonance images of the brain in patients with gliomas, *Proc. Intl. Soc. Magn. Reson. Med.* 7, 905, 1999.
13. Stark, D.D. and Bradley, W.G., Eds. *Magnetic Resonance Imaging* 2nd ed. St. Louis: Mosby Yearbook, 1992, 3–521.
14. Atlas, S.W., Ed. *Magnetic Resonance Imaging of the Brain and Spine*. New York: Raven Press, 1991, 1–128.
15. Grossman, R.I. and Yousem, D.M., *Neuroradiology*. St. Louis: Mosby Yearbook, 1994, 6–23.
16. Oatridge, A., Saeed, N., Hajnal, J.V., Puri, B.K., Mitchell, L., Holdcroft, A., and Bydder, G.M., Quantification of brain changes seen on serially registered MRI in normal pregnancy and pre-eclampsia, *Proc. Intl. Soc. Magn. Reson. Med.* 6, 1381, 1998.
17. Oatridge, A., Saeed, N., Hajnal, J.V., Puri, B.K., Holdcroft, A., Fusi L., and Bydder, G.M., Quantification of brain and ventricular size in pregnancy and pre-eclampsia, *Proc. Intl. Soc. Magn. Reson. Med.*, 7, 373, 1999.
18. Curati, W.L., Williams, E.J., Oatridge, A., Hajnal, J.V., Saeed, N., and Bydder, G.M., Use of subvoxel registration and subtraction to improve the demonstration of contrast enhancement in magnetic resonance imaging of the brain, *Neuroradiology*, 38, 717, 1996.
19. Rutherford, M.A., Pennock, J.M., Cowan, F.M., Saeed, N., Hajnal, J.V., and Bydder, G.M., Detection of subtle changes to the brain in infants and children using subvoxel registration and subtraction of serial magnetic resonance images, *Am. J. Neurorad.*, 18, 829, 1997.

20. Symms, M.R., Barker, G.J., Holmes, P., Wang, L., Yoo, D.S., Lemieux, L, Tofts, P.S., Thomas, D.J., and Stevens, J., A rapid automated system of serial changes in transient ischaemic attack using registration and subtraction of three-dimensional images, *Proc. Intl. Soc. Magn. Reson. Med.*, 5, 584, 1997.
21. Fox, N.C., Jenkins, R., Leany, S.M., Stevenson, V.L., Lorseff, N.A., Crum, W.R., Harvey, R.J., Rossor, M.N., Miller, D.H., and Thompson, A.J., Progressive cerebral atrophy in MS: a serial study using registered volumetric MRI, *Neurology*, 54, 807, 2000.
22. Oatridge, A., Newlands, E.S., Evans, H., Hajnal, J.V., Saeed, N., and Bydder, G.M., Registered serial magnetic resonance imaging of intracranial tumours, *Proc. Intl. Soc. Magn. Reson. Med.*, 4, 607, 1996.
23. Oatridge, A., Newlands, E.S., Brock, C., Evans, H., Hajnal, J.V., Saeed, N., Young, I.R., and Bydder, G.M., Assessment of growth and response to treatment in gliomas using subvoxel registration and subtraction of serial magnetic resonance images, *Proc. Intl. Soc. Magn. Reson. Med.*, 5, 97, 1997.
24. Puri, B.K., Richardson, A.J., Oatridge, A., Hajnal J.V., and Saeed, N., Cerebral ventricular asymmetry in schizophrenia: a high resolution 3D magnetic resonance imaging study, *Int. J. Psychophysol.*, 34, 207, 1999.
25. Saeed, N., Puri, B.K., Oatridge, A., Hajnal, J.V., and Young, I.R., Two methods of semi-automated quantification of changes in ventricular volume and their use in schiozophrenia, *Magn. Reson. Imaging*, 16, 1237, 1998.
26. Fox, N.C., Freeborough, P.A., and Rossor, M.N., Visualization and quantification of atrophy in Alzheimer's disease, *Lancet*, 348, 94, 1996.
27. Fox, N.C., Sachill, R.A., Crum, W.R., and Rossor, M.N., Correlation between volume of brain atrophy and cognitive disease in AD, *Neurology*, 52, 1687, 1999.
28. Oatridge, A., Kohn, A., Saeed, N., Hajnal, J.V., Puri, B.K., Smith, P.L.C, Taylor, K.M., and Bydder, G.M., Brain changes following cardiopulmonary bypass graft surgery detected by serially registered MRI, *Proc. Intl. Soc. Magn. Reson. Med.*, 1252, 2000.
29. Jager, H.E., Williams, E.J., Savage, D., Rule, S.A.J., Hajnal, J.V., Sikora, K., Goldman, J.M., and Bydder, G.M., Assessment of the brain before and after bone marrow conditioning and transplantation for chronic myeloid leukaemia using subvoxel registration and subtraction of serial magnetic resonance images, *Am. J. Neuroradiology*, 17, 1275, 1996.
30. Freeborough, P.A. and Fox, N.C., The boundary shift integral: an accurate and robust measure of cerebral volume changes from registered repeat MRI, *IEEE Trans. Med. Imaging*, 16, 623, 1997.
31. Lemieux, L., Wieshmann, U.C., Moran, N.F., Fish, D.R., and Shorvon, S.D., The detection and significance of subtle changes in mixed-signal brain lesions by serial MRI scanmatching and spatial normalization, *Med. Image. Anal.*, 2, 227–42, 1998.

8

The Role of Registration in Functional Magnetic Resonance Imaging

Mark Jenkinson and Stephen Smith

CONTENTS

8.1 Introduction to fMRI

Functional magnetic resonance imaging, or fMRI, is a noninvasive imaging technique used to investigate physiological function. It is most commonly used to study brain function by measuring blood oxygenation level, although other organs (e.g., kidneys) and other quantities (e.g., perfusion) can be studied. This chapter concentrates on using fMRI for blood oxygenation-related imaging of the brain, as image registration has become an indispensible part of the analysis of these data for research and clinical purposes.

fMRI allows the experimenter to determine which parts of the brain are activated by different types of sensory stimulation, motor activity, or cognitive activity. For instance, fMRI can be used to study responses related to visual or auditory stimulation, the movement of a subject's fingers, or the imagined rotation of 3D objects.

The subject in an fMRI experiment will lie within the magnet, and a particular form of stimulation is applied or task performed. For example, the subject may wear special glasses so that pictures can be shown during the experiment. Then, MR images of the subject's brain are taken, starting with a single high resolution scan. This is used later as an anatomical substrate for overlaying the brain areas which were activated by the stimulus. Next, a series of low resolution scans (the raw functional images) are taken, one every few seconds; normally, 100 or more such scans are obtained. During some of these scans, the stimulus (in this case the moving picture) will be presented, and during others the stimulus will be absent. These images are sensitive to changes in blood flow and/or blood oxygenation in the brain caused by brain activity. The fMRI images taken during activation can be compared with those taken during rest in order to see which parts of the brain were activated by the stimulus or activity.

Other functional neuroimaging methods exist, such as PET (positron emission tomography), EEG (electroencephalography), and MEG (magnetoencephalography). These differ from fMRI in their temporal and spatial resolutions as well as the type of physiological response measured. For instance, fMRI measures local blood oxygenation changes, PET measures either blood flow or metabolic activity (a more direct measure of activity than blood flow), EEG measures induced electrical signals on the scalp, and MEG measures induced electrical currents within the cortex. EEG and MEG have very high temporal resolution (milliseconds) but poor spatial resolution (centimeters); PET has poor temporal resolution (tens of seconds) and intermediate spatial resolution (many millimeters), while fMRI has an intermediate temporal resolution (seconds) and good spatial resolution (millimeters). PET also requires that a radioactive agent be injected into the subject, while the other methods are relatively non-invasive.

8.1.1   BOLD Contrast and Brain Function

Activity in a certain brain area causes an increase in both local blood flow rate and relative proportion of oxyhemoglobin to deoxyhemoglobin (in local blood vessels). A T2-weighted MR sequence is sensitive to this change in blood oxygenation; this is known as the BOLD (blood oxygenation level dependent) effect[9,12] and is dependent on field strengths as well as physiological and other factors. Therefore, as blood flow and oxygenation levels increase in metabolically active regions, the MR signal increases; this is used to infer neuronal activity. It is important to use an MR method which can acquire T2-weighted images very rapidly. The most commonly used method in fMRI is echo planar imaging (EPI),[10] which is capable of acquiring a full brain image every few seconds, with a typical within-slice resolution of 2 to 4 mm, and slice thickness of 3 to 8 mm.

The change in MR signal induced by the BOLD response to brain activity is typically 0.5 to 5 percent of the average image intensity within the brain. In addition, there is considerable change in the signal that is unrelated to the processes of interest (that is, not related to the given stimulus). Therefore, separation of the signal of interest from this "noise" requires sensitive statistical analysis.

To illustrate the type of statistical analysis required, consider a simple "block-design" fMRI experiment. In this example, a visual stimulation (e.g., a flashing checkerboard) is shown to the subject for a period of 10 image acquisitions followed by an equal period of "rest," where a reference stimulation (or no stimulation) is shown. This 10 ON, 10 OFF pattern is repeated several times to enable the signal-to-noise ratio (SNR) in the following statistical analysis to be large enough for activation to be detected. Given that a typical image acquisition takes 3 seconds, such a session might last 10 minutes in total.

A particular location in the brain is considered "activated" if the intensity variation follows the same pattern as the stimulus. More precisely, the intensity for each voxel, as a function of time, is compared with the stimulus function (which is 1 in the ON condition and 0 in the OFF condition) by some method, such as correlation. If the intensity and stimulus functions have a high correlation (that is, they are similar), this voxel will be classed as "active." This is quantified by converting the correlation score into a probability of the observed intensity signal occurring purely by chance (the null hypothesis); the regions with very low probability of having occurred by chance are considered "active."

8.1.2 fMRI Analysis Overview

In fMRI analysis a large number of processing stages are required before the final activation results are obtained. In-depth coverage of these stages is beyond the scope of this chapter (see Reference 11 for more detail), but it is helpful to have a broad understanding of the full analysis to appreciate the general context for the issues of motion correction and registration in fMRI.

Although no standard analysis protocol is universally accepted, a typical sequence of analysis steps for a single-session fMRI experiment is:

1. Acquire and reconstruct the individual images.
2. Phase-correct all time series for variations in timings of scanning slices within the volume scan time (TR).
3. Apply motion correction to correct for head motion.
4. Spatially smooth the data to increase SNR and precondition later statistics.

5. Filter each voxel's time series, to remove slow temporal drifts and high frequency noise.

6. Perform the statistical analysis (creating a statistical parametric map—an SPM).

7. Threshold the SPM to find the "significant activated regions."

Therefore, at the end of such an analysis, the result is a map showing the "activated" voxels or clusters of voxels (for example, see Color Figure 8.6*). These activation maps are often then subject to some higher-level analysis, such as combining the low resolution results with the subject's high resolution image or combining results across a group of subjects.

To combine images effectively, an accurate linear or nonlinear (warping) registration method is required. The transformations involved in linear registration (rigid–body or affine) have been described in Chapters 2 and 3 of this book, and nonlinear, or nonrigid, transformations are described in Chapter 13. Registration is necessary for combining low resolution statistical images with a high resolution structural image, for combining statistical results across several subjects in a group, or for transforming the results into a standard coordinate system. Moreover, for best results, the fMRI images should be corrected for geometric distortion that occurred during the functional experiment, prior to registration. In general, as the raw functional images do not have particularly good spatial resolution or contrast, accurately registering these images with standard anatomical images is quite a challenging problem.

8.2   Motion Correction

The first and most important registration issue associated with fMRI is motion correction, which attempts to eliminate intensity changes in an fMRI data set that are the result of subject motion during the experiment. This is particularly important, as all subsequent analysis requires that each voxel corresponds to a fixed location in the brain at every point in time. Since subjects often move in the scanner during the course of an experiment (which can take as long as an hour) the position of the head varies from image to image. This is particularly true for clinical patients (as opposed to "normal" subjects). Consequently, all images need to be registered to a consistent coordinate system to enable further analysis.

The motion can vary over time from small, subvoxel motion to large, obvious motion. However, even subvoxel motion has a detrimental effect on the statistical analysis—especially for smaller activations. Therefore, motion correction is required for almost all fMRI experiments.

---

* Color figures follow page 22.

As all images in an fMRI experiment are taken a few seconds apart, with the same settings, on the same scanner, and with the same subject, it is an almost ideal intrapatient, intramodality registration scenario. Consequently, rigid-body transformations with intramodal similarity measures, as described in Chapter 3, are almost universally used to model the change between one image and the next.

In addition to rigid-body motion, there are also some sources of nonrigid motion usually present. For example, pulsatile motion of the soft brain tissues occurs during the cardiac cycle. Even bulk motion of major chest organs during respiration will change the magnetic field distribution throughout the body (including the head) and will therefore affect the geometry of the scans, inducing nonrigid motion. It is possible to reduce the extent of some of these motions by using methods such as cardiac gating of the images (acquiring at the same point in the cardiac cycle each time). However, the major component of motion is due to rigid movement of the head in the scanner, and the correction of this motion will be discussed in the following sections. For more detail on physiological noise, see Hu et al. and Jezzard.[5,6]

8.2.1   A Multiple Registration Problem

The basic problem of motion correction is to align each image in the series to a consistent orientation (by registering each one to some fixed target image). Therefore, motion correction is simply a series of registrations. However, there are typically more than a hundred images to register, so speed is quite important. For instance, if each registration took 30 minutes and there were 200 images, the total motion correction time would be more than 4 days.

The standard approach taken in motion correction is to use an intramodality voxel similarity measure, such as sum of squares of differences or mean-absolute-difference, together with some optimization algorithm. The registration can be performed quite rapidly, since the resolution of the images is relatively low, the motion is usually small (so that simple local optimization will suffice), and only 6 degrees-of-freedom (DOF) transformations are used (i.e., rigid-body). For instance, a 200-image series can typically be motion corrected in less than 30 minutes—that is, less than 10 seconds per image.

The method of minimizing the cost function while varying the translation and rotation parameters is usually a standard optimization technique (such as gradient descent, Powell's method, or a simplex method—see Reference 13 for more details) or a customized version of these. It is assumed that any activation in the images does not affect the estimation of motion, and since the intensity changes due to activation are relatively low, this is probably a safe assumption.

It is necessary to choose a "target" image for motion correction. Normally this is simply an arbitrary single image from the original data. However, care needs to be exercised when choosing the target, as the first image from the sequence probably looks quite different from all subsequent images, due to MR saturation effects. Therefore, if this is used as a target, the cost function should be able to cope with the resulting changes in intensity and contrast between the target and the images registered to this target.

A more sophisticated choice of target is to take some kind of average image from across the time series. For example, re-registering ten images (selected from equally spaced points along the time series) to the first, taking the average spatial "position" of these ten images, creating an average image in this position, and then reregistering all ten to this average image results in a motion correction target which is in the "average position" for the whole time series and contains representative "average intensities." This has the benefit of minimizing the average "distance" by which all images are transformed (and therefore minimizing interpolation related blurring—see below).

8.2.2 Interpolation

After the registration phase has determined the transformation parameters required to correct for head motion, it is then necessary to transform the images to this new, consistent orientation. This requires (subvoxel) interpolation of the intensities; a critical step in motion correction, since the intensities contain the information regarding physiological response. Therefore, it is important to ensure that the least amount of artifact is introduced into the data by the interpolation stage. Consequently, choice of interpolation method is significant and, for the reasons described in Section 3.5 of Chapter 3, simple methods such as nearest neighbor or trilinear are not optimal, as they introduce unwanted blurring (spatial autocorrelation) into the data.

In contrast, the interpolation used within the initial transformation-finding phase is not particularly critical, as usually the gross features such as brain/background boundaries principally determine the transformations. Since the existence of these features is robust to the amount of blurring introduced by interpolation, the transformation parameters found are not usually very sensitive to the interpolation method chosen.

There are many different potential choices for interpolation, as discussed in Chapter 3. This also includes methods such as the use of multiple shears applied in Fourier space,[2] which are only valid for the small rigid-body transformations typical of motion correction. However, at present there is no consensus as to which method is best.

One related implementational issue worth mentioning is how areas outside the image are treated. When estimating motion parameters, this "data" outside the image should be treated as nonexistent and not of zero intensity; otherwise, the estimated parameters will be biased. However, when the end slices are of interest (i.e., they contain brain) the final applied transformation will be sensitive to the choice of outside values used by the interpolation method. It is sensible in this circumstance to "pad" (to a small extent) with a copy of the end slice. If this is not done, the slightest out-of-slice motion (including any rotation) results in unnecessary loss of information in the end slices. With padding, this problem is substantially reduced.

8.2.3   Spin History and Stimulus-Correlated Motion

Even when "perfect" alignment of the images has taken place, some motion artifact still remains in the images.[4] This is because out-of-slice movement of the brain during a scan causes nuclei in a given slice to move away from their initial slice position, changing the relative timings between the RF excitations they receive. Such timing changes are significant as they depart from the stable saturation cycle of the nuclei when there is no motion. Therefore, the signal will be artifactually increased or decreased (depending on the direction of motion), displaying saturation-like effects similar to those seen in the first few images of a scanning sequence. This is known as the spin history effect.

In the presence of such motion, the measured signal contains motion-related effects that cannot be simply corrected by spatially transforming the image. This movement of nuclei outside the slice leads to loss (or gain) of signal in some regions, typically in the order of a few percent of the mean signal. Even though these signal changes are not large, the spin history artifacts can still impair the later statistical analysis, especially when the movement is related to the stimulus. In this case the artifact induced can have a significant correlation with the stimulus input, producing artifactual statistical parameter estimates which can be much higher or much lower than expected. Even if there is no significant correlation between these residual motion-related intensity variations and the stimulus, the spin history effects will add to the noise in the model fitting process, thus reducing the significance of possible activations.

One way to deal with these unwanted intensity variations is to remove all trends from the time series that have the same form as the voxel displacement (as measured during the transformation estimation stage in motion correction). This assumes that the spin history-related artifact will be proportional to some low-order polynomial function of the displacement of the voxel from its usual position. Removal of the trend is achieved with an initial decorrelation of the data using the displacement estimates, or carried out in the later statistical analysis by using these displacements as a confound (a parameter whose estimate is not used for calculating activation) in the general model fitting procedure.[1,3]

Note that for strongly stimulus-correlated motion, the removal of these trends can drastically reduce the amount of both true and false activation. At present there is no perfect general solution to this dilemma—without much more sophisticated modeling of the physical processes involved, it is not possible to clearly disambiguate between spin history-related effects and true activation, if the motion itself is correlated with the stimulation.

In Figures 8.1 and 8.2, examples are shown of significant activation clusters resulting when different motion correction methods are used. In each figure, the top row is the result when no motion correction is applied, the middle row when standard motion correction is applied, and the bottom row when motion correction is applied, along with spin-history correction, using the

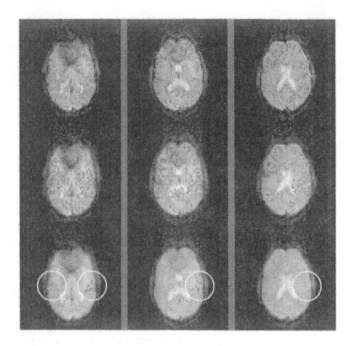

FIGURE 8.1
Significant auditory activation clusters ($Z > 2.3$, $P < 0.01$) with no motion correction (top row), standard motion correction (middle row), and motion correction with spin history correction (bottom row).

method described by Friston et al.[3] In all cases, statistical thresholding was carried out using the same significance threshold.

Figure 8.1 shows results derived from data taken during periods of auditory activation (a conversational radio program) interleaved with periods of "silence." Each row shows three consecutive slices from one of the original 3D fMRI brain images, overlaid with significant activation areas. The top row shows clear tell-tale signs of uncorrected motion around parts of the ventricles and little activation in the auditory cortex (this is the area shown as activated within the circles in the bottom row). The middle row shows the improvement in reported activation, but much "noise" remains—i.e., presumed activation well outside the auditory cortex. The bottom row shows that the spin history correction has completely removed this noise but has also greatly reduced the apparent amount of "true" activation.

Figure 8.2 shows two consecutive slices resulting from an fMRI experiment during which brief periods of painful heat were applied to the hand. There was much less overall head motion during the experiment than in the previous case; therefore there is less difference among the three sets of results. However, it is still possible (particularly within the marked circles) to see areas of activation

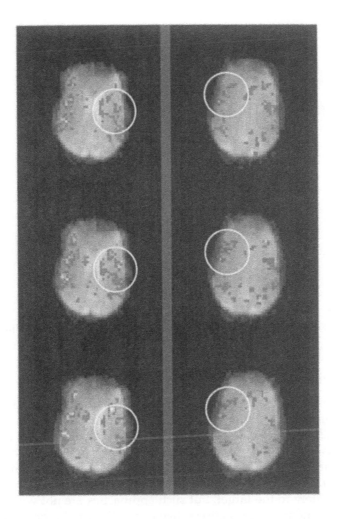

FIGURE 8.2
Significant painful heat activation clusters ($Z > 2.3$, $P < 0.01$) with no motion correction (top row), standard motion correction (middle row), and motion correction with spin history correction (bottom row). (Original data courtesy of R. Wise and I. Tracey.)

which have increased in size after basic motion correction and then decreased after motion correction with spin history correction. Figure 8.3 shows the clear correlation between the stimulation-derived model (regular peaks corresponding to time points when pain was applied) and the time series of estimated values for rotation about the x axis (thus mainly corresponding to "nodding" head movements). Given this correlation, it is to be expected that the bottom row would show less activation than the middle row, as explained above.

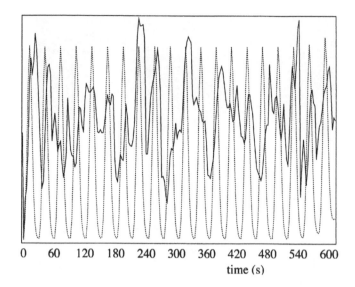

0   60   120   180   240   300   360   420   480   540   600

time (s)

FIGURE 8.3
Time series plots of stimulation model (dotted line, arbitrary units) against estimated rotation about the x axis (solid line, arbitrary units).

8.2.4   Nonrigid Motion Correction

Of course, head motion does not just occur between fMRI (multi-slice) images but also during their production, resulting in distortion of the ima-ges, as discussed in Chapter 5. Thus rigid-body motion correction is imperfect, although it is widely accepted, since the combination of the low resolution of the images and the relative speed of their capture makes the nonrigid component small. Some initial work has been undertaken[8] where each slice is registered separately to the target, but such approaches are not widely used at present. These nonrigid correction schemes are likely to become more viable as the resolution of fMRI images increases in the future.

A secondary point to note here is that if non-rigid-body motion correction is to be applied, then it is desirable to integrate the slice-timing correction (normally applied before motion correction) into this procedure. Thus, rigid-body motion, nonrigid distortions, and slice-timing effects could all be corrected at the same time.

8.3   Geometric Distortion

The acquisition of MR images is imperfect for a number of physical reasons. In particular, the magnetic field inside the head is usually inhomogeneous, even after careful shimming, and this results in geometric distortion of the image. The magnitude of distortion depends upon the parameters of the imaging

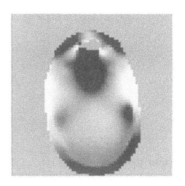

FIGURE 8.4
A field map showing typical static magnetic field variations inside the brain. Dark areas represent fields less than the external field, while bright areas represent fields higher than the external one. The total range corresponds to approximately ±0.5 ppm.

sequence used, where these parameters are chosen as a compromise between speed, contrast, and other factors. Unfortunately, EPI sequences, which are commonly used to acquire fMRI time series, are particularly susceptible to this form of geometric distortion. This is most notable near regions where there is a tissue/air interface, such as near the temporal lobes and the sinuses (see Figure 8.4).

Fortunately, a simple method is available which reduces this geometric distortion to low levels.[7] It involves acquiring a field map by appropriately combining additional images taken using different gradient echo weightings. That is, an image is produced that shows the strength of the deviation in magnetic field at each voxel. This field deviation is proportional to the amount of distortion, which principally occurs along the phase encode direction for EPI data. Therefore, by calculating the magnitude of the distortion, the image can be transformed by "warping" the distorted voxel positions to the nondistorted voxel positions.

It is also necessary to correct the intensity of unwarped voxels, as the original geometric distortion affects intensities: compressed regions get brighter and expanded regions get darker. By applying the concept of "conservation of intensity," an unwarped image can be intensity-corrected. However, there can also be a severe loss of signal associated with magnetic field inhomogeneities, due to local gradients causing spin dephasing; it is not a straightforward matter to recover this signal loss. The above considerations should ideally be taken into account when generating statistical inference during fMRI analysis, as the spatio-temporal noise structure of the images is affected by both the original distortion and the correction methods.

The resulting images then contain minimal distortion and can be better aligned with images taken with other, less distorting sequences (such as a T1-weighted structural image). Figure 8.5 shows an example of unwarping, using the field map shown in Figure 8.4; on the left is the original distorted image, and on the right is the corrected image. Note the large effect that the unwarping has on the frontal lobe. Using such geometric distortion correction, any later combination of fMRI statistics with either the same subject's high resolution scan or with other subjects' data will give more accurate results.

Before Unwarping   After Unwarping

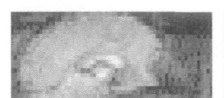 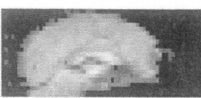

FIGURE 8.5
An example application of the unwarping transformation to remove geometric distortion.

Finally, there is the issue of interactions between head motion and geometric distortion—any head motion relative to the magnetic field will modulate the geometric distortions over time, relative to the head images. Thus, the perfect motion correction scheme would not only model rigid and nonrigid motion and slice-timing effects, but would also integrate geometric distortion modelling into the corrections.

8.4   Structural Registration

Once an activation map has been obtained, the next stage in fMRI analysis is to find out more about the nature of the activation, especially its spatial location. The activation map shares the same coordinate system as the motion-corrected raw functional images, but since these show a minimal amount of anatomical detail it is useful to register the raw functional image with another, more informative image.

Registration of the raw functional image to another image allows the information at corresponding physical locations to be compared, effectively combining the information contained in both. For instance, the location of an activation can be compared to the anatomy by registering the raw functional image to an anatomical scan of that individual. Similarly, the raw functional image can be registered to a standard template in order to assign common coordinates (such as those defined by Talairach and Tournoux[14]). Alternatively, the fMRI results from one subject can be registered to those of other subjects for multisubject statistical analysis. All of these applications will be discussed in the following sections.

8.4.1   Functional to Anatomical

The simplest application of registration for an activation map is to register it with an anatomical (structural) image of the same subject. This involves some or all of the following steps:

1. Preprocess one of the motion-corrected raw functional images, correcting for distortion (if not already done), removing bias field and/or nonbrain structures
2. Preprocess a structural image (of the same subject) to remove bias field and/or nonbrain structures
3. Register the raw functional image with the structural image
4. Apply the transformation found in the previous step to the activation image

Note that the raw functional image is registered to the structural image rather than the activation image itself. This is because the activation image only contains color "blobs" of activation (see Color Figure 8.6) which do not resemble a brain, so it is unsuitable for direct registration. However, since it shares the same coordinate system as the raw functional image, it can be transformed to the new coordinate system using the same transformation as estimated for the raw functional image.

This registration is intrasubject but intermodality. Therefore, a low DOF transformation (e.g., affine or affine plus restricted nonlinear registration, such as a few low frequency spatial basis functions) can normally be used, and is in fact desirable, since the resolution and contrast are poor in the EPI images, making them unsuitable for less restrained high DOF nonlinear registrations.

Figure 8.6 shows the results of an experiment in which both visual and auditory stimulation were applied. Because the two stimulation types were applied with different timings, statistical analysis can separate activation due to visual stimulation (red-yellow areas) from activation due to auditory stimulation (blue). The top row shows several consecutive slices from the original data with activation overlaid. This is the original resolution of the fMRI data. However, since the anatomical detail in the raw functional images is poor, it is useful to render the activation (resampled to high resolution after registration, as described above) onto the subject's high resolution structural image. This greatly assists in locating the precise anatomical regions of the activations, as shown in two example slices in the bottom row of the figure.

8.4.2 Functional to Standard Template

Another common application of registration in fMRI is the registering of activation images with a template in order to assign standard coordinates. This topic is treated in considerable detail in Chapter 14. These standard coordinates are particularly useful, as they allow the spatial locations of the activations to be reported and interpreted in a consistent, objective way. (An example of a standard coordinate system is the one proposed by

Talairach and Tournoux.[14]) Also, if a template coordinate system is associated with atlas information such as coordinate-dependent brain structure labels (e.g., "cerebellum") or functional labels (e.g., "visual area V1"), this allows automatic estimation of which brain areas have been activated. However, due to subject-subject variability and registration errors, this type of activation reporting is generally less safe than looking "by eye" at the combined activation and same-subject high resolution images, described in the previous section.

This type of registration is both an intersubject and intermodality problem. However, for fMRI, the problem can be broken down into three stages:

1. Register the raw functional image with the structural image (as above)
2. Register the structural image with the template
3. Combine the two transforms and apply to the original functional/ activation images

The reason for using a two-step registration with the structural image as the intermediary, rather than a one-step registration of the raw functional image directly to the template, is that functional images typically have poor anatomical detail, as the sequence is tuned to be fast and give good bold contrast. This, together with the fact that the raw functional images are usually low resolution, means that registrations with the template are often not very accurate, especially when large DOF transformations are used. However, when registering with the structural image of the same subject, a low DOF transformation is sufficient (usually 6 to 12 DOF), as the anatomy should be exactly the same (provided geometric scanning distortions are minimized). The structural image, which has higher resolution and better anatomical contrast, can then be registered to the template with a high DOF transformation (12 DOF or more). This allows a good match to be found despite the difference in anatomy between the individual and the template, since there is sufficient detail for the registration to utilize in the structural images.

Finally, the reason the two transforms are combined in the last step into a single transform (which takes functional data into template space) rather than applying two separate transforms is that any errors due to interpolation then occur only once rather than twice. This transformation is applied to statistical activation maps (which are originally in the same coordinate system as the functional image) so that they can be combined with structural information in standard (template) space; this allows the locations of activation sites to be reported in this standard space.

8.4.3 Group Analysis

To answer many questions about brain function, it is common to ask about activation in a group of subjects rather than in an individual. This may be in order to increase SNR, as the amount of data is increased, or, more likely, for the results to be more applicable to the population in general. In addition, it is common to use two different groups to contrast behavior, such as schizophrenics and healthy volunteers. In either case, combining results for a group analysis requires that the results from each individual be registered to a common space.

The standard image used for this registration can either be a selected member of the group, some group average, or a general template (like a Talairach-space template). Once this standard image is chosen, each of the individuals' structural images are registered to the standard, and then the activation results transformed into this space. All activation maps are then in the same coordinate system, and the locations, sizes, and statistical values of the activations can be compared across or between groups.

8.5 Conclusion

fMRI is a powerful, noninvasive imaging technique for investigating brain function. Registration plays a very important part in the analysis of fMRI experiments. First, it is used for correction of subject motion during the scanning sequence. This application is critical for avoiding detection of false, motion-related activations, which can be considerable even when the motion is subvoxel. Second, registration is used after statistical analysis to register the activation map to individual structural scans or standard spaces like Talairach space.

Since the raw functional images are tuned to be fast and give good BOLD contrast, they tend to have relatively low spatial resolution (compared to anatomical images) and poor anatomical contrast. Consequently, registration involving these images is an important and challenging task that has considerable scope for research into new methods as well as for improving and extending the existing methods.

References

1. E.T. Bullmore, M.J. Brammer, S. Rabe-Hesketh, V.A. Curtis, R.G. Morris, S.C.R. Williams, T. Sharma, and P.K. McGuire. Methods for diagnosis and treatment of stimulus-correlated motion in generic brain activation studies using fMRI. *Human Brain Mapping*, 7:38–48, 1999.
2. W.F. Eddy, M. Fitzgerald, and D.C. Noll. Improved image registration by using Fourier interpolation. *Magn. Resonance in Med.*, 36:923–931, 1996.
3. K.J. Friston, S.R. Williams, R. Howard, R.S.J. Frackowiak, and R. Turner. Movement-related effects in fMRI time-series. *Magn. Resonance in Med.*, 35:346–355, 1996.
4. J.V. Hajnal, R. Myers, A. Oatridge, J.E. Schwieso, I.R. Young, and G.M. Bydder. Artefacts due to stimulus correlated motion in functional imaging of the brain. *Magn. Resonance in Med.*, 31:283–291, 1994.

5. X. Hu, T.H. Le, T. Parrish, and P. Erhard. Restrospective estimation and correction of physiological fluctuation in functional MRI. *Magn. Resonance in Med.*, 34(2):201–212, 1995.

6. P. Jezzard. Physiological noise: strategies for correction. In C.T.W Moonen and P.A. Bandettini, Eds., *Functional MRI*. Springer-Verlag, Heidelberg, pp. 171–179, 1999.

7. P. Jezzard and R.S. Balaban. Correction for geometric distortion in echo planar images from B0 field variations. *Magn. Resonance in Med.*, 34:65–73, 1995.

8. B. Kim, J.L. Boes, P.H. Bland, T.L. Chenevert, and C.R. Meyer. Motion correction in fMRI via registration of individual slices into an anatomical volume. *Magn. Resonance in Med.*, 41:964–972, 1999.

9. K.K. Kwong, J.W. Belliveau, D.A. Chesler, I.E. Goldberg, R.M. Weisskoff, B.P. Poncelet, D.N. Kennedy, B.E. Hoppel, and M.S. Cohen. Dynamic magnetic resonance imaging of human brain activity during primary sensory stimulation. *Proc. Natl. Acad. Sci. USA*, 89(12):5675–9, 1992.

10. P. Mansfield. Multi-planar image formation using NMR spin echos. *J. of Physics C*, 10:L55–L58, 1977.

11. P.M. Matthews, P. Jezzard, and S.M. Smith, Eds. *Functional Magnetic Resonance Imaging of the Brian: Methods for Neuroscience*. Oxford University Press, 2001.

12. S. Ogawa, D.W. Tank, R. Menon, J.M. Ellermann, S.G. Kim, H. Merkle, and K. Ugurbil. Intrinsic signal changes accompanying sensory stimulation: functional brain mapping with magnetic resonance imaging. *Proc. Natl. Acad. Sci. USA*, 89(13):5951–5, 1992.

13. W.H. Press, S.A. Teukolsky, W.T. Vetterling, and B.P. Flannery. *Numerical Recipes in C*. Cambridge University Press, second edition, 1995.

14. J. Talairach and P. Tournoux. *Co-planar Stereotaxic Atlas of the Human Brain*. Thieme Medical Publisher Inc., New York, 1988.

9

Registration of MRI and PET Images for Clinical Applications

Uwe Pietrzyk*

CONTENTS

9.1 Introduction

Positron emission tomography (PET) and magnetic resonance imaging (MRI) are prominent examples of functional and morphological imaging modalities, respectively. The imaging concepts of PET and MRI are quite different, as are the images. MRI and PET are useful in conjunction precisely because they are complementary. While PET is able to provide information about a specific function

---

* Part of this work was done while the author was at the Max-Planck Institute of Neurological Research, Cologne, Germany.

such as cerebral blood flow or the density of a receptor in a certain area, MRI defines different structures or tissue types, and thus provides information about morphology and the topology of structures. Both imaging modalities are useful for clinical studies as well as for basic scientific investigations.

Once the respective images from PET and MRI have been realigned and registered, they can be fused for an integrated display, offering the opportunity to delineate function and morphology at the same time. In addition, enhanced display options can be applied to generate three-dimensionally rendered images, like the surface of the human cortex (extracted from the MR images) with activated sites (extracted from the PET images) superimposed.[1]

The clinical applications of PET-MRI registration will be discussed in this chapter with a focus on practical issues, such as methods and procedures for performing image registration with PET and MRI. Related subject matter is treated in a complementary manner in Chapter 11. The relevant question is which techniques and protocols have been shown to be applicable in a clinical setting with its specific requirements on robustness, practicability, and patient handling. While image registration has been an essential and, hence, accepted step in the analysis of multimodal brain images, especially for research purposes, only a relatively small number of publications deal with applications to other parts of the body. Limitations experienced during attempts to register nonbrain images will be outlined, as well as suggested procedures for harnessing the advantages of image registration to support the decision making process in a clinic before the start of therapy. Before images from PET and MRI are discussed in detail within the framework of image registration, the most important properties of the images from both modalities are summarized.

9.2   Properties of PET Images

Positron emission tomography employs the main features of tracer techniques developed to study the underlying mechanisms of physiological and biochemical processes in a living organism (see also Chapter 11). Labeling is obtained by exchanging one of the tracer molecule's atoms by its radioactive analogue. The radioactively labeled substance is injected intravenously and can be traced through the body using external detectors. In the case of PET, the tracer is labeled with an isotope that emits a positron. Such isotopes are available for a number of biologically relevant atoms, namely oxygen (as O-15, $t_{1/2}$ = 2.05 min), carbon (as C-11, $t_{1/2}$ = 20.4 min), and nitrogen (as N-13, $t_{1/2}$ = 10 min). In addition, fluorine (F-18, $t_{1/2}$ = 109.7 min) can be used to replace an OH-group in a molecule. Labeling with a radioactive nuclide allows the synthesis of specific tracers, which are used to determine, for example, cerebral blood flow or glucose consumption in the human brain. Hence, PET is representative of a functional imaging modality, and the primary interest in the development of PET was to quantify the three-dimensional distribution of the radioactive tracer with subsequent interpretation in a framework of physiological models.

The physical phenomenon underlying the positron emission limits the resolution of PET principally to 2 to 3 mm. During practical applications of PET imaging, the resolution is further reduced due to the limited detector size and the smoothing applied during image reconstruction. The latter is necessary to maintain sufficient signal and limit the influence of statistical noise. For further details the reader is referred to excellent reviews (see, for example, Eriksson et al.[2]) and to Chapter 5 of this book for a discussion on the influence of scanner errors.

Image registration most often relies on specific features detectable in the images, i.e., characteristic tracer uptake patterns in an organ or part of the human body. This is especially important when retrospective registration techniques are employed. PET images are stored with standard image orientation transverse to the patient's head-foot axis. A pixel represents a measurement of radioactivity concentration at a particular position inside the field of view (i.e., the volume covered by the detector system). These pixel values can be related to a physiological variable by means of an appropriate model. Usually, the radioactive tracer does not have a uniform distribution but shows a tracer-dependent-specific pattern with increased uptake, for instance, in the brain's gray matter compared to white matter, or in the heart compared to lung tissue. Different physiological processes in various organs can be investigated, such as the distribution of blood flow, oxygen utilization, protein synthesis, receptor binding, or glucose consumption. For patients with pathologies like tumors or areas of reduced perfusion due to infarction, these uptake patterns will deviate from those of normal subjects, a fact which is utilized to draw diagnoses. It must be pointed out, however, that pathologies like metastases may be missed in cases where they are not delineated from surrounding normal tissue due to similar activity concentration.[3]

From the first images produced with PET, it was obvious that PET images did not show details of anatomical structures with high resolution, if at all. This is even true for the brain when using ^{18}F-FDG (2-[^{18}F]-fluoro-2-deoxy-D-glucose) to determine the local glucose consumption. With FDG, PET images show patterns with considerable resemblance to the underlying structures known from anatomy as shown in Figure 9.1. This fact was also explored in creating a registered brain atlas based on PET and MR images.[4] There is pronounced uptake in gray matter structures compared to white matter. High uptake in the cortex, the prominent structure, with its typical irregular folding, marks the outline of the brain's surface and hence, with its easily recognizable substructures, establishes a collection of natural internal landmarks. Other important landmarks can also be identified in the central brain and correlated to anatomical structures. Similar observations can be made with tracers of cerebral blood flow.

The identification of distinct anatomical structures or landmarks can be much more difficult in cases when the tracer used during PET studies only exhibits focal uptake in a smaller part of the imaged volume. Figure 9.2 (top)

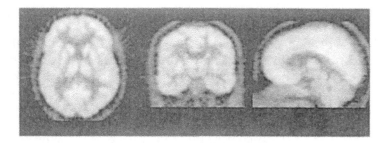

FIGURE 9.1
Example of PET-FDG brain images shown as transverse, coronal, and sagittal cuts. Although these are primarily functional tomograms, some anatomical structures are visible and this facilitates the application of automated and visual interactive registration techniques.

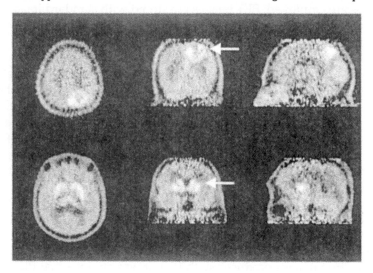

FIGURE 9.2
Example of C-11-Methionine (top) and F-18-DOPA (bottom) PET studies. Compared to Figure 9.1, much less anatomical detail is visible. These images are, however, extremely helpful for delineating pathologic areas caused by tumors (arrow, top row) or the evaluation of the dopaminergic system (arrow, bottom row). This type of image is a challenge for image registration algorithms, but can have high diagnostic utility.

shows such an example in which C-11-methionine was used to detect increased protein synthesis indicating areas where tumor tissue develops. Compared with the tumor region, C-11-methionine uptake in the remaining brain tissue is considerably lower. There are no clear outlines of the cortex or other structures as with FDG, rendering the identification of landmarks more difficult.

A similar situation is found using 6-[^{18}F]-fluoro-L-DOPA to study the pre-synaptic dopaminergic system. There is a clear concentration of the tracer accumulation in the center structures of the brain (i.e., striatum) as shown in Figure 9.2 (bottom), with some nonspecific binding of the tracer in the remaining brain tissue. Again, the outline of the outer brain surface is rather limited and not as distinct as with FDG. However, for many patients there is also tracer uptake in the skin, providing an important landmark which can be exploited during the registration process. Despite the limitations outlined above, techniques are available to cope with difficulties in correlating brain images from PET with those from MRI, as will be discussed.

For PET images from nonbrain regions (neck, thorax, heart, etc.) the task is even more complicated in regard to identification of anatomical structures. The most widely used tracer is FDG, since in oncological studies where tumors or metastases are searched for, this tracer yields the most valuable results. It has been shown, however, that reliability in tumor detection can be improved by image registration with CT or MRI.[5] The reason lies in the discriminative power between normal and pathological uptake, with clues coming from functional imaging with PET and anatomical confirmation from MRI that high PET tracer uptake in a particular structure should be interpreted as normal or pathologic. Color Figure 9.3* shows an example of a PET study with some focal uptake in the thorax. The precise localization cannot be deduced without anatomical correlation. There are further limitations in registration of PET and MR images from regions other than the brain, because the thorax or the abdomen cannot be regarded as rigid bodies. Special acquisition protocols that might help in these cases and other related issues are discussed below.

9.3 Properties of Magnetic Resonance Images

Magnetic Resonance Imaging (MRI) is a primary diagnostic tool for generating structural images of the living human body. In contrast to PET, it does not involve ionizing radiation but instead applies electromagnetic radiation with wavelength of approximately 0.3 m, hence with much lower energy than that used with x-ray computed tomography (CT) or emission tomography like PET. For obtaining tomograms, the nuclear magnetic resonance of the hydrogen nuclei (i.e., protons) is mainly used because of its intrinsic sensitivity combined with the fact that the human body is primarily composed of H_2O. Together these ensure a sufficiently strong signal. The key to MR imaging is the design of pulse sequences, which are applied in order to obtain images with desired contrast. A long list of contributions from many researchers[6] with ever more refined pulse sequences and detection techniques has led to faster image acquisition and reconstruction, providing high-resolution images of the brain or other parts of the body, with a wide variety of tissue contrasts.

An example of brain images of the same anatomy showing different contrast is given in Figure 9.4. Here the selection of appropriate echo time (TE) and repetition time (TR) changes the sequence's sensitivity to tissue properties such as T1 and T2 relaxation times, producing a differentiation among cerebral gray matter, white matter, and cerebral spinal fluid (CSF), respectively.

---

* Color Figures follow page 22.

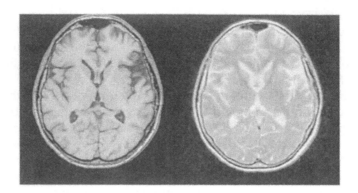

FIGURE 9.4
Example of T1 (left) and T2 (right) weighted MR images. There is an obvious difference in the contrast between these images. The left image is preferred for image registration since it shows more anatomical detail and hence establishes the basis for functional-anatomical correlation.

The first image in Figure 9.4 is T1-weighted and shows a high resemblance to a histological section and, therefore, is the first choice to obtain images with predominantly anatomical information. T2-weighted images (the second image in Figure 9.4), however, are preferred in order to detect subtle pathologies because they exhibit changes in intensity in abnormal tissues, especially in brain images. In nonbrain imaging, many pathologies are detected because of their abnormal intensity pattern or deviation from normal anatomy. In contrast to PET imaging, MRI monitors tumors by size and structural changes rather than by metabolic activity.[3]

With modern magnetic resonance imaging systems, multiple planes at arbitrary orientations can be acquired (transverse, coronal, sagittal, and oblique orientation), permitting an optimal positioning of slices relative to a particular organ or region of the body. This feature is not available with most of the other imaging techniques like PET or CT, whose primary images come in transverse orientation. Other orientations are available only by means of interpolation and reslicing of the primary images. Another predominant feature of MR images is their much higher resolution compared with PET images. This allows highly detailed morphological information to be obtained.

9.4 Problems and Solutions in MRI-PET Registration

9.4.1 General Considerations for Accurate Registration of MR and PET Images

In order to successfully perform MRI-PET registration, some specific features of each modality should be borne in mind, since a number of requirements for successful image registration procedures have to be considered. These include, among others, good image quality (resolution, contrast, no artifacts) with fields of view providing sufficient coverage of the relevant part of the body in both image sets. MR images are usually reconstructed to 256 × 256 pixel matrices with pixel size of 1 mm or less and with variable slice thickness between 1 and 10 mm, depending on the organ of investigation. Often matrices of 512 × 512 pixels are available. In addition, the image resolution (1 mm or less) which is primarily not hardware-dependent, may be optimized for a specific task by selecting the most appropriate pulse sequence. For clinical purposes often only a rather limited number of slices is acquired, so that the total measurement time is kept short, partly with the aim of avoiding the risk of motion artifacts. In these cases the slice thickness is chosen to be 4 to 6 mm for brain studies and 4 to 8 mm for nonbrain studies. The volume effectively covered by all images can be adjusted by varying the slice thickness or number of slices acquired. Also, the image orientation can be selected by the operator and adapted to obtain the best imaging result. Transverse, coronal, sagittal, and even oblique slices can be obtained. For brain studies, transverse orientation is often preferred, whereas for the thorax mostly coronal images are acquired.

Most of these properties are quite different in PET imaging: PET images are typically reconstructed into matrices with 128 × 128 pixels of size of 2 to 4 mm or even greater, with resolution of 4 to 8 mm, depending on the type of scanner. The slice thickness and number of slices are generally defined by the hardware. Also, the primary image orientation is restricted to transverse slices. The axial field of view of modern PET scanners is rather limited (16 to 25 cm), and so most of the systems offer the option to acquire a series of scans, each at a different offset of the patient bed relative to the scanner gantry. Studies with multiple bed positions thus provide image sets that may even cover the whole body, but are frequently limited to only 3 to 5 sequential positions covering up to 80 cm of the body.

The fact that PET and MR images contain different information and have different resolution, representation, and orientation complicates their comparison and interpretation. If accurate spatial registration is to be performed, pixel size and interslice distance have to be precisely known prior to starting the registration process. (It should be noted that a large pixel size leads to images prone to higher partial volume effect, i.e., averaging of signal intensities across a larger volume, leading to images with lower contrast.) It may also be necessary to correct possible geometrical distortions introduced by the imaging devices as described in Chapter 5. Another prerequisite is that the primary orientation of the images should be similar. Consider the case of coronal MR images with good in-plane resolution (pixel size 0.5 mm) but with a large slice thickness (6 mm). MR images with these properties are certainly more difficult to register to PET images, which have nearly isotropic resolution of 4 to 5 mm, than using a volumetric MR image set of 1 mm pixel size in all dimensions, or transverse images instead of coronal. Since the registration procedure usually involves reslicing of an image set by interpolation, the quality of the original coronal MR images would certainly be degraded, which might cause problems for certain image registration algorithms or for sufficient accuracy of the registration.

There also has to be sufficient commonality in the parts of the body or organ covered by the field of view of both modalities. Sometimes image sets have to be reformatted to obtain the most appropriate range of both image sets. This might, for instance, be the case when registering a multiple bed PET study covering the whole thorax with an MR image set which covers only a certain fraction of the PET volume. In brain imaging there might be excess slices acquired with MRI containing part of the neck, which is not covered with PET.

Artifacts due to unintentional patient movement cause one of the most severe problems in registration of PET and MR images. The signatures of motion artifacts are different for PET and MRI. In PET, patient movement between different steps of an acquisition protocol might, in the worst case, corrupt the images completely. Also, certain corrective steps like the correction for photon absorption based on a separate measurement, but assuming identical patient positioning, might no longer be feasible (see also Chapter 5). Patient movement of a lesser degree will cause a loss in contrast and resolution of smaller areas with enhanced intensity amplitudes of the activity distribution. A solution to this problem often applied is the splitting of the acquisition into smaller time frames, with subsequent registration and summation of individual frames and exclusion of frames where motion is evident.

The situation with motion artifacts in MR imaging is different, as it depends on the pulse sequence as to which artifacts are visible and what effect they might have. If slices are acquired sequentially, as in certain rapid imaging sequences, and the subject moves during imaging, the spatial relationship between the individual slices will be lost and the data cannot be regarded as a complete regular volume anymore. With fast, true 3D gradient echo sequences that sample a whole volume, any motion during the acquisition will tend to produce artifacts throughout the image volume, which may make the image unusable for registration. One of the pertinent motion artifacts, occurring frequently during thorax scans, is blurring and motion-induced "ghosting" caused by respiratory motion of the chest. Many MR acquisition and postprocessing techniques have been proposed to deal with the motion problem, but motion artifact remains an important source of error in the many clinical images. Therefore, one of the main efforts in designing new sequences is to achieve fast and short acquisitions covering the whole volume to be imaged.

In a clinical setting one often has to deal with a small number of slices arising from the fact that the scanning time cannot be easily prolonged without the risk of motion artifacts. This results in a tradeoff between a lower number of slices, (i.e., coarser sampling of the volume) and less motion artifacts, or very high sampling density with many slices but the risk of motion artifacts. Under clinical conditions the intention is to assure detection and precise localization of pathologies, rather than providing high-resolution morphological imaging with a large number of thin slices.

9.4.2 Techniques and Procedures Used in Clinical Applications

During the course of developing solutions to the problem of image registration many techniques have been presented, some of which are suitable for application only in very specific situations, i.e., connected to specific hardware, implemented in an exotic computing environment, or requiring very high performance computer systems. Hence, not all techniques developed to register medical images are currently optimal for usage in a clinical setting. If image registration is to be applied on a routine basis during the diagnostic decision-making process, the techniques employed have to be robust against imaging artifacts, reliable, fast, easy to use, and at least partly automated, i.e., avoiding too much user interaction and with little or no preprocessing. As will be discussed later, the technique to be chosen depends on the specific application. The main distinction concerning the techniques applied in a clinically oriented environment is again between handling brain and extracranial images. Furthermore, it is the specific application that defines the demand on precision and accuracy. For example, radiation therapy planning requires different methods than neuroscience research and development applications. Other aspects of presurgical diagnostics need a much higher accuracy than image correlation in the thorax would reasonably ask for. The former application requires an accuracy of about 1 mm or less. Based on the results from the registration step, a stereotactic intervention (the placing of a radioactive implant) is performed or the site and path of a biopsy needle is defined. A failure to accurately register the respective studies could cause unwanted damage of healthy tissue or vascular structures. In the thorax, the circumstances of image acquisition in separate scanners, using different patient beds with a different shape, and the risk of respiratory artifacts make it much more difficult to achieve an accuracy of 1 mm or less.

From a clinical point of view the techniques useful for MRI-PET registration can be classified into two main groups.[7] Some of these have been applied also to work with other types of tomographic modalities, whereas other registration techniques are dedicated developments for the registration of PET to MRI. The intention of most of these developments has been to register brain images. Unless otherwise stated, the following explanations will assume these types of images.

The first group of registration techniques represents prospective procedures designed with the intention of performing both studies (PET and MRI) following a strict dedicated protocol. An example is the application of a stereotactic head frame[8] prepared with appropriate markers visible in both modalities, and designed from materials like wood, in order to be applicable for both PET and MRI. A variety of head holders or face masks have been considered to establish a common coordinate system for both studies (e.g., Bettinardi et al.[9]). These prospective techniques focus mainly on brain imaging, although there have also been attempts to develop similar utilities for nonbrain imaging. However, these approaches tend to be demanding on both subject and operator. Depending on the patient, a face mask might not be well tolerated. Since face masks are mounted externally to the patient's head and skin, the exact placement of the devices during the imaging session has to be carefully maintained, because subsequent processing is likely to assume a fixed relationship of the marker positions with respect to the patient's head or brain. This can be problematic to achieve.

An advantage of using external markers with PET is that the markers are directly visible and so do not depend on the activity distribution of a particular tracer. As pointed out previously, PET images may display abnormal focal uptake with major anatomical landmarks much less pronounced. However, external markers can introduce imaging artifacts in the reconstruction, especially with filtered backprojection, if they have a relatively high radioactivity concentration compared to the activity of the normal tissue.

The application of external marker devices in MRI may be hampered by the fact that these devices could interfere with the standard head coils necessary for imaging. In addition, external markers are usually placed some distance from the head, where possible distortions might be largest. In any case, the position of the markers has to be accurately deduced from the images, requiring strict compliance with the imaging protocol to be adopted. The field of view must be large enough for the markers to be included in both scans, and the images must have sufficient sampling in all three dimensions to accurately locate the markers. This might be in conflict with the standard protocols, especially with MRI, when the slice thickness is usually preset to a larger value (4 to 6 mm) for practical reasons. Registration algorithms based on point markers are further discussed in Chapter 3, Section 3.4.1 and Chapter 6.

The second group of registration algorithms encompasses a variety of post-acquisition techniques with less stringent requirements in patient handling. These retrospective techniques, in general, rely solely on the information content within the images, with each pixel representing an intensity value or a physiological parameter at each particular location inside the image volume. Although both measurements (with PET and MRI) are performed independently (i.e., no special hardware enforces identical patient positioning), it is advisable to design the acquisition protocol appropriately in order to ease the subsequent registration step. This includes the proper selection of primary image orientation, pixel size, and slice thickness, whenever this is at the operator's discretion (see also Section 9.4.1 for further details).

Two subgroups of retrospective algorithms can be identified. One comprises techniques which perform the registration in an automated manner with the optimization step to find the best transformation based on similarity measures described in the literature (see Studholme et al.[10] for a recent review and discussion, and Chapters 2 and 3). Utilizing a similarity measure assumes that the images to be registered bear sufficient similarity to each other. A similarity can be based on a wide variety of properties, which need not be linearly correlated. Gray matter structures with medium intensity values on T1-weighted MR images are bound to correlate with areas of higher uptake in FDG PET images, while white matter structures (with higher intensity values on this type of MRI) correlate with relatively lower values in the PET images. This relation does not hold any longer when other tracers with a different uptake pattern are used, or when the MR pulse sequence is altered. Hence, the similarity measure has to be very robust but still sophisticated enough to cope with this problem, i.e., detect similarity without making strict assumptions about the intensity distribution in the two modalities. Other approaches explore geometrical features, such as outlines of surfaces of the head or the brain, and minimize the distance between contours extracted from the two types of image.[11] To do this, the images should allow a precise definition of surfaces; this may not be possible for certain types of images which do not allow a clear structural definition.

The alternative subgroup encompasses interactive techniques which incorporate the selection of multiple internal landmarks, the interactive definition of contours, or a combination of both.[12] Similar prerequisites regarding image orientation, image quality, etc. apply for interactive techniques as for automated registration methods. Landmark-based techniques assume the ability to define intrinsic landmarks in both image sets to be registered. Again, the situation tends to be more difficult for PET images with tracers other than FDG. As shown in Figure 9.2, images of these types pose a challenge to the operator, with the task of unambiguously identifying landmarks. When suitable features can be identified, techniques utilizing overlay and exchange of contours have been shown to be very robust for detecting even subtle misregistrations. During interactive registration the operator will use visual criteria like matching of contours around morphological structures. Multiple simultaneously controlled cursors can be applied in three dimensions to check proper alignment of isolated intrinsic landmarks. Color Figure 9.5* shows an example of a typical display used during interactive registration. Figure 9.5a displays the initial state with unregistered studies and Color Figure 9.5b shows the result after registration has been completed. It also provides an impression of what can be achieved with image registration and what forms the basis for further image analysis.

The advantage of interactive techniques is that they are widely applicable in various situations combining imaging modalities of different types and with arbitrary combinations. Also, they are not restricted to brain images, but can be applied to whole-body studies as well. Hybrid procedures are also available which draw on the strengths of both automated and interactive techniques.[13]

9.5 Discussion of Applications in a Clinical Setting

9.5.1 Introductory Remarks; Definitions

Image registration of PET and MRI is feasible and provides important additional information often not available from a single modality alone. To date, most applications have taken place under research protocols. There is, however, also

---

* Color Figures follow page 22.

an emerging trend towards accepting image registration for clinical conditions. In the scientific literature there exist different approaches both to combining images and to the interpretation of what is technically satisfactory. Therefore some preliminary definitions are required.

The terms *combination* and *correlation* of images are often used in the sense that the images have entered a combined analysis. This could mean that both studies were simply available either on radiological film or digitally on a computer network, but were not manipulated by any computer program. The physician mentally has to fuse the images and draw conclusions based on the visual interpretation of the signals evident in the images. The terms *registration, matching, alignment,* and (sometimes) *fusion* are generally used to signify that data sets were processed to obtain images that correspond spatially, i.e., on a pixel-by-pixel basis. Technically, this is most frequently solved by applying computerized algorithms and, thus, it requires the images to be readily available in digital form. Once the images are aligned, they can be fused into a single display by various techniques (overlay, checkerboard fusion, etc. — see Chapter 4).

9.5.2   Registration of PET and MR Images of the Brain

To date PET-MR image registration has been used mostly for brain images. Because of the lack of anatomical details in the images provided by the early PET systems, which had very poor spatial resolution, any aid from morphological images in defining the underlying anatomy was welcome. Image registration has entered clinical application in quite specialized areas such as presurgical workup of brain tumors, in computerized treatment planning for biopsies, open surgery, or radiation therapy, and in follow-up studies after surgery or treatment. Although not performed for strict clinical purposes, mapping of human brain function as visualized by O-15-water PET definitely required registration of PET and MR images. In fact, such activation studies may be part of the presurgical diagnosis of a patient with a tumor, for instance, in the neighborhood of areas responsible for language generation.[14] Figure 9.6 shows an example for MRI-PET registration employing a combination of retrospective techniques (interactive and automated).

9.5.3   Registration of Extracranial PET and MR Images

While the task of defining an accurate and robust protocol for registration of brain images appears relatively straightforward, the situation for other images seems to be more difficult. Usually a rigid-body transformation is the simplest approach, but certainly not the best and most accurate for body images, where exact repositioning of patients in the respective scanners is limited and motion caused by the heart cycle and by breathing may complicate the application of algorithms successfully introduced for brain images. Yet, it has been frequently noted in the literature that combining the signals from both PET and MRI may improve the interpretation of the findings and increase sensitivity and specificity in comparison to analyzing the images

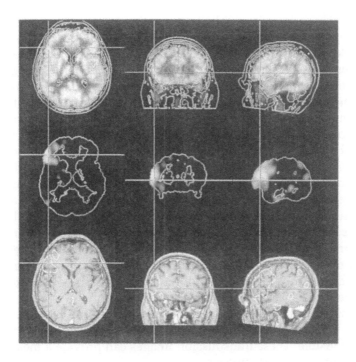

FIGURE 9.6
Result from MRI-PET registration employing automated and interactive techniques. Top row: PET-FDG study with overlaid contours derived from MRI (bottom) after interactive realignment. Middle row: result from a O-15-water PET activation study shown within the contours of the PET-FDG study after automated registration via similarity measures. Bottom row: MRI study with overlaid contours derived from activation study after interactive registration via mean image from activation study.

of both modalities independently.[5] Typical examples in which different levels of technical effort have been employed for comparing images are listed below, classified according to the definitions outlined in Section 9.5.1.

Basic combination or correlation has been performed by Braams et al.,[3] Laubenbacher et al.[15] and Jabour et al.[16] for extracranial head and neck carcinomas. The authors pointed out the definite advantage in staging the tumors although no full spatial registration was performed. In spite of the unavailability of full integration and fusion, simple visual comparison was found to be of benefit for patient treatment. Ratib et al.[17] focused on cardiac images. They did not perform exact registration, but argued that the generation of standard views based on planes oriented according to the cardiac geometry can provide a practical means to compare the images with reasonable accuracy.

Only a few groups have dealt with the problem of exact registration, (i.e., precise computerized positional matching) of PET and MRI extracranial images. Compared to neurological imaging of the brain, the exact registration of cardiac images is hampered because the heart is a nonrigid moving organ. Possible procedures for multimodal cardiac imaging have been reviewed by Gilardi et al.,[18] among them a protocol suggested by Sinha et al.,[19] who performed PET and

MRI registration of gated images by transforming to reference images acquired in the same temporal phase. They employed a surface- fitting iterative technique developed by Pelizzari et al.[11] Nekolla et al.[20] also based their registration technique on the heart surface extracted from both PET and MR images.

Other protocols for registering images from head and neck,[21,22] breast, and parts of the abdomen[23] employ interactive point-based registration techniques,[21] multiple interactive steps supported by reference to the normal tracer distribution of FDG,[22] or have relied on external and internal landmarks. Wahl et al.[23] used reconstructed transmission images from the PET examination (see Chapters 5 and 11) in the registration procedure. Indeed, Kuhl et al. had already pointed out the usefulness of transmission images for the interpretation of emission images in 1966.[24] Transmission data are routinely acquired in order to correct for photon absorption. The absorption coefficients can be reconstructed into images which resemble low-resolution x-ray CT images. Despite the relatively low resolution and the reduced sensitivity of the 511 keV photons to small variations in tissue type and density, the images show a clear body outline and gross anatomical details, especially in the thorax. They can provide the physician with enough details to help him orient the emission images obtained in the same examination, even when only a few spots with high tracer uptake scattered across the imaged volume are visible. These transmission images can provide a means to ease registration of whole body images.

Recently, Pietrzyk et al.[25] used transmission images during 3D rendering processes when no complementary morphological imaging in an appropriate orientation was available. A limitation in the combined analysis of PET emission and MR images is the absence of a body outline on most PET images. This may be overcome by including transmission images in the analysis. Figure 9.7 shows an example of such an application for images from the head and neck region, and Color Figure 9.8* shows an example in the thorax.

A further complication in combining PET and MR images is differences in the shape of the patient bed and positioning. This is not a problem for brain imaging, but is a major limitation in body imaging, where different bed shapes can lead to different positioning of the patient's spine. Also, organs under study do not remain in the same position with respect to each other once the patient has left the scanning bed or has to be moved to another imaging modality. This is demonstrated in Figure 9.7 and Color Figure 9.8. In each of these examples the range covered by the two imaging modalities is different, that of the MRI being considerably smaller. Also, as shown in Figure 9.7, the positioning of the neck may be different in the two devices, leaving the registration with some remaining systematic uncertainty. It has been recently shown by Theissen et al.[26] that a carefully designed clinical protocol can lead to successfully registered PET and MR images even in the case of extracranial images. Special care has been taken to assure identical positioning of arms in both modalities. This assumes that

---

* Color Figures follow page 22.

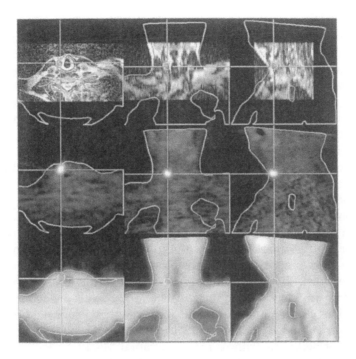

FIGURE 9.7
Images from a head and neck study of a patient with thyroid cancer. MR images acquired in the transverse plane (top), PET emission images (middle), and PET transmission images (bottom). In each row contours obtained from the PET transmission images are used as an overlay to guide the registration process. No external markers were used. There is an obvious difficulty in the fact that the range covered by the MRI is much less than that covered by the PET images. Also, the differences in positioning of the neck during the two respective studies in different devices introduce a systematic uncertainty. (Data: courtesy of Drs. Eschner, Scheidhauer, and Theissen, Nuclear Medicine, University of Cologne).

the desire to register the data from PET and MRI was known prior to both scans, which is not always the case. The actual registration was performed in an interactive fashion based on the registration of PET transmission with MR images, which were obtained as transverse slices, with subsequent image fusion of PET emission and MR images.

9.6 Conclusions

Registration of MR and PET images was one of the earliest applications of medical image registration; registration of brain images has proven to be a valuable method to enhance the diagnostic value of PET and MRI through combined analysis. This is because MR images provide detailed information about anatomical structures, and PET measures physiological parameters like glucose consumption or cerebral blood flow. Image registration has already entered clinical protocols to support radiation therapy or special surgical interventions with complementary PET/MRI information. With interactive registration techniques and automated methods based on appropriate algorithms, even PET images obtained with special tracers like [^{11}C]-methionine, which contain little anatomical detail, can be combined with MRI for clinical diagnosis or treatment planning. There are, however, many potential difficulties in the registration of MR and PET brain images, and this chapter has emphasized the importance of careful image acquisition as well as the use of a suitable algorithm for aligning the images.

For extracranial studies, exact registration is frequently hampered by the fact that many current algorithms employ rigid-body transformations, which can fail when organs move between measurements or because of cardiac or respiratory motion. However, registration of clinically acceptable accuracy seems feasible when restricted to a relatively small coverage of the body, like thorax studies. For head and neck studies, with careful positioning in both modalities, registration looks promising. PET transmission imaging has an interesting role as a link between PET emission and MR images. Little effort is involved in obtaining transmission images, since their information is needed for attenuation correction of the emission images. Recent progress in nonrigid registration algorithms, as discussed in Chapters 13 through 15 of this book, may lead to the availability of better algorithms for extracranial MR-PET registration. Such progress in combination with increasing availability of both PET and MRI in clinical settings is likely to lead to widespread application of medical image registration as a vital link in maximizing the diagnostic value of these complementary modalities in the future. In the scientific realm, the improvements in sensitivity and resolution that have been achieved for PET imaging have led to widespread use of image registration as a core component in fusing functional and anatomical data in single subjects. This increases study power by explicitly accommodating individual anatomical variability directly in functional studies.

Increasing availability and reductions in costs of the computing facilities required for image registration are also helping to stimulate more extensive use of the technique. A critical issue in all clinical applications is the validation of proposed techniques and a clear demonstration of their utility, efficiency, and cost effectiveness. The past two decades have seen extensive development of and experimentation with candidate methods and applications. The next phase of development is likely to include commercialization of standard packages and larger scale studies to provide the evidence necessary for their adoption in clinical practice.

Acknowledgments

The author is indebted for many helpful discussions with A. Thiel, M.D., Professor K. Herholz, M.D., W. Eschner, Ph.D., K. Scheidhauer, M.D., P. Theissen, M.D., F. Maes, Ph.D., Professor R. Chisin, M.D., and to H. Herzog, Ph.D., for carefully reading of this manuscript.

References

1. Toga, A.W., Ed., *Three-Dimensional Neuroimaging*, Raven Press, New York, 1990.
2. Eriksson, L., Dahlbom, M., and Widen, L., Positron emission tomography—a new technique for studies of the central nervous system, *J. Microscopy*, 1990, 157: 305–333.
3. Braams, J.W., Pruim, J., Freling, J.M., Nikkels, P.G.J., Roodenburg, J.L.N., Boering, G., Vaalburg, W., and Vermey, A., Detection of lymph node metastases of squamous cell cancer of the head and neck with FDG-PET and MRI, *J. Nucl. Med.*, 1995; 36:211–216.
4. Schifter, T., Turkington, T.G., Berlangieri, S.U., Hoffman, J.M., MacFall, A.R., Pelizzari, C.A., Tien, R.D., and Coleman, R.E., Normal brain F-18 FDG-PET and MRI anatomy, *Clin. Nucl. Med.*, 1993; 18:578–582.
5. Sailer, S.L., Rosenman, J.G., Soltys, M., Cullip, T.J., and Chen, J., Improving treatment planning accuracy through multimodality imaging, *Int. J. Radiation Oncology*, 1996; 35:117–124.
6. Elster, A.D., Gradient-echo MR imaging: techniques and acronyms, *Radiology*, 1993; 186:1–8.
7. Pietrzyk, U., Herholz, K., Schuster, A., von Stockhausen, H.-M., Lucht, H., and Heiss, W.-D., Clinical applications of registration and fusion of multimodality brain images from PET, SPECT, CT and MRI, *Eur. J. Radiol.*, 1996; 21:174–182.
8. Schad, L.R., Boesecke, R., Schlegel, W., Hartmann, G.H., Sturm, V., Strauss, L.G., and Lorenz, W.J., Three dimensional image correlation of CT, MR, and PET studies in radiotherapy treatment planning of brain tumours, *J. Compu. Assis. Tomogr.*, 1987; 11:948–954.
9. Bettinardi, V., Scardaoni, R., Gilardi, M.C., Rizzo, G., Perani, D., Paulesu, E., Striano, G., Triulzi, F., and Fazio, F., Head holder for PET, CT and MR studies, *J. Compu. Assist. Tomog.*, 1991; 15:886–892.
10. Studholme, C., Hill, D.L.G., and Hawkes, D.J., Automated three-dimensional registration of magnetic resonance and positron emission tomography brain images by multiresolution optimization of voxel similarity measures, *Med. Physics*, 1997; 24:25–35.
11. Pelizzari, C.A., Chen, G.T.Y., Spelbring, D.R., Weichselbaum, R.R., and Chen, C.-T., Accurate three-dimensional registration of CT, PET, and/or MR images of the brain, *J. Compu. Assist. Tomogr.*, 1989; 13:20–26.
12. Pietrzyk, U., Herholz, K., Fink, G., Jacobs, A., Mielke, R., Slansky, I., Würker, M., and Heiss, W.-D., An interactive technique for three-dimensional image registration: validation for PET, SPECT, MRI, and CT brain images, *J. Nucl. Med.*, 1994; 35:2011–2018.
13. Pietrzyk, U., Thiel, A., Herholz, K., and Heiss, W.-D., A hybrid image registration method employing interactive and automated techniques, *NeuroImage*, 1998; 7: S789.
14. Thiel, A., Herholz, K., von Stockhausen, H.-M., van Leyen-Pilgram, K., Pietrzyk, U., Kessler, J., Wienhard, K., Klug, N., and Heiss, W.-D., Localization of language-related cortex with O-15-labeled water PET in patients with gliomas, *NeuroImage*, 1998; 7:284–295.
15. Laubenbacher, C., Saumweber, D., Wagner-Manslau, C., Kau, R.J., Herz, M., Avril, N., Ziegler, S., Kruschke, C., Arnold, W., and Schwaiger, M., Comparison of Fluorine-18-Fluorodeoxyglucose PET, MRI and endoscopy for staging head and neck squamous-cell carcinomas, *J. Nucl. Med.*, 1995; 36:1747–1757.

16. Jabour, B.A., Choi, Y., Hoh, C.K. Rege, S.D., Soong, J.C., Lufkin, R.B., Hanafee, W.N., Maddahi, J., Chaiken, L., Bailet, J., Phelps, M.E., Hawkins, R.A. and Abemeyor, E., Extracranial head and neck: PET imaging with 2-[F-18]Fluoro-2-Deoxy-D-Glucose and MR imaging correlation, *Radiology*, 1993; 186:27–35.

17. Ratib, O., Didier, D., Chatelain, P., Righetti, A., Lerch, R., and Townsend, D., Standard views in cardiac multimodality tomographic imaging, *Am. J. Cardiac Imaging*, 1995; 9:67–76.

18. Gilardi, M.C, Rizzo, G., Savi, A., and Fazio, F., Registration of multi-modal biomedical images of the heart, *Q. J. Nucl. Med.*, 1996; 40:142–150.

19. Sinha, S., Sinha, U., Czernin, J., Porenta, G., and Schelbert, H.R., Noninvasive assessment of myocardial perfusion and metabolism: feasibility of registering gated MR and PET images, *Am. J. Roentgenol.*, 1995; 164:301–307.

20. Nekolla, S., Schricke, U., Roder, F., and Schwaiger, M., Multitracer and multimodal coregistration and fusion in static and gated cardiac studies, *J. Nucl. Med.*, 1998; 39:145.

21. Wong, W.-L., Hussain, K., Chevretton, E., Hawkes, D.J., Baddeley, H., Maisey, M., and McGurk, M., Validation and clinical application of computer-combined computed tomography and positron emission tomography with 2-[18F]Fluoro-2-Deoxy-D-glucose head and neck images, *Am. J. Surg.*, 1996; 172:628–632.

22. Uematsu, H., Sadato, N., Yonekura, Y., Tschuchida, T., Nakamura, S., Sugimoto, K., Waki, A., Yamamoto, K., Hayashi, N, and Ishii, Y., Coregistration of FDG PET and MRI of the head and neck using normal distribution of FDG, *J. Nucl. Med.*, 1998; 39:2121–2127.

23. Wahl, R.L., Quint, L.E., Cieslak, R.D., Aisen, Al.M., Koeppe, R.A., and Meyer, C.R., "Anatometaboli" tumour imaging: fusion of FDG PET with CT or MRI to localize foci of increased activity, *J. Nucl. Med.*, 1993; 34:1190–1197.

24. Kuhl, D.E., Hale, J., and Eaton, W.L., Transmission scanning: a useful adjunct to conventional emission scanning for accurately keying isotope deposition to radiographic anatomy, *Radiology*, 1966; 87:278–284.

25. Pietrzyk, U., Scheidhauer, K., Scharl, A., Schuster, A., and Schicha, H., Presurgical visualization of primary breast carcinoma with PET emission and transmission imaging, *J. Nucl. Med.*, 1995; 36:1882–1884.

26. Theissen, P., Pietrzyk, U., Dietlein, M., and Schicha, H., Image fusion between PET and MRI examinations of chest, abdomen, and pelvis. *Eur. J. Nucl. Med.*, 2000; 27:S101.

10

Registration of MR and CT Images for Clinical Applications

Derek L.G. Hill and Jozef Jarosz

CONTENTS

10.1 Introduction

During the 1980s, the tomographic imaging modalities of magnetic resonance (MR) imaging and x-ray computed tomography (CT) entered widespread clinical use, especially for imaging the brain. These two modalities are based on very different physical principles, and the images they produce have different properties. MR imaging generates images showing the distribution of protons in mobile molecules (water and fat), with the contrast between structures in the images determined by the visible proton density and the relaxation times of excited spins in the tissues and, in some cases, also by flow, diffusion, and other parameters. X-ray CT provides a map of x-ray attenuation within the body.

MR and CT scanners both produce images of anatomical structure, but the images they generate look quite different. One of the most striking differences is that cortical bone has high x-ray attenuation, so is bright in CT, whereas cortical bone contains virtually no MR visible protons, so is black in MR. MR images also tend to have better soft tissue contrast than CT. When imaging the brain, for example, MR images tend to have much higher contrast between gray matter, white matter, and cerebrospinal fluid (CSF) than do CT images. This contrast in the MR image can be manipulated in many ways by changing the timing and strength of the various radiofrequency and gradient pulses.

Although there have always been arguments for the inherent superiority of one or the other of these modalities, it has been the case for many years that both are considered essential in a well equipped modern hospital, because the information they provide is complementary. As a result, patients are frequently imaged with both for the purpose of diagnosis, or during the workup for treatment. The complementary nature of MR and CT images and the regular use of both modalities to acquire images from the same patient resulted in the combination of MR and CT images as one of the first applications of medical image registration.[1-3] All the early applications of MR-CT registration were within the head, and this remains the predominant application. Early registration methods required considerable user interaction, but MR and CT images of the head can now be registered automatically in a matter of seconds or minutes.

In this chapter, the technical issues associated with acquiring MR and CT images for registration are described, and clinical applications in which registration has been shown to have benefit are discussed. The majority of this chapter relates to registration of MR and CT images of the head, with other applications described in Section 10.3.4.

10.2 Technical Issues

10.2.1 Image Acquisition

10.2.1.1 Field of View

MR and CT images of a region in a patient frequently have quite different fields of view in the direction perpendicular to the slice plane (the "through–slice direction"). Due to the risks associated with the ionizing radiation used in CT acquisitions, the number of slices collected is kept to a minimum.

In MR, however, there is negligible risk associated with the acquisition, and modern imaging provides techniques for acquiring large numbers of slices in a short time. As a result of these differences, it is common for an MR image to have a much larger field of view in the through-slice direction than the CT image to which it is being registered.

Another important difference between MR and CT imaging is that, although MR scanners can acquire images in arbitrary slice orientations, CT scanners are limited to axial acquisitions or, by careful patient positioning and maximum tilting of the gantry, to images of the head in the coronal plane. It may, therefore, be desirable to align images acquired in different planes with the two modalities; for example, to register sagittal MR images with axial CT images. In this case, the overlapping portion of the image field of view may be considerably smaller than either image. An example set of MR and CT images of the head is shown in Figure 10.1.

The difference in field of view of MR and CT images and the restricted volume of overlap of the two images present considerable challenges to image registration algorithms. In many early applications of MR-CT registration it was essential, in order to get good registration accuracy, to acquire both images using a similar field of view and as similar as possible a slice orientation.

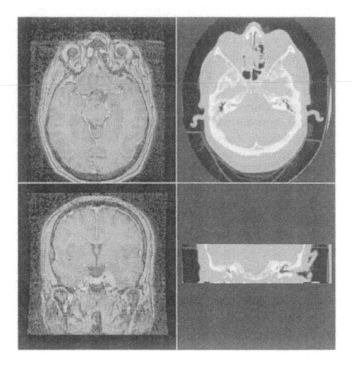

FIGURE 10.1
Example MR and CT images of the head before registration. Note the difference in field of view in the through-slice direction.

This restricted the application of MR-CT registration to small subsets of patients for whom the decision to register the image was made in advance of the acquisitions, and for whom it was acceptable to alter the image acquisition for the purposes of registration. In practice, this was rarely the case outside a small number of centers.

In the last few years, the difficulties caused by field of view have been reduced because of the widespread use, first, of spiral (or helical) CT scanning and, more recently, multislice* CT scanning. This has increased the number of slices routinely acquired. Furthermore, it is becoming more common to carry out 3D volume acquisitions with MR. These volume images tend to have larger fields of view than the multislice acquisitions and have approximately isotropic resolution, although they also tend to have fewer good contrast characteristics. As a consequence, the volume of overlap between routinely acquired MR and CT images of the same subject tends to be larger now than it was ten years ago. Despite changes in image acquisition, it is still necessary for a clinically usable MR-CT registration algorithm to be able to accurately register images with different fields of view and slice orientations.

10.2.1.2   *Resolution*

The in-plane resolution of CT images tends to be higher than that of MR images, as CT images are routinely acquired with an image matrix of 512 × 512 pixels, whereas MR images most commonly have a 256 × 256 image matrix. Also, techniques used to speed up MR acquisition frequently result in lower resolution in one in-plane direction (the phase encode direction) than this matrix size suggests. In the through-plane direction, however, the situation is often reversed, with MR having higher through-plane resolution than CT. The desire to minimize radiation dose in CT often results in the use of fewer, thicker slices than are used in MR. In traditional multislice (one slice at a time) CT acquisitions, the slice spacing can be changed part of the way through an acquisition to minimize dose. For example, slices through the skull base might be acquired with 3 mm slices and 3 mm slice spacing, but slices higher in the head where less detail is required might be acquired with 5 mm slices and 5 mm slice spacing.

These resolution factors have important implications for MR-CT registration. First, algorithms used for registration need to work with these differences in resolution. Second, care needs to be taken when combining the registered images, for example with a color overlay display. It is not possible to transform the MR image to the coordinates of the CT scan, nor the CT image to the coordinates of the MR scan, without degrading the resolution of the transformed image. Given the effort put into the original data acquisition, it seems wasteful if the registration process requires that one or another

---

* The latest generation of CT scanners can acquire about two or four slices simultaneously, rather than acquiring multiple slices one at a time; the number of slices that can be acquired simultaneously is likely to increase as the technology matures over the next few years.

image has its resolution degraded. Software for viewing the registered images needs to take this into account by providing tools for viewing the combined images in a variety of ways. For example, giving the user a choice of overlaying MR on CT (or vice versa) or allowing the images to be combined to form a new image that has higher resolution than either modality.

10.2.1.3   Image Distortion

A detailed discussion of scanner distortion is provided in Chapter 5. It is worthwhile here, however, to consider the main causes of distortion in MR-CT registration.

MR images can have distortion resulting either from errors in the gradient systems or as a result of field inhomogeneity introduced at the boundary between tissues with different magnetic susceptibility properties, such as between soft tissue and air and, to a lesser extent, between soft tissue and bone. This second type of distortion is common in the head, for example in the frontal lobe of the brain near the frontal sinus or the temporal lobes of the brain near the maxilliary and sphenoid sinuses. While methods to correct for this distortion are available,[4,5] they are seldom used clinically. Object-dependent distortion in common diagnostic MR sequences (excluding echo planar imaging) is greatest in the readout gradient direction and can be reduced, at the expense of signal-to-noise ratio, by increasing the readout gradient strength (which is under user control for scanners from some manufacturers).

Distortion in CT is quite different. While it is true that x-rays invariably travel in straight lines, the same cannot be said for the patient couch. The patient couch can bend (especially with heavy patients) as it is extended, which can lead to a variable skew distortion with slice position. There can be additional skew errors due to poorly calibrated gantry tilt. These skew errors can be substantial, leading to errors of several millimeters in some parts of the images. Another cause of distortion in spiral CT can be errors in bed speed that lead to errors in slice spacing. Errors caused by these distortions can be quite obvious in registered images, even if they are not at all apparent when viewing the images on radiographic film on a light box. Figure 10.2 shows sagittally reformatted images through a CT volume before and after correction of a 22° gantry skew. If the skew had not been corrected (for example if the file transfer process had lost this information), or if the skew were incorrectly corrected due to inaccuracies in the scanner's measurement of gantry tilt, substantial registration errors would result.

10.2.1.4   Patient Motion

Patient motion during either MR or CT acquisition makes image registration harder. Subject motion during the acquisition of a CT slice results in streaking which degrades the diagnostic quality. Patient motion between CT slice acquisitions may not reduce the diagnostic quality of the images, but motion either during or between slices can make accurate registration more difficult.

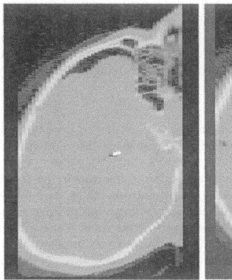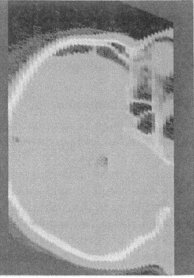

FIGURE 10.2
Reformatted sagittal view through a CT volume before (left) and after (right) correction of
a 22° gantry tilt. Any CT gantry tilt must be corrected either before or during the registration
process, or substantial errors result.

If the patient changes position during the acquisition, then for all slices
acquired before the motion the subject is in one position, and for all slices
acquired after the motion the subject is in a second position. There are, therefore, two registration transformations between this CT acquisition and an
MR acquisition: one for each patient position. A registration algorithm
might find either transformation or some average transformation, depending on the way the algorithm works. If the patient moves multiple times during an acquisition, this problem gets worse. In general, patient motion
during a CT acquisition will result in reduced registration accuracy; depending on the amount of movement, this misregistration could be a centimeter
or more.

Motion during MR acquisition is more complicated. If the acquisition is 2D
multislice, like most spin-echo acquisitions, it is normal for the scanner to
acquire several slices essentially simultaneously. When the desired number of
slices exceeds the number the scanner can collect simultaneously, multiple sets
of interleaves are acquired. Patient motion during an MR scan of this type can
result in one interleave being transformed with respect to the other. As in the
CT case, this will result in degraded registration accuracy, for example by
calculating a transformation that is some sort of average of the required
transformation for the patient in the two positions.

Motion during a CT acquisition or multislice MR acquisition can quite
easily be identified by reformatting the images in a perpendicular plane.

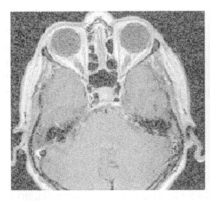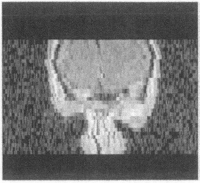

FIGURE 10.3
In this multislice spin-echo T1-weighted MR image, slices in the axial plane of acquisition are motion free (left), but motion during the study has resulted in jagged boundaries of tissues in the reformatted coronal slice (right). Motion of this type might not reduce the diagnostic value of the MR scans but can introduce unacceptably large errors into registered volumes. It is advisable always to view reformatted MR and CT images prior to registration to check for the presence of motion artifacts of this type.

For example, by reformatting axial images in the coronal or sagittal plane, motion during the scan can be easily identified. Figure 10.3 shows an example of MR image with motion between the interleaves.

Motion during a 3D volume MR acquisition will result in a ghost artifact throughout the images which will be spread out in the phase-encoded directions of the images. This is likely to be clear from inspection of any slice from the volume. Ghost artifacts in 3D acquisitions can make it hard to accurately delineate points or surfaces in the images, if these are needed for registration.

For imaging the head, the sort of motion that causes problems is normally a nodding or rolling of the head, which causes a rotation. In the abdomen or chest, breathing during the scan can cause similar problems.

For images that are to be registered, it is important to check for signs of motion as part of the routine quality assurance process; if this is not done, clinically significant errors may arise.

10.2.1.5 Data Transfer

An essential step prior to registration of MR and CT images is the transfer of both images onto the same computer. With increased use of picture archiving and communication systems (PACS), image transfer is becoming more straightforward. There are, however, many hospitals where the relevant scanners are not all networked, or compatible file formats or network protocols are not used. In these cases, the logistics of data transfer can be complicated. It may be necessary to transfer images from one computer to another using tape or removable disks, and dedicated software may be needed to convert the data to compatible formats prior to registration. This process can be very time consuming, and important data can be lost during the transfer. For example, information in the image header about whether the patient is prone or supine, or head first or feet first must be accurately transferred along with the image pixel values, if the patient's orientation within the scanner is to be known. Errors in this process can result in the left and right sides of the patient being flipped, which is potentially disastrous. The topic of data transfer is treated in more detail in Chapter 4.

10.2.2   Registration Methods

Many algorithms have been proposed for registration of MR and CT images of the head. As described in Chapter 3, these methods can be categorized into those that make use of geometrical features in the images (such as points or surfaces) and those that make use of voxel intensity values.

10.2.2.1   Registration Using Geometrical Features

The earliest techniques for registration of MR and CT images of the head were use of point landmarks[1] or stereotactic frames.[2,6,7] Point landmarks can either be point-like anatomical structures within the images visible in both modalities[1,8] or they can be external fiducial markers rigidly affixed to the skull[9] or attached to the skin.[10-12] Whether the points are anatomical features or external markers, the most common registration approach is to find the rigid-body transformation that aligns the points in the least-squares sense, as described in Chapter 3. When using external fiducial markers, the markers need to be visible in both modalities and must not introduce artifacts in the images. Fatty markers appear very bright in MR, but are a poor choice because protons in fat have a different resonant frequency from protons in water; therefore they appear displaced (in the readout direction) relative to their true position as compared to soft tissues of interest. The amount of displacement depends on the readout gradient strength, as discussed in Chapter 5. A mixture of MR contrast material and CT contrast material is a better choice,[9] but care must be taken to ensure that the markers are visible in all MR sequences of interest. Certain types of inversion recovery sequences can make features with particular relaxation times virtually invisible in the images, and if the markers have this relaxation time, they will not be visible in the images.

External fiducial markers rigidly attached to the skull have considerable advantages over point-like anatomical features for registration. First, they can appear sufficiently bright in the images to be easily identified by a user or computer algorithm. Second, it is possible to calculate the position of these features with an accuracy better than the voxel dimensions by using a center of gravity calculation,[13] provided the markers are large enough to appear in multiple voxels in all dimensions. Skin-attached markers can be identified accurately in the images, but they can move relative to features of interest in the patient, which degrades the accuracy. The identification of point-like anatomical features is more user dependent and will depend on the points selected. The disadvantage of bone-affixed external markers is that they are invasive. Also, the markers tend to be in the periphery of the MR image field of view, where distortion is likely to be greatest (see Chapter 5 for further discussion of MR distortion).

An alternative to using points in the image is to use surfaces.[3,14-16] These algorithms are described in detail in Chapter 3 and have been used for MR-CT registration for many years. For registration of MR and CT images of the head, the easiest surface to define in both modalities is the skin surface. The skin, however, tends to deform between scans as a result of differences in the shape of the head rest and head restraint between modalities. The skin surface, therefore, is not a very accurate surface to use. A better alternative would be either the inner or outer table of the skull. Both these surfaces are easy to identify in CT images, but because cortical bone is not visible in MR scans, the position of the skull surface must be inferred from adjacent structures. For T2-weighted MR images, CSF is bright, so the inner table of the skull can easily be found as the boundary of bright CSF and dark cortical bone. For T1-weighted MR images, however, CSF is dark like cortical bone, so the inner table of the skull is difficult to identify, especially in patients with atrophic brains. In this case, an alternative surface to delineate is the outer table of the skull. In T1-weighted images, the fat of the scalp is bright, so the boundary between scalp and cortical bone can be identified quite well. The problem here is that, because of the high fat content of scalp, the scalp can appear displaced in the MR image readout direction relative to structures of interest in the brain, just as fat-filled markers can be displaced. Images acquired with high readout gradient strength have less fat-water shift, so errors introduced by this can be reduced.

When registering images using surfaces, it is desirable to have as much surface visible in both images as possible. Preferably, for registration of the head, the great majority of the skull should be visible in both modalities. The skull has quite a lot of rotation symmetry, so without sufficient coverage, surface matching algorithms can easily converge to an incorrect local minimum. It is possible to increase registration accuracy in these situations by combining the use of surfaces and points.[16]

10.2.2.2 Registration Using Voxel Intensity Values

Since the mid-1990s, fully automatic algorithms have been available for registration of MR and CT images of the head by optimizing voxel similarity measures.[17-22] Van den Elsen proposed an algorithm based on correlation, in which an intensity remapping algorithm was used to make the bone in CT dark, as it is in MR.[17] An alternative approach is to correlate ridge images extracted from both MR and CT images, rather than the images themselves.[18] More recently, it has been shown that theoretical approaches such as mutual information can be used for MR-CT registration, as well as for other registration applications.[19-22] These algorithms are all described in Chapter 3. A blind multicenter study recently found that these measures based on voxel intensity values are more accurate than surface-based methods for MR-CT registration.[23]

Care must still be taken with these voxel similarity measure techniques. Although they can be fully automatic and have an accuracy comparable to bone-implanted markers,[24] they can also fail. One common cause of failure can be that the images are poorly aligned at the start. For example, if the patient is positioned very differently in the image volume for the two scans, or if the images have different slice orientations (e.g., sagittal MR and axial CT), the algorithms can fail unless a user provides a reasonably good starting estimate. A further problem for some of these algorithms is their sensitivity to the volume of overlap in the images. If one image has a much larger field of view than the other, or if the overlap between images at correct registration is a relatively small amount of the field of view of one or both original images, the algorithms can fail, even with a very good starting estimate. A solution to this problem is to use a normalized version of mutual information, which is much less sensitive to image overlap,[22] as described in Chapter 3.

10.2.2.3 Assessing Registration Accuracy

In a blind study of registration accuracy, it was shown that MR and CT images can be registered with an accuracy of better than 1 mm but algorithms can fail, resulting in errors of 1 cm or more.[24] It is, therefore, clearly important for a method of quality assurance to be used to ensure that only well-registered images are used for clinical decision making. The accuracy required for most applications of MR-CT registration is about 2 mm, as neither surgery nor radiotherapy is likely to justify better accuracy. Visual assessment of registered images can be used to check for errors, and it has been shown that trained observers can effectively distinguish between registration errors below or above accuracy thresholds of 2 to 6 mm.[25] The sensitivity and specificity of the observers to misregistration is additionally a function of the distribution of errors produced by the registration algorithm. The problem of ensuring good quality registration accuracy is discussed further in Chapter 6.

10.2.3 Viewing the Combined Images

Once the images have been registered, the combined images can be viewed in a variety of ways. These include displaying corresponding slices side by side with a linked cursor identifying corresponding points in the slices, using color overlays, or segmenting bone from the CT scan and overlaying it on the MR image to produce a combined image that has the soft tissue contrast of MR and also contains bony detail. Combined display examples are shown in Color Figure 10.4.*

It is also possible to use volume visualization techniques to render an image that combines features from the MR and CT images. An example of a rendered image is shown in Color Figure 10.5.*

---

* Color Figures follow page 22.

10.3   Applications

10.3.1   Planning Surgery of the Brain and Skull Base

The combination of MR and CT images of the head can be useful in planning certain types of neurosurgical and ENT surgical procedures. In particular, the relationship between the soft tissue contrast provided by MRI and bone detail provided by CT can be useful where a single modality is insufficient. One example is planning procedures within the posterior fossa, where CT can usefully provide information about the most suitable approach but MR is needed for soft tissue detail, because beam-hardening artifacts in the CT lead to streaks that can degrade the quality of soft tissue information. Another example application is lesions that involve bone, such as cysts in the petrous apex and glomus jugulare tumors, where soft tissue detail and bone contrast are both desirable.[8,26,27] The clinical motivation of registration is to provide the surgeon with an improved understanding of the relationship among the lesion, adjacent critical structures, and possible surgical approaches. This can result in better positioning of craniotomies, reduced craniotomy size, quicker operations with less time under anesthetic, and, consequently, improved patient outcomes.

Figures 10.4 and 10.5 show example combined MR and CT images used in planning resection of skull-base tumors. The benefits of combining multimodality information can be even greater for guiding surgical procedures, as discussed in Chapter 12.

10.3.2   Localizing Electrodes in the Brain

Functional neurosurgical procedures include implantation of mat electrodes over the surface of the brain or depth electrodes into brain parenchyma to localize an epileptogenic region or focus by subsequent neurophysiological recording in patients with intractable epilepsy. This is done to plan surgical resection of the epileptogenic area of the brain. Good anatomical localization of the electrode shown to be closest to the focus is crucial, as this will determine the success of the operation. Another type of functional neurosurgical procedure is the implantation of electrodes into the subthalamic nucleus (a small structure) in patients with Parkinson's disease, to alleviate tremor. Assessment of success of the procedure is dependent on knowing that the electrodes are satisfactorily positioned. The localization of electrodes can be achieved using CT scans, but the soft tissue contrast is relatively poor, and streak artifact from the electrodes degrades the images. While MR can be obtained with the electrodes in place, there is a potential risk from electrical current generation from changing magnetic gradients and heating from the use of electrical conductors while applying radiofrequency pulses with the MR scanner. For many patients, the risk of ionizing radiation from a CT scan may be more acceptable than the less well understood risk of an MR scan

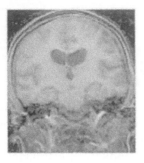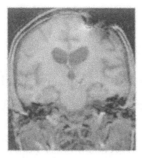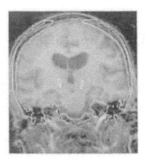

FIGURE 10.6

A coronal slice through an MR volume dataset acquired from a patient with a motor disorder to undergo functional surgery (note motion artifact), together with a registered post-implantation MR scan (center) and the pre-implantation MR overlaid with high density features (bone and electrodes) from a post-implantation CT scan (right). The combined pre-implantation MR and CT avoids the susceptibility artifacts and potential risk to the patient resulting from post-electrode implantation MR scanning.

with electrodes in place. The electrodes also cause some distortion of the MR image.

Figure 10.6 shows an example coronal MR slice acquired post-implantation of depth electrodes alongside a pre-implantation MR image in the same position with the outline of the bone and electrodes imaged in post-implantation CT overlaid.

A difficulty in registration of pre-implantation MR scans to post-implantation CT scans is that the brain can deform substantially between these procedures,[28] as it does during other neurosurgical procedures.[12,29,30] Brain deformation remains poorly understood, but it is likely that deformation will be greater if a large craniotomy is required (e.g., for insertion of electrode mats on the surface of the brain), or if large amounts of CSF are lost during a procedure. When deformation of more than about 1 mm arises, a rigid-body registration algorithm is insufficient for accurately aligning the MR and CT images. In this case a nonrigid algorithm could be used. Nonrigid registration algorithms are described in Chapter 13, but these are primarily used for intramodality applications; reliable nonrigid registration of images from very different modalities has not yet been demonstrated.

10.3.3 Radiotherapy Planning

The recent development of 3D CT-based radiotherapy planning has involved the use of multiple CT slices to show a tumor in all three dimensions.[31] This allows "conformal" radiotherapy to be planned, where multiple radiation beams are used, configured as tightly as possible to the contour of a tumor to spare adjacent potentially radiosensitive normal tissues from damage. This technique has been of most use in the head and skull base and to preserve brain and optic nerves, and has also been applied to the prostate. MR images would seem ideal for the purposes of planning. The much greater soft tissue contrast of MR allows better definition of the boundaries of a tumor from adjacent normal tissues and structures.[32] In the brain, MR techniques such as functional studies or perfusion imaging can also provide information about eloquent areas of the brain which would have significant consequences for the patient if damaged, or the physiology of an already treated tumor, which may influence whether further treatment is required. When a tumor is irradiated, the margins of the radiation beams carefully and precisely calculated on the planning images must correspond exactly spatially to the beams used to irradiate the patient. The images used for planning purposes must be geometrically accurate or as free from distortion as possible. MR is subject to distortions to a greater extent than CT as described in Chapter 5. CT has a further important advantage over MR in that the intensities of image voxels (measured in Hounsfield units) represent electron density and can be used to calculate dose distributions directly. These two factors have limited the use of MR scans so far for radiotherapy planning. Registration of CT and MR images provides one way of overcoming these problems and utilizing the different information from both modalities to optimize treatment.[6,26,33,34]

10.3.4   Applications outside the Head

Techniques for registering MR and CT images are almost invariably restricted to finding a rigid-body or affine transformation. Outside the head, a nonrigid transformation is normally necessary because of soft tissue deformation resulting from change in patient positioning, respiration, etc. When registering MR or CT images with PET or SPECT images, some parts of the body such as the pelvis can be treated as rigid bodies because careful patient positioning can make tissue deformation smaller than the resolution of the PET or SPECT images. For MR-CT registration, this assumption is not valid. There is nevertheless considerable interest in registration of MR and CT outside the head for staging cancer and planning radiotherapy; for example, in the spine and prostate.

10.4   Conclusions

The registration of MR and CT images was one of the first applications of medical image registration. Despite a large number of algorithms devised for MR and CT registration, these algorithms are not used routinely outside a small number of highly specialized centers. Furthermore, the applicability of MR-CT registration is restricted primarily to the head by current algorithms that can only determine rigid-body or affine transformations. MR-CT registration is likely to become more widely used in the future. The driving factors are fully digital x-ray departments that make access to the data more straightforward, increasing use of image-guided surgery and stereotactic radiosurgery systems that include registration software, and greater use of MRI and CT as interventional modalities. When MR or CT is used as an interventional modality, it can nevertheless be desirable to have access to accurately registered pre-intervention images of other modalities; incorporating registration algorithms into the workstation controlling the interventional modality can make this straightforward. Future developments in nonrigid registration algorithms, discussed elsewhere in this book, are likely to make these applicable to MR-CT registration, which will open up many new applications, including planning of surgery and radiotherapy outside the head.

References

1. G.T.Y. Chen, M. Kessler, and S. Pitluck, Structure transfer between sets of three dimensional medical imaging data, in *Computer Graphics 1985*, pp. 171–175, Dallas: National Computer Graphics Association, 1985.
2. T.M. Peters, J.A. Clark, A. Olivier, E.P. Marchand, G. Mawko, M. Dieumegarde, L. Muresan, and R. Ethier, Integrated stereotaxic imaging with CT, MR imaging, and digital subtraction angiography, *Radiology*, vol. 161, pp. 821–826, 1986.
3. D.N. Levin, C.A. Pelizzari, G.T.Y. Chen, C.-T. Chen, and M.D. Cooper, Retrospective geometric correlation of MR, CT, and PET images, *Radiology*, vol. 169, pp. 817–823, 1988.
4. T.S. Sumanaweera, G.H. Glover, S.M. Song, J.R. Adler, and S. Napel, Quantifying MRI geometric distortion in tissue, *Magn. Reson. Med.*, vol. 31, pp. 40–47, 1994.
5. H. Chang and J.M. Fitzpatrick, A technique for accurate magnetic resonance imaging in the presence of field inhomogeneities, *IEEE Trans. Med. Imaging*, vol. 11, pp. 319–329, 1992.
6. L.R. Schad, R. Boesecke, W. Schlegel, G.H. Hartmann, V. Sturm, L.G. Strauss, and W.J. Lorenz, Three dimensional image correlation of CT, MR, and PET studies in radiotherapy treatment planning of brain tumors, *J. Comput. Assist. Tomogr.*, vol. 11, pp. 948–954, 1987.
7. J. Zhang, M.F. Levesque, C.L. Wilson, R.M. Harper, J. Engel, Jr., R. Lufkin, and E.J. Behnke, Multi-modality imaging of brain structures for stereotactic surgery, *Radiology*, vol. 175, pp. 435–441, 1990.
8. D.L.G. Hill, D.J. Hawkes, J.E. Crossman, M.J. Gleeson, T.C.S. Cox, E.E.C.M.L. Bracey, A.J. Strong, and P. Graves, Registration of MR and CT images of skull base surgery using point-like anatomical features, *Br. J. Radiol.*, vol. 64, pp. 1030–1035, 1991.
9. C.R. Maurer, Jr., J.M. Fitzpatrick, M.Y. Wang, R.L. Galloway, Jr., R.J. Maciunas, and G.S. Allen, Registration of head volume images using implantable fiducial markers, *IEEE Trans. Med. Imaging*, vol. 16, pp. 447–462, 1997.
10. P.A. van den Elsen, M.A. Viergever, A.C. Van Huffelen, W. Van der Meij, and G.H. Wieneke, Accurate matching of electromagnetic dipole data with CT and MR images, *Brain Topogr.*, vol. 3, pp. 425–432, 1991.
11. E.P. Sipos, S.A. Tebo, S.J. Zinreich, D.M. Long, and H. Brem, *In vivo* accuracy testing and clinical experience with the isg viewing wand, *Neurosurgery*, vol. 39, pp. 194–202, 1996.
12. N.L. Dorward, O. Alberti, B. Velani, F.A. Gerritsen, W.F.J. Harkness, N.D. Kitchen, and D.G.T. Thomas, Postimaging brain distortion: magnitude, correlates, and impact on neuronavigation, *J. Neurosurg.*, vol. 88, pp. 656–662, 1998.

13. M.Y. Wang, C.R. Maurer, Jr., J.M. Fitzpatrick, and R.J. Maciunas, An automatic technique for finding and localizing externally attached markers in CT and MR volume images of the head, *IEEE Trans. Biomed. Eng.*, vol. 43, pp. 627–637, 1996.
14. C.A. Pelizzari, G.T.Y. Chen, D.R. Spelbring, R.R. Weichselbaum, and C.-T. Chen, Accurate three-dimensional registration of CT, PET, and/or MR images of the brain, *J. Comput. Assist. Tomogr.*, vol. 13, pp. 20–26, 1989.
15. H. Jiang, R.A. Robb, and K.S. Holton, A new approach to 3-D registration of multimodality medical images by surface matching, *Visualization in Biomed. Computing 1992*, vol. Proc. SPIE 1808, pp. 196–213, 1992.
16. C.R. Maurer, Jr., R.J. Maciunas, and J.M. Fitzpatrick, Registration of head CT images to physical space using a weighted combination of points and surfaces, *IEEE Trans. Med. Imaging*, vol. 17, pp. 753–761, 1998.
17. P.A. van den Elsen, E.-J.D. Pol, T.S. Sumanaweera, P.F. Hemler, S. Napel, and J.R. Adler, Grey value correlation techniques used for automatic matching of CT and MR brain and spine images, *Visualization in Biomed. Computing 1994*, vol. Proc. SPIE 2359, pp. 227–237, 1994.
18. P.A. van den Elsen, J.B.A. Maintz, E.-J.D. Pol, and M.A. Viergever, Automatic registration of CT and MR brain images using correlation of geometrical features, *IEEE Trans. Med. Imaging*, vol. 14 pp. 384–396, 1995.
19. W.M. Wells, III, P. Viola, H. Atsumi, S. Nakajima, and R. Kikinis, Multi-modal volume registration by maximization of mutual information, *Med. Image Anal.*, vol. 1, pp. 35–51, 1996.
20. C. Studholme, D.L.G. Hill, and D.J. Hawkes, Automated 3D registration of MR and CT images of the head, *Med. Image Anal.*, vol. 1, pp. 163–175, 1996.
21. F. Maes, A. Collignon, D. Vandermeulen, G. Marchal, and P. Suetens, Multimodality image registration by maximization of mutual information, *IEEE Trans. Med. Imaging*, vol. 16, pp. 187–198, 1997.
22. C. Studholme, D.L.G. Hill, and D.J. Hawkes, An overlap invariant entropy measure of 3D medical image alignment, *Pattern Recogn.*, vol. 32, pp. 71–86, 1999.
23. J.B. West, J.M. Fitzpatrick, M.Y. Wang, B.M. Dawant, C.R. Maurer, Jr., R.M. Kessler, and R.J. Maciunas, Retrospective intermodality techniques for images of the head: surface-based versus volume-based, *IEEE Trans. Med. Imaging*, pp. 144–150, 1999.
24. J.B. West, J.M. Fitzpatrick, M.Y. Wang, B.M. Dawant, C.R. Maurer, Jr., R.M. Kessler, R.J. Maciunas, C. Barillot, D. Lemoine, A. Collignon, F. Maes, P. Suetens, D. Vandermeulen, P.A. van den Elsen, S. Napel, T.S. Sumanaweera, B. Harkness, P.F. Hemler, D.L.G. Hill, D.J. Hawkes, C. Studholme, J.B.A. Maintz, M.A. Viergever, G. Malandain, X. Pennec, M.E. Noz, G.Q. Maguire, Jr., M. Pollack, C.A. Pelizzari, R.A. Robb, D. Hanson, and R.P. Woods, Comparison and evaluation of retrospective intermodality brain image registration techniques, *J. Comput. Assist. Tomogr.*, vol. 21, pp. 554–566, 1997.
25. J.M. Fitzpatrick, D.L.G. Hill, Y. Shyr, J. West, C. Studholme, and C.R. Maurer, Jr., Visual assessment of the accuracy of retrospective registration of MR and CT images of the brain, *IEEE Trans. Med. Imaging*, vol. 17, pp. 571–585, 1998.
26. D.L.G. Hill, D.J. Hawkes, M.J. Gleeson, T.C.S. Cox, A.J. Strong, W.-L. Wong, C.F. Ruff, N.D. Kitchen, D.G.T. Thomas, J.E. Crossman, C. Studholme, A.J. Gandhe, S.E.M. Green, and G.P. Robinson, Accurate frameless registration of MR and CT images of the head: applications in surgery and radiotherapy planning, *Radiology*, vol. 191, pp. 447–454, 1994.

27. A.J. Gandhe, D.L.G. Hill, C. Studholme, D.J. Hawkes, C.S. Ruff, T.C.S. Cox, M.J. Gleeson, and A.J. Strong, Combined and three-dimensional rendered multimodal data for planning cranial base surgery: a prospective evaluation, *Neurosurgery*, vol. 35. pp. 463–470, 1994.

28. D.L.G. Hill, A.D. Castellano Smith, A. Simmons, C.R. Maurer, T.C.S. Cox, R. Elwes, M.J. Brammer, D.J. Hawkes, and C.E. Polkey, Sources of error in comparing functional magnetic resonance imaging and invasive electrophysiology recordings, *J. Neurosurg.*, vol. 93, pp. 214–223, 2000.

29. D.L.G. Hill, C.R. Maurer, Jr., R.J. Maciunas, J.A. Barwise, J.M. Fitzpatrick, and M.Y. Wang, Measurement of intraoperative brain surface deformation under a craniotomy, *Neurosurgery*, vol. 43, pp. 514–528, 1998.

30. D.W. Roberts, A. Hartov, F.E. Kennedy, M.I. Miga, and K.D. Paulsen, Intraoperative brain shift and deformation: a quantitative analysis of cortical displacement in 28 cases, *Neurosurgery*, vol. 43, pp. 749–758, 1998.

31. J.A. Purdy, 3D treatment planning and intensity-modulated radiation therapy, *Oncology (Huntington)*, vol. 13, pp. 155–68, 1999.

32. V.S. Khoo, MRI-magic radiotherapy imaging for treatment planning? *Br. J. Radiol.*, vol. 73, pp. 229–233, 2000.

33. M.L. Kessler, S. Pitluck, P. Petti, and J.R. Castro, Integration of multimodality imaging data for radiotherapy treatment planning, *Int. J. of Radiation Oncology, Biol., Physics*, vol. 21, pp. 1653–67, 1992.

34. J.G. Rosenman, E.P. Miller, G. Tracton, and T.J. Cullip, Image registration: an essential part of radiation therapy treatment planning, *Int. J. of Radiation Oncology, Biol. Physics*, vol. 40, pp. 197–205, 1998.

11

Image Registration in Nuclear Medicine

Dale L. Bailey

CONTENTS

11.1 Introduction

Nuclear medicine is a functional imaging modality. It uses radionuclides labeled to target molecules, or *radiotracers*, for diagnostic studies and for delivering *in vivo* radiation therapy. The biodistribution of a radiotracer in the body depends on the delivery to and functional uptake by the organ or pathway under examination. The great advantage of nuclear medicine lies in the premise that functional changes precede anatomical changes in all cases apart from trauma. Thus, appropriate radiotracers are able to demonstrate changes due to disease long before there are macroscopic manifestations.

Phelps and Coleman[1] recently characterized the fundamental principles of diagnostic nuclear medicine as:

- The development and use of radiolabeled molecules to image or measure the molecular basis of disease for early detection, accurate

234   *Medical Image Registration*

characterization, treatment planning, and assessment of therapeutic outcomes

- The design and development of radionuclide imaging and measurement devices for performing molecular examinations of patients
- The use of the tracer technique to perform these procedures with minimal or no mass effects that could alter the biological process being imaged or measured
- The ability to measure molecular concentrations and rates of biological processes involving substrate concentrations down to micromoles to femtomoles per gram of tissue

Nuclear medicine images demonstrate function, rather than anatomy. Some of the limitations of nuclear medicine imaging studies include limited spatial resolution, poor signal-to-noise ratio, and frequently poor uptake of the radiotracer in the diseased condition. Registration with a structural or anatomical image can be useful in addressing a number of these issues. The main applications at present are

- **Intramodality and intermodality spatial registration**—intramodality registration in positron emission tomography (PET) and single photon emission computed tomography (SPECT), e.g., PET-PET, SPECT-SPECT, and intermodality registration with other functional or structural data such as from x-ray CT and magnetic resonance imaging (MRI), e.g., PET-MRI
- **Correcting nuclear medicine emission data**—correction for photon attenuation and scattering, partial volume correction to compensate for limited spatial resolution, and guiding image reconstruction algorithms where anatomical priors can be used to "encourage" a reconstruction towards a particular solution, based on the known biodistribution of the radiotracer
- **Intersubject registration (spatial normalization)**—standardizing the geometric conformation of uptake in an organ for comparisons with normal databases or for use in cohort studies

The methods used to achieve the above, and examples of their use, are the subject of this chapter. Some discussion of MR-PET registration is included here, but this topic is treated in more detail in Chapter 9.

11.2   Early Uses of Image Registration in Nuclear Medicine

Functional images do not necessarily follow anatomy, and therefore nuclear medicine studies have often benefited from the use of patient or organ outlines from other imaging devices as anatomical guides. As long ago as 1966,

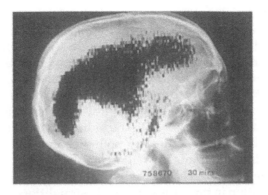

FIGURE 11.1
An early example of coregistration of anatomical and functional data in nuclear medicine. The scan shows the intracerebral ventricular system after an intrathecal injection of ^{131}I-HSA superimposed on a lateral skull x-ray. Both imaging systems produced life-size images, making alignment relatively straightforward. (Image courtesy of Professor Henry N. Wagner, Jr., Johns Hopkins School of Hygiene and Public Health, Baltimore).

Kuhl et al. reported using a chest x-ray and a [^{99m}Tc]-sulphur colloid liver scan to detect pleural effusions. By overlaying the gamma camera image with the x-ray and drawing the boundaries of the diaphragm they could identify the fluid collections.[2] Similarly, Anger and McRae used chest x-rays in conjunction with liver and lung scans to demonstrate discrepancies which would indicate a subphrenic collection between the liver and the diaphragm. They also detected pericardial effusions by overlaying a gamma camera transmission image (analogous to a low resolution x-ray) on the nuclear medicine blood pool image.[3,4] These are some of the earliest uses of image registration as a complement to the conventional nuclear medicine scan. An example is shown in Figure 11.1. From the late 1960s, nuclear medicine devices have had the ability to measure transmission as well as the emission distribution of the radiotracer.[5-10] This is now standard, with sophisticated transmission systems using scanning line sources[11] or stationary sources[12,13] available on most gamma cameras. More recently, dedicated purpose-built dual imaging devices incorporating x-ray CT with either PET or SPECT detectors in a single scanner have been developed and will be discussed later.[14,15]

11.3 Spatial Registration of Nuclear Medicine Images

Possibly the best known application of image registration in nuclear medicine today is that of spatially coregistering nuclear medicine emission scans with other radionuclide scans or with anatomical images. This can be performed on two-dimensional planar or three-dimensional volumetric data. A simple example shown in Color Figure 11.2* is of an x-ray of the hand coregistered with the corresponding bone scan. In this example the bone scan was performed to detect sites of increased radiotracer accumulation in the small bones of the hand, and to localize this as accurately as possible.[16] Small fractures may be present and detected in this way when they are not apparent on x-ray alone. To perform such a registration, the patient's hand is placed in a rigid frame for both the radiograph and the gamma camera images. Fiducial markers, visible on both the x-ray and gamma camera, are incorporated into the frame thus allowing the *retrospective* realignment and scaling of the data, which, for these purposes, are taken to be a rigid object. The registration in this case is relatively straightforward: the operator uses an interactive computer program to identify the corresponding markers in the two images and the registration algorithm determines the scaling, translation, and rotation degrees of freedom to align the markers (see the description of the Procrustes algorithm in Chapters 2 and 3 for more details of this approach). Once registered, any bone which has abnormal uptake can be accurately localized. Most registration tasks, however, are more complicated than this example. The majority of registrations involve three-dimensional volumetric data, often between different modalities. Many of the early algorithms developed for spatial registration were intended for use with different modalities, e.g., PET and MRI.[17]

Spatial registration provides an anatomical framework in which to interpret the functional emission data arising from SPECT and PET. Combining functional PET data with structural MRI data in neuroscience research was one of the first applications for PET-MRI registration that achieved widespread routine use. In a paper in 1993, Watson et al. demonstrated, for the first time in man accurate spatial localization of the functional locus of an area of the brain outside the primary visual cortex which was predominantly interested in visual motion alone[18] known as "V5." Given the limited spatial resolution of the PET blood flow studies, it would have been difficult to localize, as precisely as was done in this paper, the exact location of the functional area V5 in the parieto-occipital cortex without the aid of accurately registered MRI. The data were registered with an automated algorithm where the parameter that was optimized, also known as *cost function*, was the partitioned image uniformity (PIU) measure,[17] described in Chapter 3. Today it is standard to represent areas of change in cerebral activity measured with PET or functional MRI (fMRI) superimposed with a high resolution structural MRI scan. This approach also has application in coregistering brain scans containing lesions with, for example, [^{18}F]-DG (PET) or [^{99m}Tc]-HmPAO (SPECT) scans. The registration problem in the case of the human brain is simplified in that it can be treated as a rigid body, and therefore a transformation allowing only for six degrees of freedom (three translations and three rotations) plus

---

* Color Figures follow page 22.

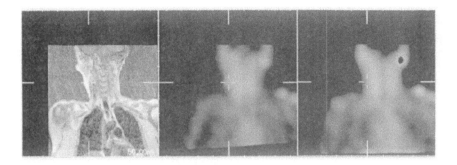

FIGURE 11.4
MRI (left), [^{111}In]-Octreotide (center), and [^{99m}Tc]-DMSA(V) (right) coregistration. The SPECT studies were aligned to the MRI scan by using fiducial markers, which were visible on both the MRI and SPECT studies. The fiducial markers are not visible in the MR slice shown, as they lie in a different plane.

scaling, in some cases, is all that is usually required. Two examples of inter-modality automated registrations are shown in Color Figure 11.3*.

Figure 11.4 shows an example of an MRI scan of the head and neck coregistered with SPECT reconstructions of the uptake of [^{111}In]-octreotide, which maps somatostatin receptors on certain types of cancer cells, and [^{99m}Tc]-DMSA(V) which can demonstrate calcification in medullary tumors. The registration problem in this case is not a trivial one, as the reconstructed volumes are vastly different in nature. The registration was done with a point-landmark method using fiducial markers visible on both the SPECT and MRI scans. In the absence of the MRI, it would be difficult to interpret precisely where the uptake is localized on the SPECT scan. The MRI scan, of course, gives no indication of the functional status of the receptors expressed by this cancer. An alternative method for registration would be to use the transmission scans acquired simultaneously with the SPECT scans, automatically coregister the reconstructed anatomical scans to the MRI to derive the transformation matrix, and apply these transformations to the SPECT emission data.[19]

Coregistration between PET or SPECT and anatomical modalities outside the brain has been less accurate. This is mainly due to the range of different conformations the body can assume on a scanning bed, as well as internal movement of organs within the chest and abdomen. For example, x-ray CT scans of the chest are usually taken with a breath-holding maneuver. This raises the diaphragm and affects not only the thoracic contents but abdominal contents as well. By contrast, nuclear medicine scans are usually acquired over minutes or tens of minutes, and therefore the patient will normally breath tidally. This tends to blur the organ boundaries and will cause an intrinsic misregistration internally even if the outside boundary of the patient were exactly

---

* Color Figures follow page 22.

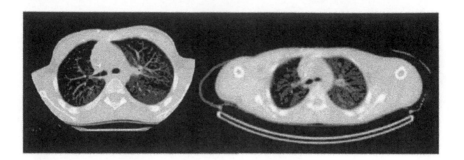

FIGURE 11.5
CT scan of the same subject acquired on a conventional fast scanner with breath hold (left) and low dose CT scan on newly developed multi-modality SPECT/PET CT device acquired over 14 seconds (GE Medical Systems, Hawkeye, right). The images demonstrate the large differences in the body shape between the different studies. Note that the subject's arms are resting at the side in the Hawkeye image. As the image on the right will match the corresponding emission scan far more closely, this image emphasises the intrinsic difficulties in coregistering scans from different devices under the different conditions. (Images courtesy of Professor Ora Israel, Rambam Medical Centre, Israel).

matched. Registration in this example requires not just translations and rotations but also additional degrees of freedom to take account of tissue deformation. An example of a large deformation is seen in Figure 11.5. Methods for nonrigid registration of images are described in Chapter 13, but this remains an area of intense investigation, especially for intermodality registration.

There is growing interest in the development of multimodality devices combining structural and functional measurements. These include human scanners capable of PET or SPECT with x-ray CT,[14,15] small animal scanning combining PET and MRI,[20] and a functional spectroscopic device combining PET and nuclear magnetic resonance spectroscopy (NMRS) for studying acute changes in an isolated rat heart model.[21] The appeal of these devices is that they acquire the different data at the same time, or at least in the same scanning session, and therefore minimize the problems of tissue deformation and any other sources of variation. When using dynamic scanning, simultaneous acquisition also provides temporal registration of the image sequences, which may be extremely difficult to achieve retrospectively. The PET-CT[14] and SPECT-CT[15] scanners for human use provide structural data from the CT scan that can be used for attenuation and scatter correction of the emission data, resolution recovery operations (discussed in the next section), and, of course, correlative imaging. It has also been suggested that they will have a future role in radiotherapy treatment planning and interventional procedures such as CT-guided biopsy. An example of a PET-CT scan performed with a prototype dual modailty scanner at the University of Pittsburgh is shown in Color Figure 11.6*.

Another application of image registration is in quantitative evaluation of serial scans. PET studies using [^{18}F]-labeled deoxyglucose ([^{18}F]-DG) are becoming increasingly available as PET scanners and gamma cameras modified to

---

* Color Figures follow page 22.

operate in coincidence mode, so called gamma camera PET (GC-PET), are more widely installed. [18F]-DG is an analogue of glucose which is potentially useful for monitoring the response of tumors to anticancer therapy. The [18F]-DG scans permit the assessment of any change in the pattern of uptake by the tumors in response to the therapy. To do so in a quantitative manner, it is desirable to realign the patient's scans so that regions of interest placed over the tumors on the initial study can be used to assess the change in [18F]-DG uptake over time in subsequent studies. Typical time courses for these studies are to scan the subject before treatment (baseline) and in the weeks and months after therapy. [18F]-DG is particularly promising, as early changes in uptake may indicate the efficacy (or not) of a particular therapy regimen. The alternatives to [18F]-DG scans are x-ray CT or MRI, where change in tumor size is taken as the measure of efficacy of treatment. Change in size, however, may take many months to occur and therefore the nuclear medicine scan can give a much earlier indication of the treatment's effectiveness.

In a collaborative study with the Oncology Imaging Group from the Royal Free Hospital in London, image registration techniques have been employed to half-body, attenuation-corrected [18F]-DG scans acquired with a gamma camera PET system in patients with advanced cancers undergoing novel anticancer therapy.[22] The aim of the work is to assess changes in [18F]-DG uptake. The patients are scanned at baseline and at 28 and 56 days after treatment. The first step in the processing is to correct each data set for differences in the injected amount of radioactivity and variations in normal physiological uptake. This is done by normalizing the reconstructed data to a reference tissue which is taken as being invariant over the different studies. As this is a study using antibody-directed therapy, the liver has been chosen as the reference tissue against which to normalize all [18F]-DG uptake in the body. After this normalization the data are realigned to the baseline scan using the mutual information algorithm of Studholme et al.,[23] described in Chapter 3. This fully automated algorithm operates on the volumetric half-body [18F]-DG scan and produces coregistered data for further analysis. Regions of interest placed over the tumors on the baseline scan are then transferred to the subsequent studies in the identical locations to provide an objective assessment of the change in [18F]-DG uptake. This removes any operator bias in defining regions of interest on individual studies. The assessment will, of course, be complicated if the tumor has changed in size over this time; however, in this approach an attempt has been made to assess objectively the quantitative uptake by the tumors in the same region. An example of one of these studies is shown in Figure 11.7.

11.4 Image Registration for Correction of Nuclear Medicine Emission Data

Nuclear medicine images suffer from a number of degrading effects. These include limited resolution, poor signal-to-noise ratio, and spatially varying loss or corruption of signal due to photon interaction with matter. Anatomical

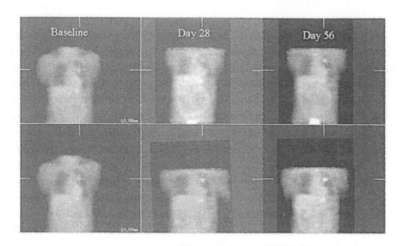

FIGURE 11.7
An example of coregistration of [^{18}F]-DG scans obtained with a gamma camera PET system is shown. The top row shows the raw, reconstructed data before realignment and the bottom row shows the studies on days 28 and 56 realigned to the baseline scan. The data were realigned with a fully automated algorithm using mutual information criteria for matching.[23] The patient had a primary cancer of the bowel with a large (2 cm) secondary lesion in the left lung (indicated by the crosshairs on the baseline scan). The lung lesion showed a 20% increase in [^{18}F]-DG uptake at day 28 compared with the baseline study and 50% increase at day 56. Note the differences in the images in the bladder (days 28 and 56) and the starting and stopping points for the scans. In spite of these differences, the automated routine performed extremely well.

images can help to correct a number of these processes and are discussed in this section.

11.4.1 Scatter and Attenuation Correction

Photons emitted from radionuclides *in vivo* have a relatively high likelihood of undergoing attenuation or scattering within the body. In emission tomography, where the task is to reconstruct a three-dimensional volume from multiple one- or two-dimensional projections, photon attenuation and scattering are confounding factors in the projection data which need to be corrected in order to produce accurate, distortion-free quantitative images. The origin of attenuation and scattering is the interaction of the photons with the tissues of the body, and this is dependent in part on the electron density of the tissues. Electron density can be measured with x-rays or gamma rays. Consequently, many investigators have used planar, line, or point sources of radionuclides and the gamma camera or PET camera to measure photon transmission[7,9,10,24,25] to provide correction factors to be used with the emission data. The use of x-ray CT scans has also been suggested.[26] Fleming et al. used x-ray CT images to produce attenuation correction factors for attenuation correction of SPECT emission data.[27] For a recent review of transmission scanning in nuclear medicine, see Bailey.[28]

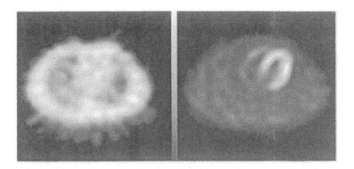

FIGURE 11.8
Simultaneous structural (transmission) and functional (emission) cardiac scan on a modern SPECT camera using scanning line sources of [153]Gd for the transmission scan and [^{99m}Tc]-tetrofosmin for the emission scan.

The structural images of electron density and the emission data need to be spatially coregistered before correcting for attenuation and scattering. If the transmission data are acquired on the gamma camera simultaneously with the emission data, registration is virtually guaranteed. However, data from x-ray CT will usually be recorded by a separate scanner on a different occasion and therefore needs to be registered to the emission data before generating the correction factors to be applied to the emission data. In addition, as x-rays are (a) usually of lower energy than the gamma rays used in nuclear medicine imaging, and (b) polychromatic (i.e., composed of a continuum of photon energies rather than a discrete single energy), some adjustments are needed to scale the attenuation coefficient (μ) to the appropriate energy for the emission nuclide.[29] Once the data have been spatially registered and scaled to the appropriate μ value they can be incorporated into the reconstruction process. An example of simultaneously acquired SPECT emission and transmission data is shown in Figure 11.8. The transmission scan not only provides a means for generating attenuation correction factors, but also an anatomical framework to aid interpretation of the emission data.

More recently, attenuation data have been incorporated into scatter correction techniques in both PET and SPECT. Coregistered SPECT attenuation and emission projection data have been used to estimate the amount of scatter (*scatter fraction*) with which to scale the scatter distribution estimate (the emission projections convolved with an appropriate scatter kernel).[30,31] The data are usually acquired in a simultaneous emission-transmission scan. A similar approach has been used with reconstructed emission and attenuation data.[32] The use of information about the body density as well as the distribution of the radiotracer permits more sophisticated estimations of the scatter, including methods based on Monte Carlo realizations[33] or direct calculation of the scatter using the physics of photon scattering cross-sections

(Klein-Nishina equation). In PET, Ollinger[34] and Watson[35] used the reconstructed emission and attenuation data to directly calculate the scatter that would be expected given the object density and radiotracer distribution. These methods have been shown to be highly accurate. All of these methods, of course, rely on spatially registered data sets. The dual-modality PET-CT and SPECT-CT systems also can use the x-ray CT data in scatter correction algorithms.

The attenuation data from simultaneous emission-transmission scans have uses beyond providing attenuation and scatter correction factors. They have been used in respiratory research in SPECT to define differences between lung volume and distribution patterns of radioactively labeled aerosols.[36-38] In the heart, Iida et al. used the reconstructed attenuation images to estimate tissue bulk in an effort to correct for resolution limitations in PET myocardial perfusion studies to produce a "perfusable tissue index," a measure of the viable tissue.[39] More sophisticated methods for partial volume correction are discussed in the next section.

11.4.2   Partial Volume Correction

Nuclear medicine images do not exhibit the same high spatial resolution that is seen in x-ray CT or MRI. Generally, the main reasons for this are limited photon flux (to minimize the radiation dose to the patient) and restrictions imposed by the physical limitations in detecting high energy gamma radiation with scintillation crystals. The typical spatial resolution in emission tomography varies from 2 to 4 mm for high resolution PET scanners to approximately 12 to 18 mm for SPECT systems. This leads to a characteristic known as the partial volume effect. This "blurring," due to limited spatial resolution, causes an object to appear larger than it is if its true size is less than approximately three times the system resolution.[40] While the **total** reconstructed counts within the object are conserved, the count **density** is decreased from the true value because the data are "smeared" over a larger area. A simple method to estimate the true count density is to take the total counts in the "blurred" representation of the object (organ, tumor, etc.) and normalize the count density to the actual area of the object as measured by x-ray CT or MRI. More sophisticated approaches use the anatomical data to perform a pixel-by-pixel correction of the emission data, with *a priori* knowledge of the expected biodistribution patterns.[41] An example is shown in Figure 11.9.

These procedures work, in general, in the following way. The structural and functional data are first coregistered to the same space with a suitable algorithm. Next, the structural scan is segmented into a number of discrete, homogeneous compartments between which radiotracer uptake is known to differ (e.g., differences between gray and white matter uptake in the brain reflecting differences in glucose metabolism, blood flow, or receptor density). A probability is then assigned to a photon arising from each of the different compartments (say 4:1:0 for gray matter:white matter:CSF, skull or

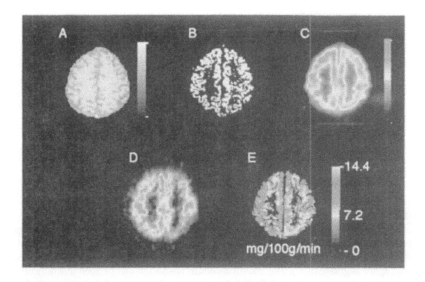

FIGURE 11.9
Partial volume effect correction in an iterative reconstruction algorithm. The images show
A) segmented MRI scan, B) extracted gray matter compartment, C) FDG PET scan, D) partial
volume corrected FDG PET scan, and E) the partial volume corrected PET scan superimposed on the structural MRI scan. (Images courtsey of Dr Claire Labbé, University Hospital
of Geneva and CERMEP.)

outside the brain in this example), and the relative "spill-in" and "spill-out" for
each compartment calculated. This process may be performed iteratively using
updated estimates of the radiotracer distribution at each step. There are many
variations on this general approach (see, for example, Rousset et al.[42]).

11.4.3 Anatomically Guided Reconstruction

New developments in reconstruction algorithms, which apply partial volume correction in an earlier step in the processing sequence, incorporate
knowledge of the object's boundaries into the reconstruction in an attempt
to improve upon the limited spatial resolution by restoration of the emission data during reconstruction.[43–45] Much prior information can be built into
iterative reconstruction schema, such as photon attenuation, scattering, and
an intrinsic correction for the blurring or limited spatial resolution of the
measuring systems.[46] The underlying idea behind so called "anatomically
guided reconstruction" is that the functional image is strongly correlated
with the anatomical distribution of known sites of radiopharmaceutical
uptake, e.g., receptors, tumors, boundaries of organs, the cerebral gray/white
matter interface, etc. These algorithms produce a probabilistic estimate of the
likely distribution which has given rise to the two-dimensional projection
data measured, test this against the actual measured projection data, modify
the estimated reconstruction in some deterministic way, and then again test

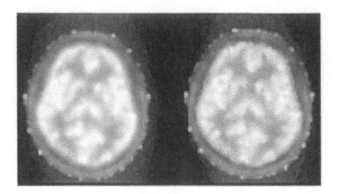

FIGURE 11.10
One slice of a PET [^{18}F]-DG scan of the brain is shown. The image on the left was reconstructed with a conventional iterative reconstruction algorithm and the image on the right
was reconstructed using anatomical priors (gray matter, white matter, skull, CSF, and sub-
rachnoid space segmentation). The improvement in resolution can be seen in the "guided"
reconstruction. (Image courtesy of Dr Babek Ardekani, University of Technology, Sydney).

it against the measured projection data. This procedure is performed iteratively until a match between the measured and the estimated data is
achieved. The simplest example of such a guide is to use the outline of the
patient's body, which can be measured in a variety of ways (Compton scatter
window,[47] transmission scan, CT scan, etc.). By "encouraging" the solution to
match in some prescribed way the known anatomical boundaries of the
object, higher resolution reconstructions can be achieved.[48,49] To do this it is
necessary to have coregistered, segmented data which have been classified
according to the expectation of their functional uptake of the radiotracer.[50] An
example of the improvement achievable using anatomically guided reconstruction is shown in Figure 11.10.

11.5   Spatial Normalization

Spatial normalization refers to a type of intersubject registration involving the
transformation of images into a common, predefined standard space, which
often implies a distortion of the original organ. The purpose of doing this is to
be able to compare data from one subject with those from the same subject
studied at a different time, or against other subjects. An important application for this is to compare a patient scan against a database of normals having
the same scan. For this application, the data need to be transformed into a
standard representation.

One of the first uses of spatial normalization applied to nuclear medicine
images was in the analysis and display of myocardial perfusion scans. This is
one of the most frequently performed diagnostic tests in clinical nuclear medicine. The aim of the test is to assess areas of compromised blood flow in the

a. A scan at resting work rate and therefore basal myocardial perfusion, and

b. A scan at peak stress where the radiotracer is injected as the patient is undergoing a paradigm designed to increase myocardial perfusion, either by physical exertion or pharmacological stress on the heart.

A common clinical question asked of this scan is whether areas of decreased blood flow at stress are normally perfused at rest: this "reversibility" indicates compromised blood flow in the arteries supplying the myocardium, but normal underlying myocardial tissue. This may be improved by surgical intervention. The fact that the rest scan is normal indicates that the underlying myocardium is still functionally viable. In this example, therefore, the study at stress and the study at rest need to be realigned to detect differences. Visual inspection of the aligned images is often sufficient to report the scan. However, a valuable tool to assess the change quantitatively is to compare both the stress and rest studies with normal databases from subjects who have undergone the same scan but with proven low likelihood of any myocardial perfusion deficit. As the shape and size of different individuals' hearts will vary, a spatial normalization step is required to "transform" each heart to a standardized representation.

To illustrate this, a pair of stress/rest scans of a subject are shown in Figure 11.11. The data are from a SPECT study using [^{99m}Tc]-tetrofosmin. The top rows show the stress and rest scans coregistered using an automated routine.[51] Next, myocardial perfusion throughout the left ventricle is determined and plotted as a function of angle around the circular sections of the myocardium seen in the scan. In an idealized scan, a profile generated over 360° around the myocardium in the short axis views would produce a constant count. Due to normal variations in myocardial thickness and perfusion the profile is not necessarily constant. This process is repeated for all of the slices through the short axis projections and therefore the entire left ventricular myocardium is mapped to a series of profiles of perfusion. A common method for displaying these profiles in a compressed manner is the so called "polar plot" display.[52] Each profile is mapped from the base of the heart to the apex onto a series of concentric rings as if the three-dimensional ellipsoid of the left ventricle has been "squashed." Once in this format, the data are now represented in a standard, spatially normalized space and can be compared against other individuals' scans. These can be seen in the lower pair of images in Figure 11.11. Some larger clinical centers have generated normal databases in this manner which consist of a series of subjects' count profiles.[53] Individual subjects can be compared statistically against the normal population profiles to objectively assess changes which may be outside the normal range. This is one of the first examples in nuclear medicine of the use of spatial transformations for cohort studies. By virtue of the simplification of a three-dimensional ellipsoidal distribution into a single image, the polar plot has

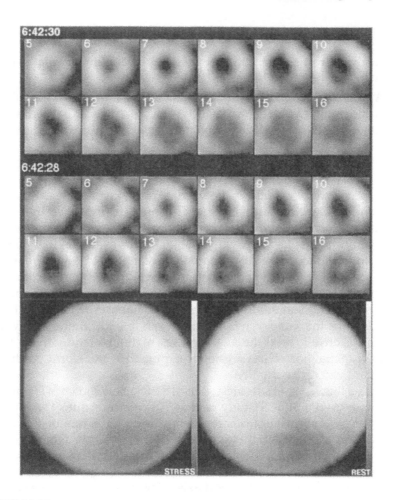

FIGURE 11.11
A SPECT stress/rest myocardial perfusion study (upper rows), spatially normalized and displayed as a polar plot (lower two images) for all slices, is shown. The top two rows show reconstructed sections through the left ventricle of the heart when the tracer was injected while the heart was being stressed. The sections are sliced from apex towards the base of the heart (the valve plane). The next two rows show the same heart after the tracer has been injected at rest. The polar plots on the bottom for stress (left) and rest (right) condense the multiple slices into a single display, where the apical slices are located in the center of the image and the basal slices are at the edges. There is a small "notch" of decreased perfusion at stress in the upper section of the reconstructions (labeled 7–10, top row) which corresponds to the anterior myocardial wall, and which is normal at rest. This is seen in the top half, center, of the polar plots. Once the data are in this standard representation, they can be compared with a data base of "normals" to assess the significance of the defects. The large dark area at the lower right half of the polar plots corresponds to the valve plane of the heart where there is little myocardium, and is a normal appearance.

achieved popularity. It has been used widely in myocardial imaging in both SPECT (perfusion) and PET (myocardial blood flow, [^{18}F]-DG uptake, adreno-receptors). The method has also been applied for the comparison of PET and SPECT cardiac data in the same subject.[54]

Spatial normalization is not only used in myocardial scanning. A common application in neuroscience research is to assess the change in a functional parameter (cerebral perfusion, cerebral glucose metabolism) in response to some challenge or stimulation such as a motor, cognitive, or sensory task. These "cerebral activation" studies demonstrating functional anatomy have been widely reported in both the scientific and popular literature and are discussed in Chapter 14. As in the case of myocardial perfusion scanning, the data need to be spatially normalized to a standard space to permit comparisons with scans from other individuals. Friston et al. chose a neuro-anatomical atlas of a normal brain published by Talaraich and Tournoux[55] as the standard space for their PET scan analysis.[56] Much effort has gone into producing high quality standard atlases for neuroimaging,[57–59] and much of this work continues. Functional anatomical studies of the brain now employ such diverse measurement devices as SPECT, PET, functional MRI (fMRI), ERP (event-related potential measured using EEG), and magneto-encephalography (MEG). Standardization of the space for reporting the data from all of these devices is necessary to provide a common platform for discussing results in this new, emerging field. A standard model has also been developed for the airways of the lung,[60] which has application in the modeling of the distribution of inhaled radioactively labeled particles throughout the airways.[61] The aim of standardization in these applications is to aid in targeting drugs to specific generations of the airways.

11.6 Conclusions and Future Directions

Coregistration with images from complementary modalities has been employed in nuclear medicine for many decades. It acts as an adjunct to interpretation of the functional nuclear medicine images, as well as offering the ability to overcome some intrinsic limitations in nuclear medicine images. We are currently witnessing an increasing convergence in the combination of structural and functional data, most notably in the development of dual modality imaging devices. Even with single modality devices, we will see further developments of algorithms and software to enhance the information provided in combination with other complementary data.

The applications and use of image registration in nuclear medicine in the near future will include:

- Correlative image interpretation
- Attenuation correction

- Scatter correction
- Correction for limited resolution
- Improving reconstruction accuracy in emission tomography
- Coregistration of serial functional studies
- Transformation to standard space for comparison with normal studies
- Transformation to standard space for comparison with data from other modalities (multiparametric functional imaging)
- Conformal radiotherapy treatment planning
- Functionally guided biopsy

There will, no doubt, be many more applications as the devices and algorithms become more widely available and researchers and clinicians develop innovative approaches to diagnosing and treating human disease. The future will see developments in the use of multiparametric mapping combining functional and structural data from a wide variety of measuring systems. Nuclear medicine can only benefit from such evolving integration, in which image registration plays a central role.

Acknowledgment

I am grateful to my colleague Richard Lewis for providing a number of the examples shown in this chapter, and for proofreading the drafts.

References

1. Phelps, M.E. and Coleman, R.E., Nuclear medicine in the new millennium. *J. Nucl. Med.* 2000; 41(1):1–4.
2. Kuhl, D.E., Hale, J., and Eaton, W.L., Transmission scanning: a useful adjunct to conventional emission scanning for accurately keying isotope deposition to radiographic anatomy. *Radiology* 1966; 87:278.
3. Anger, H.O. and McRae, J., Transmission scintiphotography. *J. Nucl. Med.* 1968; 9(6):267–269.
4. McRae, J. and Anger, H.O., Transmission scintiphotography and its applications, in: *Medical Radioisotope Scintigraphy*; Salzburg: Intl. Atomic Energy Agency; 1968. p. 57–69.
5. Sorenson, J.A., Briggs, R.C., and Cameron, J.R., ^{99m}Tc point source for transmission scanning. *J. Nucl. Med.* 1969; 10(5):252–253.

6. Tothill, P. and Galt, J.M., Quantitative profile scanning for the measurement of organ radioactivity. *Phys. Med. Biol.* 1971; 16:625–634.

7. Morozumi, T., Nakajima, M., Ogawa, K., and Yuta, S., Attenuation correction methods using the information of attenuation distribution for single photon emission CT. *Med. Imag. Tech.* 1984; 2:20–28.

8. Macey, D. and Marshall, R., Absolute quantitation of radiotracer uptake in lungs using a gamma camera. *J. Nucl. Med.* 1984; 23:731–735.

9. Malko, J.A., Van Heertum, R.L., Gullberg, G.T., and Kowalsky, W.P., SPECT liver imaging using an iterative attenuation correction algorithm and an external flood source. *J. Nucl. Med.* 1986; 27:701–705.

10. Bailey, D.L., Hutton, B.F., and Walker, P.J., Improved SPECT using simultaneous emission and transmission tomography. *J. Nucl. Med.* 1987; 28(5):844–851.

11. Tan, P., Bailey, D.L., Meikle, S.R., Eberl, S., Fulton, R.R., and Hutton, B.F. A scanning line source for simultaneous emission and transmission measurements in SPECT. *J. Nucl. Med.* 1993; 34(10):1752–1760.

12. Tung, C-H., Gullberg, G.T., Zeng, G.L., Christian, P.E., Datz, F.L., and Morgan, H.T. Non-uniform attenuation correction using simultaneous transmission and emission converging tomography. *IEEE. Trans. Nucl. Sci.* 1992; 39(4):1134–1143.

13. Celler, A., Sitek, A., Stoub, E., Lyster, D., and Dykstra, C., Development of a multiple line-source array for SPECT transmission scans. *J. Nucl. Med.* 1997; 38(5)(Supplement):215P–216P.

14. Townsend, D.W., Kinahan, P.E., and Beyer, T., Attenuation correction for a combined 3D PET/CT scanner. *Physica Medica* 1996; XII (Suppl 1):43–48.

15. Lang, T.F., Hasegawa, B.H., Liew, S.C., Brown, J.K., Blankespoor, S.C., Reilly, S.M., et al. Description of a prototype emission-transmission computed tomography imaging system. *J. Nucl. Med.* 1992; 33(10):1881–1887.

16. Hawkes, D.J., Robinson, L., Crossman, J.E., Sayman, H.B., Mistry, R., Maisey, M.N., et al. Registration and display of the combined bone scan and radiograph in the diagnosis and management of wrist injuries. *Eur. J. Nucl. Med.* 1991; 18(9):752–756.

17. Woods, R.P., Mazziotta, J.C., and Cherry, S.R., MRI-PET Registration with automated algorithm. *J. Comput. Assist. Tomogr.* 1993; 17(4):536–546.

18. Watson, J.D.G., Myers, R., Frackowiak, R.S.J., Hajnal, J.V., Woods, R.P., Mazziotta, J.C., et al. Area V5 of the human brain: evidence from a combined study using positron emission tomography and magnetic resonance imaging. *Cereb. Cortex.* 1993; 3(2):79–94.

19. Sipila, O., Nikkinen, P., Savolainen, S., Granstrom, M-L., Gaily, E., Poutanen, V-P., et al. Transmission imaging for registration of ictal and interictal single-photon emission tomography, magnetic resonance imaging and electroencephalography. *Eur. J. Nucl. Med.* 2000; 27(2):202–205.

20. Shao, Y., Cherry, S.R., Farahani, K., Slates, R., Silverman, R.W., Meadors, K., et al. Development of a PET detector system compatible with MRI/NMR systems. *IEEE. Trans. Nucl. Sci.* 1997; NS-44:1167–1171.

21. Marsden, P.K., Shoa, Y., Cherry, S.R., Cave, A., Parkes, H.G., Silverman, R.W., et al. Simultaneous acquisition of PET Images and NMR spectra in a high field magnet. *J. Nucl. Med.* 1997; 38(5[Supplement]):45P.

22. Bailey, D.L., Adamson, K.L., Francis, R.J., Green, A.J., and Begent, R.H.J., A method for longitudinal quantitative assessment of response to anti-cancer therapy with FDG and hybrid PET. *J. Nucl. Med.* 2000; 41(5(Suppl)):183P.

23. Studholme, C., Hill, D.L.G., and Hawkes, D.J., Automated 3D registration of MR and PET brain images by multi-resolution optimisation of voxel similarity measures. *Med. Physics* 1997; 24:25–35.

24. Karp, J.S., Muehllehner, G., Qu, H., and Yan, X-H., Singles transmission in volume-imaging PET with a ^{137}Cs source. *Phys. Med. Biol.* 1995; 40:929–944.

25. deKemp, R.A. and Nahmias, C. Attenuation correction in PET using single photon transmission measurement. *Med. Phys.* 1994; 21(6):771–778.

26. Moore, S.C., Attenuation compensation, in: Ell, P.J., Holman, B.L., Eds. *Computed Emission Tomography.* London: Oxford University Press; 1982. p. 339–360.

27. Fleming, J.S., A technique for using CT images in attenuation correction and quantification in SPECT. *Nucl. Med. Commun.* 1989; 10:83–97.

28. Bailey, D.L., Transmission scanning in emission tomography. *Eur. J. Nucl. Med.* 1998; 25(7):774–787.

29. Beyer, T., Kinahan, P.E., Townsend, D.W., and Sashin, D., The use of X-ray CT for attenuation correction of PET data, in: Trendler, R.C., Ed. *IEEE Nuclear Science Symposium and Medical Imaging Conference;* 1994; Norfolk, VA: Inst of Electrical and Electronic Engineers; 1994. p. 1573–1577.

30. Bailey, D.L., Hutton, B.F., Meikle, S.R., Fulton, R.R., and Jackson, C.B., Iterative scatter correction incorporating attenuation data. *Eur. J. Nucl. Med.* 1989; 15:452 (Abstract).

31. Meikle, S.R., Hutton, B.F., and Bailey, D.L., A transmission dependent method for scatter correction in SPECT. *J. Nucl. Med.* 1994; 35(2):360–367.

32. Welch, A., Gullberg, G.T., Christian, P.E., and Datz, F.L., A transmission-map-based scatter correction technique for SPECT in inhomogeneous media. *Med. Phys.* 1995; 22(10):1627–1635.

33. Ljungberg, M. and Strand, S-E., Scatter and attenuation correction in SPECT using density maps and Monte Carlo simulated scatter functions. *J. Nucl. Med.* 1990; 31:1560–1567.

34. Ollinger, J.M., Model-based scatter correction for fully 3D PET. *Phys. Med. Biol.* 1996; 41(1):153–176.

35. Watson, C.C., Newport, D., and Casey, M.E., A single scatter simulation technique for scatter correction in 3D PET, in: Grangeat, P. and Amans, J-L., Eds. *Three-Dimensional Image Reconstruction in Radiology and Nuclear Medicine.* Dordrecht: Kluwer Academic; 1996. p. 255–268.

36. Phipps, P.R., Gonda, I., Bailey, D.L., Borham, P.W., Bautovich, G.J., and Anderson, S.D., Comparison of planar and tomographic scintigraphy to measure the penetration index of inhaled aerosols. *Am. Rev. Resp. Dis.* 1989; 139: 1516–1523.

37. Phipps, P.R., Gonda, I., Anderson, S.D., Bailey, D.L., and Bautovich, G.J. Regional deposition of saline aerosols of different tonicities in normal and asthmatic subjects. *Eur. Respir. J.* 1994; 7(8):1474–1482.

38. King, G.G., Eberl, S., Salome, C.M., Meikle, S.R., and Woolcock, A.J., Airway closure measured by a technegas bolus and SPECT. *Am. J. Respir. Crit. Care. Med.* 1997; 155(2):682–688.

39. Iida, H., Rhodes, C.G., de Silva, R., Yamamoto, Y., Araujo, L.I., Maseri, A., et al. Myocardial tissue fraction—correction for partial volume effects and measure of tissue viability. *J. Nucl. Med.* 1991; 32:2169–2175.

40. Sorenson, J.A., and Phelps, M.E., *Physics in Nuclear Medicine.* Orlando: Harcourt Brace Jovanovich; 1987.

41. Labbé, C., Froment, J.C., Kennedy, A., Ashburner, J., and Cinotto, L., Positron emission tomography metabolic data correction for cortical atrophy using magnetic resonance imaging. *Alzheimer. Dis. & Assoc. Disord.* 1996; 10:141–170.
42. Rousset, O.G., Ma, Y., and Evans, A.C. Correction for partial volume effects in PET: principle and validation. *J. Nucl. Med.* 1998; 39(5):904–11.
43. Leahy, R. and Yan, X., Incorporation of anatomical MR data for improved functional imaging with PET, in: Colchester, A.C.F. and Hawkes, D.J., Eds. *Information Processing in Medical Imaging.* New York: Springer-Verlag; 1991. p. 105–120.
44. Ouyang, X., Wong, W.H., Johnson, V.E., Hu, X., and Chen, C-T., Incorporation of correlated structural images in PET image reconstruction. *IEEE Trans. Med. Imag.* 1994; MI-14(4):627–640.
45. Ardekani, B.A., Braun, M. and Hutton, B.F., Improved quantification with the use of anatomical information in PET image reconstruction, in: Uemura, K., Lassen, N.A., Jones, T., and Kanno, I., Eds. *Quantification of Brain Function: Tracer Kinetics and Image Analysis in Brain PET:* Elsevier; 1993. p. 351–362.
46. Lange, K. and Carson, R., EM reconstruction algorithms for emission and transmission tomography. *J. Comput. Assist. Tomogr.* 1984; 8:306–316.
47. Jaszczak, R.J., Chang, L.T., and Stein, N.A., Whole body single photon emission computed tomography using large field of view scintillation cameras. *Phys. Med. Biol.* 1979; 24:1123–1143.
48. Ardekani, B.A., Braun, M., Hutton, B.F., and Kanno, I., Minimum cross-entropy reconstruction of PET images using prior anatomical information obtained from MR, in: Myers, R., Cunningham, V.J., Bailey, D.L., and Jones, T., Eds. *Quantification of Brain Function Using PET.* San Diego: Academic Press; 1996. p. 113–117.
49. Hsu, C.H.L. and Leahy, R.M., PET Image reconstruction incorporating anatomical information using segmented regression, in: *Medical Imaging 97*, SPIE; 1997; Newport Beach CA, 1997.
50. Ardekani, B.A., Braun, M.I.K., and Hutton, B.F., Automatic detection of intradural spaces in MR images. *J. Comput. Assist. Tomogr.* 1994; 18(6):963–969.
51. Slomka, P.J., Hurwitz, G.A., Stephenson, J., and Cradduck, T., Automated alignment and sizing of myocardial stress and rest scans to three-dimensional normal templates using an image registration algorithm. *J. Nucl. Med.* 1995; 36(6):1115–1122.
52. DePascquale, E.E., Nody, A.A., and DePuey, E.G., Quantitative rotational thallium-201 tomography for identifying and localizing coronary artery disease. *Circulation* 1988; 77:316–327.
53. Kiat, H., VanTrain, K., and Berman, D. Quantitative analysis of SPECT—Thallium-201 reversibility: development and preliminary validation of an objective method. *J. Nucl. Med.* 1989; 1989:739.
54. Gilardi, M.C., Rizzo, G., Savi, A., Landoni, C., Bettinardi, V., Rossetti, C., et al. Correlation of SPECT and PET cardiac images by a surface matching registration technique. *Comput. Med. Imag. Graphics* 1998; 22(5):391–398.
55. Talairach, J. and Tournoux, P., *Co-Planar Stereotactic Atlas of the Human Brain: 3-Dimensional Proportional System: An Approach to Cerebral Imaging.* Stuttgart: Georg Thieme Verlag; 1988.
56. Friston, K.J., Ashburner, J., Frith, C.D., Poline, J-B., Heather, J.D., and Frackowiak, R.S.J., Spatial registration and normalisation of images. *Human Brain Mapping* 1995; 2:165–189.

57. Evans, A.C., Marrett, S., Neelin, P., Collins, L., Worsley, K., Dai, W., et al. Anatomical mapping of functional activation in stereotactic coordinate space. *Neuroimage* 1992; 1(1):43–53.
58. Mazziotta, J.C., Toga, A.W., Evans, A., Fox, P., and Lancaster, J., A probabilistic atlas of the human brain: theory and rationale for its development. The International Consortium for Brain Mapping (ICBM). *Neuroimage* 1995; 2(2):89–101.
59. Thompson, P.M., MacDonald, D., Mega, M.S., Holmes, C.J., Evans, A.C., and Toga, A.W., Detection and mapping of abnormal brain structure with a probabilistic atlas of cortical surfaces. *J. Comput. Assis. Tomog.* 1997; 21(4):567–581.
60. Sauret, V., Goatman, K.A., Fleming, J.S., and Bailey, A.G., Semi-automated tabulation of the 3D topology and morphology of branching networks using CT: application to the airway tree. *Phys. Med. Biol.* 1999; 44(7):1625–1638.
61. Fleming, J.S., Halson, P., Conway, J., Moore, E., Nassim, M.A., Hashish, A.H., et al. Three-dimensional description of pulmonary deposition of inhaled aerosol using data from multimodality imaging. *J. Nucl. Med.* 1996; 37(5):873–877.

12

Guiding Therapeutic Procedures

Philip J. Edwards, David J. Hawkes, Graeme P. Penney,
and Matthew J. Clarkson

CONTENTS

12.1 Introduction

Just over two months after the discovery of x-rays, a bromide print was used to aid in the surgical removal of a needle from a woman's hand.[1] In conventional clinical practice today, the wide range of medical imaging modalities available are largely used for diagnosis or monitoring the progression of disease. During an intervention, images showing the pathology and surrounding anatomy may be displayed on a light box, but the correspondence between image and patient is established entirely in the mind of the clinician, using knowledge of anatomy and surgical appearance accrued over many years of training. In many procedures it would be desirable if this correspondence between image and patient could be achieved by some more accurate and ergonomic method, providing the interventionist with aligned radiological data showing the position of the target and surrounding critical structures. The goal is to make procedures less invasive, faster, and safer.

Alignment of therapeutic equipment to the patient using radiological data has long been a routine part of radiotherapy and frame-based stereotactic neurosurgery. With the advent of 3D volume imaging techniques there has been increasing interest in wider application of image guidance using more flexible alignment processes and improved visualization to enhance the data available to the interventionist. Here, rather than registering different imaging modalities, the technical aim is to take preoperative images and align them to the physical space of the patient.

The use of imaging during a procedure has created the discipline of interventional radiology. In this scenario both the target and the therapeutic device are visible in the real-time images. Examples of this include fluoroscopic guidance of stent placement and ultrasound-guided breast biopsy. Endoscopic procedures, such as laparoscopic surgery, also have the target and the surgical tool visible in the same optical image. Though these interventions may be termed "image-guided," there is no registration issue, and as such we will not consider these procedures in this chapter. We are interested in the incorporation of images taken before an intervention, which must be aligned to the patient. Real-time imaging may have a role in this process, however, with preoperative images enhancing the real-time view or the intraoperative images aiding in the registration process.

The registration problem can be stated as follows. We have a detailed 3D description of patient anatomy and perhaps physiology from preoperative imaging modalities. In the treatment room we have a position measurement, imaging, or treatment device which defines a coordinate system in 3D physical space. We wish to align the preoperative images to physical space in order to present the clinician with the preoperative data correctly aligned to the patient.

It would be impossible to cover in depth the full range of existing and potential clinical applications of image guidance in a single chapter. Our account will be confined to the more common applications in which we have some experience, and those that raise particular algorithmic problems. We start by examining methods employed in the more conventional tracked pointer systems and then move on to consider areas of research in intraoperative registration using real-time imaging such as ultrasound, fluoroscopy, video, and MRI. Applications in both improving rigid registration and compensating for tissue deformation are discussed. Finally, we look at visualization and interaction of the therapist with the guidance data.

12.2 Technical Issues

A number of technical problems must be solved to provide image guidance. First, a 3D coordinate system in the treatment room must be defined. The patient must then be immobilized or tracked with respect to this coordinate system. Finally, corresponding features need to be identified in the preoperative image, and physically on the patient.

If an intraoperative or perioperative imaging device is to be used to find these features on the patient, there are further technical considerations. The imaging device must be calibrated to relate the image coordinates to 3D space. The registration problem then becomes that of alignment of the intraoperative and preoperative images. This can be achieved either by extraction of salient features or using a voxel intensity-based method.

The term *perioperative imaging* is sometimes used to describe imaging immediately prior to the procedure or immediately after its completion. It also covers procedures where the operation must stop while imaging takes place. The term *intraoperative* will be used to cover all imaging at the time of the operation.

12.2.1 Defining the Operating Room Coordinate System

To align images to the patient, it is first necessary to define a coordinate system within the operating room (OR). A number of coordinate measuring devices have been developed for this purpose. Errors in tracking will first be considered, and then each of these devices will be briefly described.

12.2.1.1 *Error in Registration of Images to Physical Space*

The clinical accuracy requirement of image guidance is one of the most important criteria when deciding which technology to apply to a particular application. Engineers use the word "error" to define the limits to accuracy of a system. Surgeons prefer "accuracy" because of the wider connotation of the word "error" in surgery. Some insist that their system never introduces any error. In this chapter we stick with the engineers' definition.

Different definitions of registration error have caused some confusion in the past, so before introducing the different technologies it is worth defining the relevant measures of error. The terms used here were introduced in Section 3.4.1.2 of Chapter 3, and discussed in detail in Section 6.2.1 of Chapter 6. Image-guided surgery relies on identifying corresponding features both in preoperative images and the physical space of the patient in the operating room or interventional suite. An error will be associated with locating these features in the images. There will also be an error in identifying the physical location of these points in the patient. If these features are defined as points in both, such as the centers of spheres or cylinders[2,3] or intersection of two lines,[4] the error in correspondence is often referred to as the fiducial localization error (FLE).[5] The corresponding features are used to compute a coordinate transformation between the images and physical space. This coordinate transformation is then used to predict where a point in physical space—the "target," indicated, for example, with a hand-held pointer—is located in the preoperative images.

The error in predicting location of the target in the preoperative image is often referred to as target registration error (TRE). Fitzpatrick et al. have derived a formula for TRE from the point distribution in fiducial point-based registration assuming that the FLE is isotropic and randomly distributed.[5] Point-based registration using the orthogonal Procrustes method also computes a residual root-mean-square (RMS) error on aligning the points, which is sometimes termed the fiducial registration error (FRE). It is important to remember that FRE does not estimate TRE. In particular, discarding points until the FRE drops below some threshold is a very poor way of ensuring a good TRE.

A number of sources of error contribute to the overall system error of any surgical navigation system. These include:

- Error in locating features for registration in the images. This is determined by the size and shape of the features and the spatial and contrast resolution of the images.
- Scaling errors and other geometric distortions in the images.
- Error in locating the same features in the physical space of the patient.
- Any relative movement of these features between imaging and intervention. For example, skin is mobile, so skin markers can move.

- The breakdown of assumptions inherent in the type of transformation used. Almost all image guidance assumes a six degree of freedom rigid-body transformation between images and physical space, so any tissue deformation, voluntary or involuntary, by the patient, or tissue distortion caused by the intervention itself will lead to error.

12.2.1.2 Mechanical Localizers

The first frameless neuronavigation device to be widely used was the Faro arm (Faro Technologies Inc., Florida, U.S.), a mechanical device that is attached to the side of the surgical table. Encoders on each of the axes of the arm enable calculation of the tip position. Problems with such a device are that range of movement is somewhat limited, and any movement of the head clamp requires reregistration. Moreover, the inherent accuracy was found to be somewhat lower than other methods. Marketed as the ISG Viewing Wand, this mechanical localizer started the regular use of frameless image guidance, finding applications in ear, nose, and throat (ENT) surgery[6] and neurosurgery.[7-10]

12.2.1.3 Ultrasound Transducers in Air

The first example of frameless navigation was the system developed by Roberts et al.[11] This system used a microscope to register the images to the patient and provide the guidance information. The localization system was based on ultrasonic "spark-gap" transducers attached to the microscope. These emit a very short ultrasound pulse which can be detected by three or more microphones in the operating room. The time delay for the sound pulse to reach each microphone gives a measure of distance and hence localizes the spark gap. Others have developed this technology for conventional pointer-based guidance,[12] where the transducers are attached to a wand. Some problems have been encountered due to variations of the speed of sound with temperature and air flow which led to a significant fiducial localization error of several millimeters, but research is still being carried out to refine the method.[13]

12.2.1.4 Radio Frequency Tracking

Another technology that has been proposed for surgical tracking is radio frequency (RF) coils. Three large orthogonal coils are used to transmit a signal that is picked up by three smaller orthogonal coils inside a tracker attached to the patient or pointing device. The signal received by each of the receiver coils can be used to calculate the position and orientation of the tracker. These devices suffer from inaccuracies when brought close to metal due to distortion of the RF field. This distortion can lead to FLEs of several centimeters, and there is usually no way of knowing that the accuracy has been compromised in this way. For neurosurgery, a wooden or plastic operating table needs to be constructed. Interference with other devices in the operating theater has also been reported.

12.2.1.5 Active/Passive Optical Tracker

With three linear cameras or two 2D cameras, if a point can be located in each view, the 3D position of the point relative to the cameras can be calculated. This is the basis of a number of tracking systems. The localized points are either active (bright infrared-emitting diodes, IREDs) or passive (highly reflecting spheres). In smaller camera systems such as the Polaris from Northern Digital Inc. (Ontario, Canada) or Flashpoint from Image-Guided Technologies (Colorado, U.S.), each IRED or reflecting sphere can be localized with a FLE of 0.2 to 0.4 mm. With the Optotrak, a larger and more expensive version from Northern Digital, accuracy is 0.1 to 0.2 mm. The main difficulty with optical tracking is that line of sight between the cameras and tracked objects must be maintained. An additional possible error source with the reflecting sphere system is partial obscuration of the sphere or contamination with blood, which may shift the measured location. Nevertheless, the high accuracy and stability of these systems has meant that optical tracking is now the technology of choice for most commercial image-guided surgery systems.

12.2.2 Immobilization Techniques

Having defined a coordinate system for the room, we now want to describe physical points inside the patient. To define accurate coordinates within a patient, the subject must be rigidly fixed with respect either to a tracker or the coordinate measurement device itself.

12.2.2.1 Stereotactic Frames

Stereotactic frames have been used in neurosurgery since the 1950s. These devices are rigidly attached to the patient's skull prior to imaging. High contrast imaging markers relate the frame to a trajectory and target defined from the images. The therapeutic device, usually a biopsy needle or electrode, is then mounted on the frame, for example via an isocentric arc system. The angles on the arc are calculated to give the required trajectory. Since the frame inherently defines a coordinate system, there is no need for any of the tracking technologies described in the previous section.

Stereotactic frames have the advantage that they have been used for many years and are well understood by surgeons. They are also considered by many clinicians to be the most accurate guidance method and have been measured as providing registration accuracies of better than 1 mm.[14] There have, however, been some suggestions that the accuracy is overstated.[15] The disadvantages are that only a single point target and trajectory can be defined, the frame is invasive and uncomfortable for the patient as the device has to remain fixed to the patient's skull from imaging to surgery, and the bulky device hampers any kind of complex surgical approach. These factors limit the application of stereotactic frames primarily to biopsies and placement of cannulae or electrodes.

12.2.2.2 Head Clamp

The most common method of immobilization recommended by commercial systems is to attach a tracker to a head clamp, such as the Mayfield head clamp (Ohio Medical Instrument Company Inc., Cincinnati, Ohio). These clamps are often used in neurosurgery and have the advantage over stereo-tactic frames that they are not required during imaging and allow much freer access to the patient for open surgery. With a Mayfield clamp or similar device, a process of registration is required at the beginning of the proce-dure. A tracking device can be attached to the clamp when the patient is positioned to track any movement of the clamp and, hence, the head during the procedure.

12.2.2.3 Molded Devices

An alternative method to screwing a device firmly into the bone of the patient's skull during imaging and therapy is to use a patient-specific mold that can be accurately removed and replaced. In radiotherapy, for example, a cast of the patient's head is taken and a plastic mold is made. This device is used to ensure that the patient is immobilized and placed correctly in a simulator room where the images are taken that will be used to plan the treat-ment. The same mold is then used to position the patient in the treatment room.

The accuracy of guidance using these devices is determined by the repeat-ability and stability of the patient position with respect to the mold. A head mold covers the skin of the face and accuracy is therefore limited by move-ment of the patient's skin. Such masks are generally considered to give ther-apy accurate to 3 to 5 mm.[16] For surgery guidance, a significantly higher accuracy is needed. Blocks molded to fit the patient's upper teeth have been proposed as a more accurate method.[17,18] Such blocks allow free movement of the patient's head, which is desirable in ENT surgery, and also place the tracker close to the target volume. Target registration errors of 1 to 2 mm RMS have been achieved with such devices.[18]

In spinal surgery, a mold of the relevant vertebra may be made by stero-lithography from a CT scan of the patient. The desired trajectory of pedicle screws in the spinous processes can be marked as part of the planning pro-cess and, guide holes made in the prototyped block. During surgery this block is simply clipped into place on the correct vertebra and the screws inserted through the guide holes.[19]

12.3   3D Image-to-Physical Space Registration

Having defined a coordinate system within the patient, it is now necessary to align the preoperative images to this space. The process essentially consists of identifying features in the preoperative images which can also be found on the patient using the localization device.

While there are some similarities between image-to-image registration and image-to-physical registration, there are specific problems associated with image acquisition and identifying the physical features on the patient in the operating room.

12.3.1   Preoperative Image Preparation and Planning

Care has to be taken in the acquisition of images for image guidance. The images must be acquired with sufficient spatial resolution for the guidance task. In practice, for CT and MRI this means that the slice thickness must be sufficiently small. It is not unusual to need a slice thickness of 3 mm or less in CT or MRI. The slice thicknesses of 5 mm or more in diagnostic imaging will make it hard, if not impossible, to identify features with the submillimetric accuracy necessary for certain image guidance applications.

Geometric image calibration is required as part of the quality assurance of the imaging device, and steps may need to be taken to reduce geometric distortions in MRI. CT gantry tilt should be known accurately and compensated for if nonzero. Image guidance is one of the most demanding applications for the geometric integrity of medical images. A 2% error in scaling over 200 mm will result in a relative displacement of 4 mm, well outside the accuracy of modern localizing devices. While CT and MRI manufacturers still quote accuracies worse than this figure in their formal specifications, methods exist to calibrate scanners with a high degree of accuracy.[20]

While there are advantages in terms of reduced cost, radiation dose, and time in using previously acquired images, in practice lack of access to the digital data and the problems in image quality outlined above often mean that repeat scans are required specifically for image guidance. This adds significantly to the cost of image-guided procedures. Issues of image preparation and artifact reduction are covered in more detail in Chapters 4 and 5.

Most image guidance entails a planning step, which may be as simple as identifying a single target or may involve delineation and labeling of complete structures such as a tumor in neurosurgery or individual bones in computer-assisted orthopedic surgery. This process of segmentation is one of the weakest links in image-guided-surgery. Software tools are improving, but fast and accurate image segmentation software that requires minimal intervention is still not available for most applications.

The software may also allow some planning or even rehearsal of the surgical procedure. Craniotomies and trajectories in neurosurgery can be planned to avoid critical structures. In image-guided total hip replacement, a computer-assisted orthopedic surgical procedure, implant size and orientation and acetabular cup orientation can be defined by manipulation of the preoperative images.[21] In maxillofacial surgery, the surgeon may rehearse the cutting and movement of segments of bone to achieve the desired surgical outcome.

12.3.2 Point-Based Registration

The most common method used in commercial systems to perform registration is to find corresponding point landmarks in the images and on the patient. Such points are generally termed fiducials. These may be anatomical landmarks, skin-affixed markers, or bone-implanted fiducials. The algorithm normally used is the orthogonal Procrustes solution described in Chapter 3, Section 3.4.

Our experience suggests that anatomical landmarks can be found with a FLE of 3 to 5 mm. Published data suggest that skin-affixed fiducials can be accurate to around 2 mm if used with care, the main source of inaccuracy being the fact that the skin can move.[22] Bone-implanted markers are by far the most accurate fiducials, allowing each marker to be located both in the image and on the patient to within 0.7 mm.[2,3]

12.3.3 Contour Registration

Linear features of an object could be used to provide registration. These could be specific geometric features such as lines of maximum curvature, watershed, or crest lines.[23] Marking linear features with a tracked pointer would be rather difficult, so such contour registration has only been proposed for use in conjunction with an intraoperative imaging device (see Section 12.4.2).

12.3.4 Surface Registration

A further method implemented in most commercial systems is to match a number of points on the surface of the patient's skin to the same surface extracted from the preoperative scans. Physical points are marked by dragging a hand-held pointer over the skin. Unfortunately, skin is soft and may deform. Brainlab (Munich, Germany) uses a laser point light source swept over the skin surface, which avoids skin distortion due to physical contact. However, there may still be some deformation due to muscle movement or changes in patient positioning between scanning and intervention. To get accurate rigid registration it is therefore desirable to mark points on the bone surface and match this to the bone surface extracted from CT. These surface points can be registered to the image surface using one of the surface-matching algorithms described in Chapter 3, such as the iterative closest point (ICP) algorithm.[24]

Rigid movement can occur within a surface of nearly constant curvature without any penalty to a cost function that minimizes the distance of physical points to the surface. It is therefore important to include points on surfaces which have variable and high curvature to provide a good registration. Combination of both landmark and surface points has been suggested as a way of overcoming this difficulty. It has been shown that a single landmark improved multiple surface registration accuracy from 1.5 to 1.0 mm (mean).[25]

12.3.5 Intensity-Based Registration

Algorithms that register two images based solely on the gray level intensity of corresponding voxels, such as maximization of mutual information, have become the method of choice for 3D-to-3D image alignment. If an intraoperative image is available, such methods may also be applicable to therapy guidance. The relevance of intensity-based registration to intraoperative images will be examined in the next section.

12.4 Intraoperative Imaging

The value of using a tracked pointer or similar device is limited in that only a single point is marked at any one time, and any points must be on the surface of the patient. However, a wealth of potential information is available from real-time imaging in the operating room that does not suffer from these limitations. The imaging modalities and methods of alignment to preoperative images will be considered in this section.

With intraoperative imaging, one needs to address two technical issues—calibration and registration. Calibration of the imaging device relates the image data to 3D space. It is important to consider the spatial integrity of the image data and the accuracy with which calibration can be achieved. A reference object of known dimensions is generally used to perform calibration. The device may be tracked by one of the methods described in Section 12.2.1, or may define the intraoperative coordinate system itself.

For alignment, data extraction is required if features such as landmark points or lines are to be identified in the intraoperative image. Direct intensity-based methods circumvent the need for such segmentation, as alignment is achieved using the image data directly.

With any method, it is important to consider the speed of the algorithm. Results must be obtained within a few seconds, or at least a minute or two, to be useful during a surgical procedure. For the intraoperative imaging modalities described in this section we will look at calibration, registration, and the accuracy and computational efficiency with which these can be achieved.

12.4.1   Video

Video provides real-time images of the exposed surface of the patient. This may be skin surface or exposed bone or soft tissue. Though the data in a single camera image is 2D, 3D information is potentially available from the use of perspective. By taking multiple camera images from different positions, a better estimation of 3D location can be achieved.

12.4.1.1   *Perspective Calibration*

The camera gives a perspective projection of 3D space into a 2D image. It is standard to use the pinhole camera model (Figure 12.1). Calibration generally involves taking a camera image of an object with high-contrast markings at known 3D positions. The image is then transferred to a computer for analysis using a framegrabber. The 2D positions of the markers are usually found automatically. The corresponding 2D and 3D points are used as the input data for the calibration.

In this section only the full perspective model will be discribed. Simpler projection models have been proposed, such as weak or parallel projection, which enable easier mathematical formulation at the expense of some inaccuracy. The full perspective model is accurate in the presence of negligible geometric distortion.

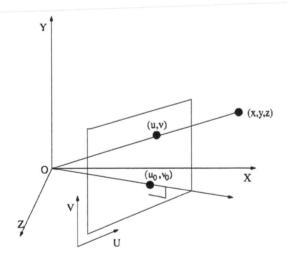

FIGURE 12.1
The general perspective projection model. The effective pinhole of the camera is at O. Pixel coordinates in the image plane are (U, V) and (u_0, v_0) is the nearest point on the image plane to O. A general 3D point (x, y, z) projects to (u, v) by Equation 12.1.

A general perspective projection can be described by (see Chapter 3):

$$
\gamma \begin{pmatrix} u \\ v \\ 1 \end{pmatrix} = \begin{pmatrix} k_u & 0 & u_0 & 0 \\ 0 & k_v & v_0 & 0 \\ 0 & 0 & 1 & 0 \end{pmatrix} T_{rigid} \begin{pmatrix} x \\ y \\ z \\ 1 \end{pmatrix} \tag{12.1}
$$

where the vectors $(x, y, z, 1)^T$ and $(u, v, 1)^T$ are the homogeneous coordinates of a 3D point and its 2D projection. The term γ represents the distance from the effective pinhole along the optical axis (the Z axis in the above formulation). Division by γ to calculate u and v provides the perspective effect of more distant objects being smaller. There are ten camera parameters, four intrinsic—(k_u, k_v) are the pixel sizes relative to the focal length and (u_0, v_0) is the perpendicular projection of the origin—and the six extrinsic parameters of the rigid-body transformation. A general 3×4 matrix can be decomposed into these ten parameters.[26] The most widely used calibration method is that developed by Tsai,[27] where an iterative scheme is used to calculate the ten parameters. Tsai also incorporates a polynomial radial distortion model.

12.4.1.2 Video Registration

The use of calibrated stereo video with patterned light, either a regular grid from a laser or a speckled pattern to provide high frequency details and high contrast, can rapidly produce a large number of surface points. These can then be matched to the same surface from the preoperative scan.[4]

A method which can potentially match a single video image to a preoperative scan surface was originally proposed by Viola and Wells.[28] A rendering of the 3D surface is produced and compared to the video image. The 3D rigid transformation of the preoperative surface is iteratively updated, and the mutual information (MI) between the normal vectors in the model and the video frame calculated. Tracking with such a method can be enhanced by the use of texture mapping[29] and has improved efficiency by rendering using OpenGL.[30]

Single view algorithms invariably suffer from inaccuracies along the optical axis of the camera. While it is possible to resolve to better than 1 mm perpendicular to the optical axis, errors increase to 3–5 mm at best along the line of sight.[28] Using two or more cameras enables must better 3D resolution.[31]

A new method which can be used with two or more video images has been proposed by Clarkson et al.[32] This method requires the surface visible in the video images, such as a skin or bone surface, to be segmented from the preoperative image. The algorithm uses a similarity measure termed photoconsistency. The measure takes each point on the segmented surface and calculates the image intensity where this point projects in each video image. Assuming a fixed light source and a Lambertian reflectance, the intensity value in each video image should be the same at registration. The photoconsistency measure is based on the variance of the difference between the intensity values in both video images. Minimizing this cost function to solve for the pose of the modeled object gave an accurate (1.27 mm) and robust registration for four images of a volunteer's face.

Video can provide tracking and registration without attaching any device to the patient, though this requires a large area of skin to be visible. As a result, the method is probably most applicable to initial registration for surgery before draping, or for radiotherapy.

12.4.2 X-ray Fluoroscopy

A fluoroscopy set provides real-time x-ray images of the patient. The perspective geometry is the same as that of a camera, except the patient is placed between the pinhole (x-ray source) and the imaging plane. Also, x-rays project through the patient, so fluoroscopy images contain information about internal structure in particular bony detail.

12.4.2.1 Calibration

The projection geometry of an x-ray set is essentially the same as that of a video camera and hence the methods of calibration are the same. The only difference is that the 3D calibration object must have x-ray visible markers, usually lead or aluminium balls, placed in known relative positions. These positions can be defined during manufacture or measured using a CT scan.

12.4.2.2 Registration

Several methods for registration of a 3D preoperative scan to the 2D x-ray projection have been proposed. Contour-based algorithms have been proposed in which the projection of a segmented surface from the preoperative scan is matched to the outline of the same structure in the x-ray image.[33–35] These algorithms tend to use physical measurements, such as the mean distance between the 2D x-ray projection and a projection of the 3D segmented surface, as a similarity measure. Such algorithms are efficient to run after feature extraction has occurred. However, automatic, fast, and accurate feature extraction from a complex scene, such as an interventional fluoroscopy image, is a difficulty task[35] and the final registration result is susceptible to errors in segmentation.[34,36]

Algorithms based on image intensity require little or no feature extraction but rely on production of digitally reconstructed radiographs (DRRs) from the preoperative CT scan.[36,37] The similarity measures used by these algorithms compare the pixel intensities in the fluoroscopy image and the DRR. They are usually statistically based, e.g., cross correlation.[37] Recent development of the similarity measure has resulted in cost functions such as pattern intensity[38] or gradient difference,[39] that have been shown to be robust to both low frequency intensity gradients caused by overlying soft tissue structures and the presence of interventional instruments such as a catheter

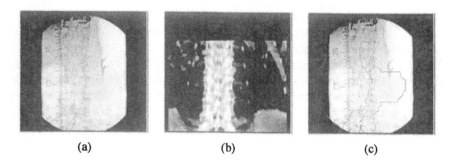

(a)   (b)   (c)

FIGURE 12.2
Registration of preoperative CT to intraoperative fluoroscopy. A fluoroscopy image of the lumbar spine showing a measurement catheter and a ruler which is used to define positions during the intervention (a), a DRR produced from the CT volume at the final registration position (b), and overlay of the segmented aorta from the CT scan (c).

or needle.[39] Figure 12.2 illustrates registration of fluoroscopy and CT images from a patient with an aortic aneurysm.

The accuracy of registration from a CT image to a single x-ray has similar problems to video, i.e., translations along the source-detector axis of the fluoroscopy set are poorly resolved. Tests on a spine phantom showed that translation accuracy of 1 mm is achieved parallel to the imaging plane, rising to 10 mm along the optical axis and rotational errors below 1°.[39] However, by using biplanar x-rays it is possible to register all six rigid-body degrees of freedom accurately.

12.4.3   Ultrasound Imaging

Ultrasonic imaging uses high frequency sound waves, typically 3 to 10 MHz (cf. < 100 KHz for coordinate defining ultrasound in air). A short pulse is produced and reflections from tissue boundaries are measured. Real time 1D (A-mode) or 2D (B-mode) information can be provided. An ultrasound A-mode trace can be used to identify an interface between two tissue types, for example the external bone surface. Ultrasound B-mode provides a 2D slice through the patient's anatomy. A calibrated probe can be used to provide 3D data when tracked by one of the methods described in Section 12.2.1. The calibration process will be considered first.

12.4.3.1   Calibration

Figure 12.3 shows the requirements for ultrasound calibration. For A-mode, we want to find a mapping from time along the A-mode trace, t, to a 3D point, P, with respect to the tracker on the probe:

$$P = P_0 + d\hat{n},$$

$$d = \frac{ut}{2}$$

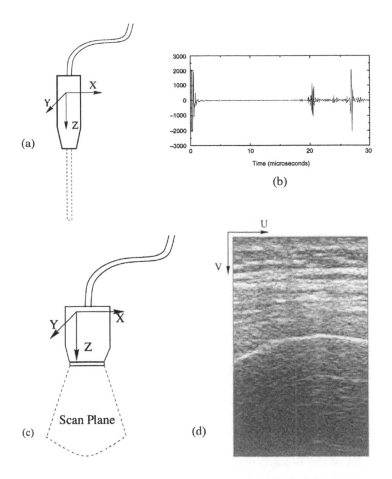

FIGURE 12.3
Ultrasound calibration. A tracked A-mode probe (a) has an associated 3D coordinate system. The calibration challenge is to relate the position along the A-mode time axis (b) to a point in 3D. For the B-mode probe (c), we want to relate 2D coordinates (u, v) in the B-mode scan (d) to 3D space.

where u is the speed of sound in tissue, P_0 is the position of the transducer, and $\hat{n}$ is the unit vector along the beam direction. The calibration process involves finding P_0 and $\hat{n}$. A method to achieve this using multiple scans of a steel ball is described by Maurer et al.[40]

B-mode calibration relates a 2D image pixel, (u, v), to a 3D point, P, with respect to a tracker on the probe. Prager[41] describes the transformations as follows:

$$P = T_{C \leftarrow T} T_{T \leftarrow R} T_{R \leftarrow P} x \tag{12.2}$$

where $x = (s_u u, s_v v, 0, 1)^T$, $T_{R \leftarrow P}$ is the rigid transformation from x to the probe tracker, $T_{T \leftarrow R}$ is from probe tracker to tracking device coordinates, and $T_{C \leftarrow T}$ transforms tracking coordinates to the reconstruction or calibration volume. The pixel scalings (in mm) of the B-scan are given by s_u and s_v.

For the calibration we are interested in calculating eight parameters, six for the rigid-body transformation $T_{R \leftarrow P}$ plus s_u and s_v. A number of phantoms have been proposed, which have an associated constrained set of P coordinates. The simplest is a crosswire.[42] The origin of the calibration volume is set to be at the crosswire, so $P = (0, 0, 0, 1)^T$ in homogeneous coordinates. The position of the crosswire in the B-scan and the tracking of the probe are measured for a number of scans giving measurements of (u, v) and $T_{T \leftarrow R}$. An iterative search can then give the desired parameters. A crosswire is a rather laborious calibration phantom, since holding the probe still is awkward and the position in the B-mode scan usually needs to be marked manually. A flat plane can also be used, however. In this case $P = (x, y, 0, 1)^T$ if we define the plane as perpendicular to the z axis. With an ingeniously manufactured device known as the Cambridge phantom, Prager manages to create a virtual plane with a surface that remains largely perpendicular to the probe throughout the range of required movements.[41] This provides a quick and accurate calibration.

A further method is to use a 3D calibration object with multiple features of known shape. These could either be measured using 3D scan of the phantom or accurately manufactured. Taking a number of B-scans of the phantom and their associated tracking matrices, it is possible to iterate over the eight calibration parameters to achieve the best match between the 3D model and the set of B-scans. Using normalized mutual information (NMI)[43] described in Section 3.4.8 of Chapter 3, as a similarity measure and employing a hierarchical search strategy, this approach has been shown to provide accurate calibration.[44] Advantages of this method include the fact that no segmentation of the B-scans is required and that the phantom can be made from tissue-equivalent gel rather than using water. Both this method and the Cambridge phantom have provided calibration accuracy of better than 1 mm on a 10 MHz probe.

12.4.3.2 Ultrasound Registration

A-mode ultrasound can provide a number of points on the interface between two tissue types. These can be matched to the same interface from a preoperative scan using a points-to-surface matching algorithm such as iterative closest point.[24] The proposed application of a calibrated A-mode probe is location of points on the skull surface for noninvasive registration to bone for image-guided neurosurgery.[40]

A calibrated B-mode probe can also provide points on the interface between bone and soft tissue if this surface is segmented from the B-mode scans. These points can be matched to a preoperatively segmented dataset in the same way. This has been proposed as a method of registration for pedicle screw implantation in the spine.[45,46]

These methods of matching to bone assume the rigid-body transformation. Ultrasound also provides potentially useful data about the position of soft tissue structures deep below the operative surface that have deformed since the preoperative scan (see Section 12.5).

12.4.4 Interventional MRI

With interventional MRI (iMRI) a fast-imaging modality with 3D capabilities is available in the operating room. One may ask why registration is necessary if we have an instant 3D image of the patient. There can be, however, much information in preoperative scans unlikely to be available from iMRI, for example functional data or the precise location of bone. Also, the quality of preoperative images from a diagnostic scanner is likely to be much higher in terms of contrast, signal-to-noise ratio, and geometric distortion.

Tracking of instruments relative to the most recent iMRI scan is also an issue that may involve a registration process. The iMRI scans could be taken at regular intervals throughout the procedure, with real time tracking of a pointer or tool to provide guidance in between the scans. This would most likely include marking of fiducials or surface points as described in Section 12.3. If the procedure is performed entirely within the scanner and the patient does not move, it is also possible that such alignment could be achieved by scanner calibration.

Volumetric intensity-based registration, especially with the use of mutual information as a similarity measure, has become the most popular and robust method for alignment of multiple 3D images.[43] It seems likely that such methods will also prove useful in the operating theater for alignment of preoperative scans to iMRI.[47] iMRI should prove particularly useful in generating updated 3D images which compensate for soft tissue motion during interventions (see Section 12.5).

12.5 Tissue Deformation Correction

Nonrigid registration is the subject of Chapters 13 to 15. Image to physical registration for therapy guidance poses specific problems in this area. If the surgery or treatment plan is created using a preoperative image, this should ideally be updated according to any movement of the patient, whether rigid or nonrigid.

One way of tackling this problem is to create a physical model that closely matches the tissue properties, measure only the required physical parameters to constrain this model, and update the registration accordingly. Use of the finite element method to create approximations to tissue mechanics, for example by using linear elastic elements, has been attempted.[48] Up to 70% of the deformation of the brain could be recovered merely by using the direction of gravity as input. This approach is described in greater detail in Chapter 15.

To achieve results in a time frame that is useful during surgery, however, a simpler model is likely to be required. For spinal surgery, a method which provides a smooth deformation between the rigid vertebrae has been proposed.[49,50] To incorporate fluid regions we have also proposed a simplified tissue model with rigid, fluid, and deformable components.[51]

In this active area of research, it is important to consider the clinical application when developing an algorithm. The tissue model does not necessarily have to be physically accurate. Intraoperative imaging can provide much input data about the current position and shape of the patient's anatomy, and this information may be sufficient to constrain a much simplified tissue model. The model also needs to be only as accurate as the application requires.

An algorithm based on approximating B-splines[52] has been used to align immediate pre- and post-intervention MR images for a range of neurosurgical procedures. The resulting deformation fields have been used to determine how much brain tissue has distorted or moved as a result of the intervention.[53]

Ultrasound is being developed as less expensive alternative intraoperative imaging modality to update preoperative images. A method has been proposed that involves extraction of contours from the B-scans, which are converted to deformation vectors that are linearly interpolated throughout the volume.[54] This method provided registration accuracies of better than 2 mm on a phantom designed to mimic the brain and ventricular structures for image-guided neurosurgery. King et al.[55] have recently proposed a Bayesian method to use intraoperative ultrasound to update the location of contours of structures delineated in preoperative MR images.

12.6 Clinical Applications

Registration of images to the patient in the treatment room provides the clinician with accurately aligned data to ensure that treatment is given in accordance with the preoperative plan. Benefits to the patient include smaller entry wounds (e.g., craniotomies), lower failure rate (e.g., pedicle screw placement), and less morbidity, due to avoidance of critical structures. Current applications of preoperative image alignment to the patient tend to assume the rigid-body transformation. The registration accuracy is limited by the amount of soft tissue deformation. This limits surgical applications to those near bone, such as skull base surgery,[56] spinal surgery,[45,46] or orthopedics.[21]

Alignment of images to the patient using stereotactic frames has long been a part of neurosurgery. It is in the field of neurosurgery that the first frameless surgical navigation device was developed.[11] The first system in regular clinical use was the mechanical version of the ISG viewing wand. A range of commercial systems is now available, most of which use optical tracking. A number of clinical trials have established the efficacy of image guidance in adult neurosurgery,[7-9,22,57] pediatric neurosurgery,[10] and ENT.[6] The method is rapidly gaining acceptance.

Image-guided surgery is also well established in computer-assisted orthopedic surgery. Systems are available for image-guided reconstructive hip surgery, knee reconstruction and ligament surgery, trauma surgery, and spinal surgery. In total hip replacement, image guidance allows accurate alignment of the femoral head implant and orientation of the acetabular cup using a computer model of the pelvis derived from CT. This is the basis of the HipNav™ system.[21] Either bone-implanted markers visible on CT or the surface of the bones of the pelvis are used for intraoperative registration. In the latter, a pointer is used to palpate the bone during surgery, and an algorithm similar to the ICP algorithm described in Chapter 3 is used for registration. The results of total hip replacements in 100 patients show improved clinical outcomes and reduced soft tissue damage and incision length.[58] The KneeNav™ system for total knee replacement and anterior cruciate ligament reconstruction has been developed using the same principles as HipNav.

Robotic devices such as the ROBODOC™ [59] are being introduced to provide good registration, greater stability during cutting of the bone, and improved accuracy of cutting. The ROBODOC pinless system uses a thin pointer to collect bone surface points percutaneously on the distal femur[60] and the exposed proximal surface. The ROBODOC system drills the bone very accurately according to the plan. As of April 1999, 2000 ROBODOC operations had been undertaken successfully at BGU, Frankfurt, and as of September 2000 over two dozen systems were in operation in Germany.

In spinal surgery, image guidance methods allow accurate pedicle screw placement. The pedicle is the strongest part of the vertebrae and therefore ideal for screw type anchoring. Unfortunately, insertion of screws without guidance has a high risk (10 to 40%) of incorrectly placed screws. One hundred consecutive patients were randomly assigned to image-guided pedicle screw insertion or the conventional manual method. For those with image guidance, 0.4% (1/219) had pedicle perforation, compared with 11.5% (32/277) using the conventional method.[61]

Interventional radiology attempts to provide surgery that is minimally invasive by using small approach incisions and accurate guidance by intraoperative imaging. If the guidance is by fluoroscopy, there may be features visible in a preoperative CT scan that are not readily visible in the x-ray image. These data can be overlaid on the fluoro image to aid the interventionist. This process is shown in Figure 12.2, where an overlay of the aorta can be used to help guide a catheter.

Radiotherapy does not require interactive display for the therapist, but accurate alignment to the patient is vital for treatment to be given in accordance with the plan. Immobilization in a molded plastic mask is the most common technique to ensure that the patient is in the same position as he was in the simulator room. Accuracy becomes even more important when planning is performed using 3D scans in conjunction with techniques such as conformal therapy or radiosurgery. Video registration may provide a means to track the patient without the need for immobilization. This is only relevant if we have a treatment machine capable of adjusting for small movements. In the meantime, tracking methods may be able to detect patient movement and abort treatment when necessary.

For surgery away from bone, it will be necessary to solve the problem of nonrigid tissue movement. For surgery of the thorax or abdomen there will be considerable movement of tissue, and this must be compensated for. The use of surface registration techniques has been proposed to allow preoperative CT images to help guide liver resections.[62] Tracked ultrasound, by providing real time image data about underlying structures, may become a significant tool for this purpose. Interventional MRI, which gives volumetric data in close to real time, will also play a useful role as the cost of this emerging technology comes down.

12.6.1   Clinical Accuracy Requirements

It is important to consider what accuracy is required for a given application. It has become the holy grail of neurosurgical guidance that the accuracy of any system should be ~1 mm. The accurate placement of a small craniotomy, however, probably does not require accuracy much better than about 5 mm,[57] and for some procedures in the thorax and abdomen it may be possible to tolerate even larger errors.

12.6.2   Visualization

Alignment of the preoperative images to the patient is not the end of the story for image-guided therapy. The preoperative data still need to be presented to the clinician in a useful way. In standard commercial neuronavigation systems, image guidance is provided using a tracked pointer or probe, and the position of this is shown as orthogonal slices, or perhaps surface-rendered view on a computer monitor (Figure 12.4a). This has the disadvantage that

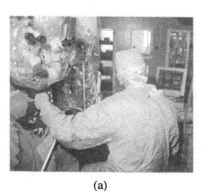
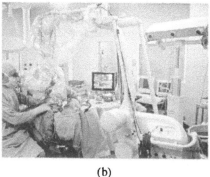

(a)   (b)

FIGURE 12.4
Pointer based guidance (a) showing the need to look away from the surgical field, and augmented reality guidance (b) with overlays directly on the surgical view.

information about only one point is provided, and the surgeon needs to look away from the surgical field to a computer screen.

A better method is to provide overlays directly on the surgical view (Figure 12.4b). For neurosurgery, the use of the operating microscope for this purpose was originally proposed by Kelly[63] and continued by Roberts.[11] Simple outlines or trajectories in one eyepiece have now become standard. The use of separate overlays in the left and right eyepieces can further enhance the surgeon's ability to relate preoperative image data to the intraoperative scene. We have demonstrated such a stereo system in which segmented structures from a preoperative scan can be perceived by most people to be sitting beneath the viewed surface as though the tissue is transparent.[56]

An alternative approach is to place a reflecting screen over the patient. A system proposed in 1938 used x-rays to place a small light source opposite a bullet or fragment of shrapnel so that the reflection in a half-silvered mirror could guide the surgeon to the target.[64] Peuchot has developed this method to incorporate two reflecting surfaces at slightly different angles to enable projection of stereo graphics onto the patient for spinal surgery.[65] Stereoscopic graphics can also be produced using a polarized light, switched by an active filter screen over the monitor or glasses, to direct a different view to each eye. Such screens have been proposed for use in preoperative planning[66] and surgical guidance.[67]

With any image guidance application it is important to consider how the therapist will view and interact with the data. Treatment room ergonomics is an important factor, especially in the already crowded operating room. With interactive image guidance it is vital not only that the information is presented in a simple and easy to interpret manner, but also that the clinician is made aware of possible inaccuracies in the system.

12.7 Conclusions

The applications of therapy guidance using data from images taken before an intervention have been examined. Simple tracking of pointers or tools has been presented, along with the enhancement of registration using readily available intraoperative imaging modalities—video, fluoroscopy, ultrasound, and iMRI.

As the abundance and quality of data available from intraoperative imaging increases, one may wonder whether alignment of preoperative images to the patient has a future. However, images from diagnostic scanners are also developing apace, with higher resolution, better contrast, and more functional data becoming feasible. Applications such as functional MRI, where considerable scanning and processing time is required, provide information that cannot currently be acquired in real time during treatment, and which may more appropriately be obtained prior to treatment when the patient is alert and there is sufficient time for a comprehensive set of functional tests.

To provide the best available information to an interventionist, the problem must be tackled from both ends: developing intraoperative imaging technology to provide immediate data, and improving registration with pretreatment images, particularly in the presence of tissue deformation. Therapy guidance will continue to provide challenges to the medical image analysis community for some years to come.

References

1. S. Webb. *The Physics of Medical Imaging*. IOP Publishing Ltd., Bristol, 1988.
2. C. Maurer, M.J. Fitzpatrick, M.Y. Wang, R.L. Galloway, R.J. Maciunas, and G.S. Allen. Registration of head volume images using implantable fiducial markers. *IEEE Trans. on Med. Imaging*, 16(4):447–461, 1997.
3. F.C. Vinas, L. Zamorano, R. Bucic, Q.H. Li, F. Shamsa, Z. Jiang, and F.G. Diaz. Application accuracy study of a semipermanent fiducial marker system for frameless stereotaxis. *Computer-Assisted Surgery*, 2:257–263, 1997.
4. A.C.F. Colchester, J. Zhao, S.K. Holton-Tainter, C.J. Henri, N. Maitland, P.T.E. Roberts, C.G. Harris, and R.J. Evans. Development and preliminary evaluation of VISLAN, a surgical planning and guidance system using intraoperative video imaging. *Med. Image Anal.*, 1(1):73–90, 1996.
5. M.J. Fitzpatrick, J.B. West, and C. Maurer. Predicting error in rigid-body point-based registration. *IEEE Trans. on Med. Imaging*, 17(5):694–702, 1998.
6. S.J. Zinreich, S.A. Tebo, D.M. Long, H. Brem, D.E. Mattox, M.E. Loury, C.A. Vanderkolk, W.M. Koch, D.W. Kennedy, and R.N. Bryan. Frameless stereotaxic integration of CT imaging data—accuracy and initial applications. *Radiology*, 188(3):735–742, 1993.
7. E. Watanabe, Y. Mayanagi, Y. Kosugi, S. Manaka, and K. Takakura. Open surgery assisted by the neuronavigator, a stereotaxic, articulated, sensitive arm. *Neurosurgery*, 28:792–800, 1991.
8. D.R. Sandeman, N. Patel, C. Chandler, R.J. Nelson, H.B. Coakham, and H.B. Griffith. Advances in image-directed neurosurgery—preliminary experience with the ISG viewing wand compared with the Leksell-G frame. *Br. J. Neurosurgery*, 8(5):529–544, 1994.
9. J.G. Golfinos, B.C. Fitzpatrick, L.R. Smith and R.F. Spetzler. Clinical use of a frameless stereotaxic arm—results of 325 cases. *J. Neurosurgery*, 83(2):197–205, 1995.
10. J.M. Drake, J. Prudencio, S. Holowka, J.T. Rutka, H.J. Hoffman, and R.P. Humphreys. Frameless stereotaxy in children. *Ped. Neurosurg.*, 20(2):152–159, 1994.
11. D.W. Roberts, J.W. Strohbehn, J.F. Hatch, W. Murray, and H. Kettenberger. A frameless stereotaxic integration of computerized tomographic imaging and the operating microscope. *J. Neurosurg.*, 65:545–549, 1986.
12. H.F. Reinhardt, G.A. Horstmann, and O. Gratzl. Sonic stereometry in microsurgical procedures for deep-seated brain tumors and vascular malformations. *Neurosurgery*, 32(1):51–57, 1998.
13. G. Alusi, A.C. Tan, A.D. Linney, K. Raoof, and Wright A. Three dimensional tracking with ultrasound for augmented reality applications in skull base surgery. In J. Troccaz, W.E. Grimson, and R. Mijsges, Eds., *Proceedings of CVRMed-MRCAS*, LNCS 1205, Springer-Verlag, Heidelberg, pages 511–517, 1997.

14. M.S. Alp, M. Dujovny, M. Misra, F.T. Charbel, and J.I. Ausman. Head registration techniques for image-guided surgery. *Neurolog. Res.*, 20:31–37, 1998.
15. R.J. Maciunas, R.L. Galloway, and J.W. Latimer. The application accuracy of stereotactic frames. *Neurosurgery*, 35(4):682–694, 1994.
16. C. Weltens, K. Kesteloot, G. Vandevelde, and W. Vandenbogaert. Comparison of plastic and Orfit^R masks for patient head fixation during radiotherapy—precision and costs. *Int. J. Radiat. Oncol. Biol. Phys.*, 33(2):499–507, 1995.
17. R. Hauser, B. Westermann, and R. Probst. Non-invasive tracking of patients' head movements during computer-assisted intranasal microscopic surgery. *Laryngoscope*, 211:491–499, 1997.
18. M.R. Fenlon, A.S. Jusczyzck, P.J. Edwards, and A.P. King. Locking acrylic resin dental stent for image-guided surgery. *J. of Prosthetic Dentistry*, 83:482–485, 2000.
19. K. Martens, K. Verstreken, J. van Cleyenebreugel, K. van Brussel, J. Goffin, G. Marchal, and P. Seutens. Image-based planning and validation of C1–C2 transarticular screw fixation using personalized drill guides. In *MICCAI 99: LNCS 1679*, C. Taylor and A. Colchester, Eds., Springer-Verlag, Heidelberg, pages 860–867, 1999.
20. D.L.G. Hill, C.R. Maurer, Jr., C. Studholme, J.M. Fitzpatrick, and D.J. Hawkes. Correcting scaling errors in tomographic images using a nine degree of freedom registration algorithm. *J. of Comp. Assisted Tomogr.*, 22(2):317–323, 1998.
21. A.M. DiGioia, B. Jaramaz, M. Blackwell, D.A. Simon, F. Morgan, J.E. Moody, C. Nikou, B.D. Colgan, C.A. Aston, R.S. Labarca, E. Kischell, and T. Kanade. Image guided navigation system to measure intraoperatively acetabular implant alignment. *Clinic. Orthopaedics and Related Res.*, 355:8–22, 1998.
22. J.P. Wadley, N.L. Dorward, M. Breeuwer, F.A. Gerritsen, N.D. Kitchen, and D.G.T. Thomas. Neuronavigation in 210 cases: Further development of applications and full integration into contemporary neurosurgical practice. In *Proceedings of Computer-Assisted Radiology and Surgery 1998*, H. Lemke, M. Vannier, K. Inamura, and A. Farman, Eds., Elsevier, Amsterdam, pages 635–640, 1998.
23. J. Declerck, G. Subsol, J.P. Thirion, and N. Ayache. Automatic retrieval of anatomic structures in 3D medical images. In N. Ayache, Ed., *Computer Vision, Virtual Reality and Robotics in Medicine*, LNCS 905, Springer-Verlag, Heidelberg, pages 153–159, 1995.
24. P.J. Besl and N.D. McKay. A method for registration of 3-D shapes. *IEEE Trans. on Pattern Anal. And Machine Intell.*, 14(2):239–256, 1992.
25. C. Maurer, R.J. Maciunas, and M.J. Fitzpatrick. Registration of head CT images to physical space using a weighted combination of points and surfaces. *IEEE Trans. on Med. Imaging*, 17(5):753–761, 1998.
26. S. Ganapathy. Decomposition of transformation matrices for robot vision. *Pattern Recogn. Lett.*, 2:401–412, 1984.
27. R.Y. Tsai. A versatile camera calibration technique for high-accuracy 3D machine vision metrology using off-the-shelf tv cameras and lenses. *IEEE J. of Robotics and Automation*, 3(4):323–344, 1987.
28. P. Viola and W.M. Wells III. Alignment by maximization of mutual information. *Int. J. of Comp. Vision*, 24(2):137–154, 1997.
29. M.J. Clarkson, D. Rueckert, A.P. King, P. J. Edwards, D.L.G. Hill, and D.J. Hawkes. Registration of video images to tomographic images by optimising mutual information using texture mapping. In *MICCAI 99: LNCS*, N. Ayache, Ed., Springer-Verlag, Heidelberg, pages 579–588, 1999.

30. N. Hata, M. Wells, W.M. Halle, S. Nakajima, P. Viola, R. Kikinis, and F.A. Jolesz. Image guided microscopic surgery system using mutual-information based registration. In K.H. Hone and R. Kikinis, Eds., *Visualization in Biomedical Computing*, LNCS 1131, Springer-Verlag, Heidelberg, pages 317–326, 1996.

31. M.I. Miga, K.D. Paulsen, P.J. Hoopes, F.E. Kennedy, Jr., A. Hartov, and D.W. Roberts. *In vivo* quantification of a homogeneous brain deformation model for updating preoperative images during surgery. *IEEE Trans. Biomed. Engineering*, 47(2):266–273, Feb. 2000.

32. M.J. Clarkson, D. Rueckert, D.L.G. Hill, and D.J. Hawkes. A multiple 2D video-3D medical image registration algorithm. In *Proc. SPIE Medical Imaging 2000*, volume 3979, pages 342–352, 2000.

33. J. Feldmar, N. Ayache, and F. Betting. 3D-2D projective registration of free-form curves and surfaces. *Comp. Vision and Image Understanding*, 65(3):403–424, March 1997.

34. A. Gueziec, P. Kazanzides, B. Williamson, and R.H. Taylor. Anatomy-based registration of CT-scan and intraoperative x-ray images for guiding a surgical robot. *IEEE Trans. on Med. Imaging*, 17(5):715–728, 1998.

35. S. Lavallée and R. Szeliski. Recovering the position and orientation of free-form objects from image contours using 3D distance maps. *IEEE Trans. On Pattern Anal. And Machine Intell.*, 17(4):378–390, 1995.

36. L.M. Brown and T.E. Boult. Registration of planar film radiographs with computed tomography. In *Proc. of the IEEE Workshop on Mathematical Methods in Biomed. Image Anal.*, pages 42–51, 1996.

37. L. Lemieux, R. Jagoe, D.R. Fish, N.D. Kitchen, and D.G.T. Thomas. A patient-to-computed-tomography image registration method based on digitally reconstructed radiographs. *Med. Physics*, 21(11):1749–1760, November 1994.

38. J. Weese, G.P. Penney, P. Desmedt, T.M. Buzug, D.L.G. Hill, and D.J. Hawkes. Voxel-based 2-D/3-D registration of fluoroscopy image and CT scans for image- guided surgery. *IEEE Trans. on Biomed. Eng.*, 1(4):284–293, December 1997.

39. G.P. Penney, J. Weese, J.A. Little, P. Desmedt, D.L.G. Hill, and D.J. Hawkes. A comparison of similarity measures for use in 2D-3D medical image registration. *IEEE Trans. on Med. Imaging*, 17(4):586–595, 1998.

40. C.R. Maurer, R.P. Gaston, D.L.G. Hill, M.J. Gleeson, M.G. Taylor, M.R. Fenlon, P.J. Edwards, and D.J. Hawkes. Acoustick: a tracked a-mode ultrasonography system for registration in image-guided surgery. In *MICCAI 99: LNCS 1679*, C. Taylor and A. Colchester, Eds., Springer-Verlag, Heidelberg, pages 953–962, 1999.

41. R.W. Prager, R.N. Rohling, A.H. Gee, and L. Berman. Rapid calibration for 3-D freehand ultrasound. *Ultrasound in Med. and Biol.*, 24(6):855–869, 1998.

42. C.D. Barry, C.P. Allott, N.W. John, P.M. Mellor, P.A. Arundel, D.S. Thomson, and J.C. Waterton. Three-dimensional freehand ultrasound: image reconstruction and volume analysis. *Ultrasound in Med. and Biol.*, 23:1209–1224, 1997.

43. C. Studholme, D.L.G. Hill, and D.J. Hawkes. An overlap invariant entropy measure of 3D medical image alignment. *Pattern Recogn.*, 32(1):71–86, 1999.

44. J.M. Blackall, D. Rückert, C.R. Maurer Jr., G.P. Penney, D.L.G. Hill, and D.J. Hawkes. An image registration approach to automated calibration for freehand 3D ultrasound. In *MICCAI 2000: LNCS*, Springer-Verlag, Heidelberg, pages 462–471, 2000.

45. S. Lavallée, J. Troccaz, P. Sautot, B. Mazier, P. Cinquin, P. Merloz, and J.P. Chirossel. Computer-assisted spinal surgery using anatomy-based registration. In R.H. Taylor, S. Lavallée, G.C. Burdea, and R.W. Mosges, eds., *Registration for Computer Integrated Surgery: Methodology, State of the Art*, pages 425–449. Cambridge, MA: MIT Press, 1995.
46. J.L. Herring, B.M. Dawant, C. Maurer, D.M. Muratore, R.L. Galloway, and M.J. Fitzpatrick. Surface-based registration of CT images to physical space for image-guided surgery of the spine: A sensitivity study. *IEEE Trans. on Med. Imaging*, 17(5):743–752, 1998.
47. N. Hata, T. Dohi, S. Warfield, W.M. Wells, R. Kikinis, and F.A. Jolesz. Multimodality deformable registration of pre- and intraoperative images for MRI-guided brain surgery. In *MICCAI 99: LNCS*, W.M. Wells, A. Colchester, and S. Delp, Eds., Springer-Verlag, Heidelberg, pages 1067–1074, 1998.
48. M. Leventon, W.M. Wells III, W.E.L. Grimson. Multiple View 2D-3D Mutual Information Registration. In *Image Understanding: Proceedings of the DARPA Workshop 1997*, Morgan Kaufmann Publishers, San Francisco, 1997.
49. J. Little, D.L.G. Hill, and D.J. Hawkes. Deformations incorporating rigid structures. *Comp. Vision Image Understanding*, 66:223–232, 1997.
50. G.P. Penney, J.A. Little, J. Weese, D.L.G. Hill, and D.J. Hawkes. Deforming a preoperative volume to represent the intraoperative scene. In *Proc. SPIE Med. Imaging 2000*, volume 3979, pages 482–492, 2000.
51. P.J. Edwards, D.L.G. Hill, J.A. Little, and D.J. Hawkes. A three component deformation model for image-guided surgery. *Med. Image Analysis*, 2(4):355–367, 1998.
52. D. Rueckert, L.I. Sonoda, C. Hayes, D.L.G. Hill, M.O. Leach, and D.J. Hawkes. Nonrigid registration using free-form deformations: application to breast MR images. *IEEE Trans. on Med. Imaging*, 18(8):712–721, 1999.
53. C.R. Maurer, D.L.G. Hill, A.J. Martin, H.Y. Liu, M. McCue, D. Rueckert, D. Lloret, W.A. Hall, R.E. Maxwell, D.J. Hawkes, and C.L. Truwit. Investigation of intraoperative brain deformation using a 1.5-T interventional MR system: Preliminary results. *IEEE Trans. on Med. Imaging*, 17(5):817–825, 1998.
54. R.M. Comeau, A.F. Sadikot, A. Fenster, and T.M. Peters. Intraoperative ultrasound for guidance and tissue shift correction in image-guided neurosurgery. *Med. Physics*, 37(4):787–800, 2000.
55. A.P. King, J.M. Blackall, G.P. Penney, P.J. Edwards, D.L.G. Hill, and D.J. Hawkes. Bayesian estimation of intraoperative deformation fi image-guided surgery using 3-D ultrasound. In *MICCAI 2000: LNCS*, Springer-Verlag, Heidelberg, pages, 588–597, 2000.
56. P.J. Edwards, A.P. King, C.R. Maurer, J., D.A. de Cunha, D.J. Hawkes, D.L.G. Hill, R.P. Gaston, M.R. Fenlon, A. Jusczyzck, A.J. Strong, C.L. Chandler, and M.J. Gleeson. Design and evaluation of a system for microscope-assisted guided interventions (MAGI). *IEEE Trans. on Med. Imaging*, 19(11):1082–1093, 2000.
57. N.L. Dorward, O. Alberti, J.D. Palmer, Kitchen N.D., and Thomas D.G.T. Accuracy of true frameless stereotaxy: *in vivo* measurement and laboratory phantom studies. *J. of Neurosurg.*, 90(1):160–168, 1999.
58. T.J. Levison, J.E. Moody, B. Jaramaz, C. Nikou, and A.M. Digioia. Surgical navigation for THR: a report on clinical trials utilising HipNav. In *MICCAI 2000: LNCS*, Springer-Verlag, Heidelberg, pages 1184–1187, 2000.

59. W.L. Barger, A. Bauer, and M. Borner. Primary and revision total hip replacement using the ROBODOC^R system. *Clin. Orthopaedics and Related Res.*, pages 82–91, 1998.

60. U. Wiesel, A. Lahmer, and M. Börner. ROBODOC^R at BGU, Frankfurt—experiences with the pinless system. In A.M. DiGioia and L.P. Nolte, eds., *Proc. Comp. Assisted Orthopaedic Surg. (CAOS 1999)*, pages 113–117, 1999.

61. T. Laine, T. Lund, M. Ylikoski, J. Lohikoski, and D. Schlenzka. Accuracy of pedicle screw insertion with and without computer assistance—a randomised clinical study in 100 consecutive patients. In *Proc. Comp. Assisted Orthopaedic Surg. (CAOS 2000)*, pages 27–31, 2000.

62. A.J. Herline, J.L. Herring, J.D. Stefansic, W.C. Chapman, R.L. Galloway, and B.M. Dawant. Surface registration for use in interactive, image-guided liver surgery. *Comp. Aided Surg.*, 5(1):11–17, 2000.

63. P.J. Kelly, G.J. Alker, and S. Goerss. Computer-assisted stereotactic laser microsurgery for the treatment of intracranial neoplasms. *Neurosurgery*, 10:324–331, 1982.

64. H. Steinhaus. Sur la localisation au moyen des rayons x. *Comptes Rendus de L'Academie des Science*, 206:1473–5, 1938.

65. B. Peuchot, A. Tanguy, and M. Eude. Virtual reality as an operative tool during scoliosis surgery. In N. Ayache, ed., *Computer Vision, Virtual Reality and Robotics in Medicine*, LNCS 905, Springer-Verlag, Heidelberg, pages 549–554, 1995.

66. R.A. Kockro, L. Serra, Y. Tseng-Tsai, C. Chan, S. Yih-Yian, C. Gim-Guan, E. Lee, L.Y. Hoe, N. Hern, and W.L. Nowinski. Planning and simulation of neurosurgery in a virtual reality environment. *Neurosurgery*, 46:118–135, 2000.

67. M. Blackwell, C. Nikou, A.M. DiGioia, and T. Kanade. An image overlay system for medical data visualization. In *MICCAI'98*: LNCS, Springer-Verlag, Heidelberg, pages 232–240, 1998.

Section III

Techniques and Applications of Nonrigid Body Registration

13

Nonrigid Registration: Concepts, Algorithms, and Applications

Daniel Rueckert

CONTENTS

13.1 Introduction

The previous chapters in this book have focused on rigid transformations for image-to-image and image-to-physical space registration. In many applications a rigid transformation is sufficient to describe the spatial relationship between two images. For example, brain images of the same subject can be related by a rigid transformation since the motion of the brain is largely constrained by the skull. However, there are many other applications where nonrigid transformations are required to describe the spatial relationship between images adequately. For example, in intrasubject registration non-rigid transformations are required to accommodate any tissue deformation due to interventions or changes over time. Similarly, in intersubject registration, nonrigid transformations are often required to accommodate the substantial anatomical variability across individuals.

In contrast to rigid registration techniques, nonrigid registration techniques are still the subject of significant ongoing research activity. The goal of this chapter is to give an overview of the different nonrigid registration techniques and the current state of the art in this fast-moving area. A recent overview of hierarchical approaches to nonrigid registration can be found in Lester and Arridge.[1]

13.2 Techniques

Any nonrigid registration technique can be described by three components: a transformation which relates the target and source images (images A and B as defined in Chapter 3), a similarity measure which measures the similarity between target and source image, and an optimization which determines the optimal transformation parameters as a function of the similarity measure. The main difference between rigid and nonrigid registration techniques is the nature of the transformation. The goal of rigid registration is to find the six degrees of freedom (three rotations and three translations) of transformation $\mathbf{T} : (x, y, z) \mapsto (x', y', z')$ which maps any point in the source image into the corresponding point in the target image. An extension of this model is the affine transformation model which has twelve degrees of freedom and allows for scaling and shearing:

$$\mathbf{T}(x, y, z) = \begin{pmatrix} x' \\ y' \\ z' \\ 1 \end{pmatrix} = \begin{pmatrix} a_{00} & a_{01} & a_{02} & a_{03} \\ a_{10} & a_{11} & a_{12} & a_{13} \\ a_{20} & a_{21} & a_{22} & a_{23} \\ 0 & 0 & 0 & 1 \end{pmatrix} \begin{pmatrix} x \\ y \\ z \\ 1 \end{pmatrix} \qquad (13.1)$$

These affine or linear transformation models are often used for the registration of images for which some of the image acquisition parameters are unknown, such as voxel sizes or gantry tilt,[2,3] or to accommodate a limited amount of shape variability.[4] By adding additional degrees of freedom (DOF), such a linear transformation model can be extended to nonlinear transformation models. Figure 13.1 shows some examples of the different types of transformations commonly used for image registration.

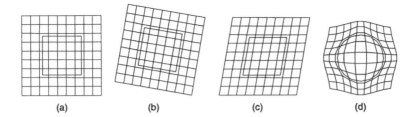

FIGURE 13.1
Example of different types of transformations of a square: (a) identity transformation,
(b) rigid transformation, (c) affine transformation, and (d) nonrigid transformation.

For example, the quadratic transformation model is defined by second order polynomials

$$
\mathbf{T}(x, y, z) = \begin{pmatrix} x' \\ y' \\ z' \\ 1 \end{pmatrix} = \begin{pmatrix} a_{00} & \cdots & a_{08} & a_{09} \\ a_{10} & \cdots & a_{18} & a_{19} \\ a_{20} & \cdots & a_{28} & a_{29} \\ 0 & \cdots & 0 & 1 \end{pmatrix} \begin{pmatrix} x^2 \\ y^2 \\ \vdots \\ 1 \end{pmatrix} \tag{13.2}
$$

whose coefficients determine the 30 degrees of freedom of the transformation. In a similar fashion this model can be extended to higher order polynomials such as third (60 DOF), fourth (105 DOF), and fifth-order polynomials (168 DOF).[5] However, their ability to recover anatomical shape variability is often quite limited since they can model only global shape changes and cannot accommodate local shape changes. In addition, higher order polynomials tend to introduce artifacts such as oscillations;[6] therefore, they are rarely used for nonrigid registration.

13.2.1 Registration Using Basis Functions

Instead of using a polynomial as a linear combination of higher order terms, one can use a linear combination of basis functions θ_i to describe the deformation field:

$$
\mathbf{T}(x, y, z) = \begin{pmatrix} x' \\ y' \\ z' \\ 1 \end{pmatrix} = \begin{pmatrix} a_{00} & \cdots & a_{0n} \\ a_{10} & \cdots & a_{1n} \\ a_{20} & \cdots & a_{2n} \\ 0 & \cdots & 1 \end{pmatrix} \begin{pmatrix} \theta_1(x, y, z) \\ \vdots \\ \theta_n(x, y, z) \\ 1 \end{pmatrix} \tag{13.3}
$$

A common choice is to represent the deformation field using a set of (orthonormal) basis functions such as Fourier (trigonometric) basis functions[7,8] or wavelet basis functions.[9] In the case of trigonometric basis functions this corresponds to a spectral representation of the deformation field where each basis function describes a particular frequency of the deformation. Restricting the summation in Equation (15.3) to the first N terms (where $1 < N < n$) has the effect of limiting the frequency spectrum of the transformation to the N lowest frequencies.

13.2.2   Registration Using Splines

The term spline originally referred to the use of long flexible strips of wood or metal to model the surfaces of ships and planes. These splines were bent by attaching different weights along their length. A similar concept can be used to model spatial transformations. For example, a 2D transformation can be represented by two separate surfaces whose height above the plane corresponds to the displacement in the horizontal or vertical direction. An example of such a transformation is shown in Figure 13.2.

Many registration techniques using splines are based on the assumption that a set of corresponding points or landmarks can be identified in the source and target images. This is analogous to the use of point landmarks for rigid or affine registration using the Procrustes method described in Chapter 3. These corresponding points are often referred to as *control points*. At these control points, spline-based transformations either interpolate or approximate the displacements which are necessary to map the location of the control point in the target image into its corresponding counterpart in the source image. Between control points, they provide a smoothly varying displacement field. The interpolation condition can be written as

$$\mathbf{T}(\phi_i) = \phi_i' \qquad i = 1,\ldots,n \qquad\qquad (13.4)$$

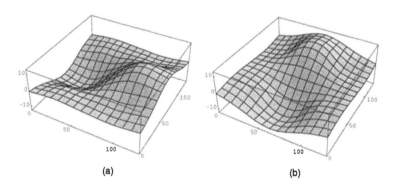

(a)   (b)

FIGURE 13.2
An example of a nonrigid transformation required to warp a square into a circle. The corresponding transformation is shown as two separate surfaces defining (a) the displacement in the horizontal direction and (b) the displacement in the vertical direction.

where ϕ_i denotes the location of the control point in the target image and ϕ'_i denotes the location of the corresponding control point in the source image. There are a number of different ways to determine the control points. For example, anatomical or geometrical landmarks which can be identified in both images can be used to define a spline-based mapping function, which maps the spatial position of landmarks in the source image into their corresponding position in the target image.[10] In addition, Meyer et al.[11] suggested updating the location of control points by optimization of a voxel similarity measure such as mutual information. Alternatively, control points can be arranged with equidistant spacing across the image, forming a regular mesh.[12] In this case the control points are only used as a parameterization of the transformation and do not correspond to anatomical or geometrical landmarks. Therefore they are often referred to as *pseudo-* or *quasi-*landmarks.

13.2.2.1 Thin-Plate Splines

Thin-plate splines are part of a family of splines that are based on radial basis functions. They have been formulated by Duchon[13] and Meinguet[14] for the surface interpolation of scattered data. In recent years they have been widely used for image registration.[10,15,16] Radial basis function splines can be defined as a linear combination of n radial basis functions $\theta(s)$.

$$t(x, y, z) = a_1 + a_2 x + a_3 y + a_4 z + \sum_{j=1}^{n} b_j \theta(|\phi_j - (x, y, z)|) \quad (13.5)$$

Defining the transformation as three separate thin plate spline functions $\mathbf{T} = (t_1, t_2, t_3)^T$ yields a mapping between images in which the coefficients a characterize the affine part of the spline-based transformation, while the coefficients b characterize the nonaffine part of the transformation. The interpolation conditions in Equation (13.4) form a set of $3n$ linear equations. To determine the $3(n + 4)$ coefficients uniquely, 12 additional equations are required. These 12 equations guarantee that the nonaffine coefficients b sum to zero and that their crossproducts with the x, y and z coordinates of the control points are likewise zero. In matrix form this can be expressed as

$$\begin{pmatrix} \Theta & \Phi \\ \Phi^T & 0 \end{pmatrix} \begin{pmatrix} b \\ a \end{pmatrix} = \begin{pmatrix} \Phi' \\ 0 \end{pmatrix} \quad (13.6)$$

Here a is a 4×3 vector of the affine coefficients a, $\mathbf{b}$ is a $n \times 3$ vector of the nonaffine coefficients b, and Θ is the kernel matrix with $\Theta_{ij} = \theta(|\phi_i - \phi_j|)$. Solving for a and b using standard algebra yields a thin-plate spline transformation which will interpolate the displacements at the control points.

The radial basis function of thin-plate splines is defined as

$$\theta(s) = \begin{cases} |s|^2 \log(|s|) & \text{in 2D} \\ |s| & \text{in 3D} \end{cases} \quad (13.7)$$

A wide number of alternative choices for radial basis functions including multiquadrics and Gaussians exists.[17,12] Modeling deformations using thin-plate splines has a number of advantages. For example, they can be used to incorporate additional constraints such as rigid bodies[18] or directional constraints[19] into the transformation model, and they can be extended to approximating splines where the degree of approximation at the landmark depends on the confidence of the landmark localization.[20]

13.2.2.2 B-Splines

In general radial basis functions have infinite support. Therefore each basis function contributes to the transformation and each control point has a global influence on the transformation. In a number of cases the global influence of control points is undesirable since it becomes difficult to model local deformations. Furthermore, for a large number of control points the computational complexity of radial basis function splines becomes prohibitive. An alternative is to use freeform deformations (FFDs) which have been widely used for animations in computer graphics. FFDs based on locally controlled functions such as B-splines are a powerful tool for modeling 3D deformable objects[21] and have been used successfully for image registration.[22-24] The basic idea of FFDs is to deform an object by manipulating an underlying mesh of control points. The resulting deformation controls the shape of the 3D object and produces a smooth and C^2 continuous transformation. In contrast to radial basis function splines which allow arbitrary configurations of control points, spline-based FFDs require a regular mesh of control points with uniform spacing.

A spline-based FFD is defined on the image domain $\Omega = \{(x, y, z) \mid 0 \leq x < X, 0 \leq y < Y, 0 \leq z < Z\}$ where Φ denotes an $n_x \times n_y \times n_z$ mesh of control points $\phi_{i,j,k}$ with uniform spacing δ. In this case the displacement field $\mathbf{u}$ defined by the FFD can be expressed as the 3D tensor product of the familiar 1D cubic B-splines:[25]

$$\mathbf{u}(x, y, z) = \sum_{l=0}^{3} \sum_{m=0}^{3} \sum_{n=0}^{3} \theta_l(u) \theta_m(v) \theta_n(w) \phi_{i+l,\, j+m,\, k+n} \qquad (13.8)$$

where $i = \lfloor \frac{x}{\delta} \rfloor - 1, j = \lfloor \frac{y}{\delta} \rfloor - 1, k = \lfloor \frac{z}{\delta} \rfloor - 1, u = \frac{x}{\delta} - \lfloor \frac{x}{\delta} \rfloor, v = \frac{y}{\delta} - \lfloor \frac{y}{\delta} \rfloor, w = \frac{z}{\delta} - \lfloor \frac{z}{\delta} \rfloor$, and θ_l represents the l-th basis function of the B-splines:[25]

$$\theta_0(s) = (1 - s)^3/6$$

$$\theta_1(s) = (3s^3 - 6s^2 + 4)/6$$

$$\theta_2(s) = (-3s^3 + 3s^2 + 3s + 1)/6$$

$$\theta_3(s) = s^3/6$$

As mentioned previously, FFDs are controlled locally, which makes them computationally efficient even for a large number of control points. In particular, the basis functions of cubic B-splines have a limited support, i.e., changing control point $\phi_{i,j,k}$ affects the transformation only in the local neighborhood of that control point.

13.2.3 Elastic Registration

Elastic registration techniques were proposed by Bajcsy et al.[26] for matching a brain atlas with a CT image of a human subject. The idea is to model the deformation of the source image into the target image as a physical process which resembles the stretching of an elastic material such as rubber. This physical process is governed by two forces. The first term is the *internal* force which is caused by the deformation of elastic material (i.e., stress) and counteracts any force which deforms the elastic body from its equilibrium shape. The second term corresponds to the *external* force which acts on the elastic body. As a consequence, the deformation of the elastic body stops if both forces acting on it form an equilibrium solution. The behavior of the elastic body is described by the Navier linear elastic partial differential equation (PDE):

$$\mu\nabla^2\mathbf{u}(x, y, z) + (\lambda + \mu)\nabla(\nabla \cdot \mathbf{u}(x, y, z)) + \mathbf{f}(x, y, z) = 0 \quad (13.9)$$

Here $\mathbf{u}$ describes the displacement field, $\mathbf{f}$ is the external force acting on the elastic body, ∇ denotes the gradient operator, and ∇^2 denotes the Laplace operator. The parameters μ and λ are Lamé's elasticity constants which describe the behavior of the elastic body. These constants are often interpreted in terms of Young's modulus E_1, which relates the strain and stress of an object, and Poisson's ratio E_2, which is the ratio between lateral shrinking and longitudinal stretching:

$$E_1 = \frac{\mu(3\lambda + 2\mu)}{(\lambda + \mu)} \qquad E_2 = \frac{\lambda}{2(\mu + \lambda)} \quad (13.10)$$

The external force $\mathbf{f}$ is the force which acts on the elastic body and drives the registration process. A common choice for the external force is the gradient of a similarity measure such as a local correlation measure based on intensities,[26] intensity differences,[27] or intensity features such as edge and curvature.[28] An alternative choice is the distance between the curves[29] and surfaces[30] of corresponding anatomical structures.

The PDE in Equation (13.9) may be solved by finite differences and successive over relaxation (SOR).[31] This yields a discrete displacement field for each voxel. Alternatively, the PDE can be solved for only a subset of voxels which correspond to the nodes of a finite element model.[28,32] These nodes form a set of points for which the external forces are known. The displacements at other voxels are obtained by finite element interpolation. An extension of the elastic registration framework has been proposed by Davatzikos[33] to allow for spatially varying elasticity parameters. This enables certain anatomical structures to deform more freely than others.

13.2.4 Fluid Registration

Registration based on elastic transformations is limited by the fact that highly localized deformations can not be modeled, since the deformation energy caused by stress increases proportionally with the strength of the deformation. In fluid registration these constraints are relaxed over time, which enables the modeling of highly localized deformations including corners. This makes fluid registration especially attractive for intersubject registration tasks (including atlas matching) which have to accommodate large defor-mations and large degrees of variability. At the same time the scope for misregistration increases, as fluid transformations have a vast number of degrees of freedom.

Elastic deformations are often described in a *Lagrangian* reference frame, i.e., with respect to their initial position. In contrast to that, fluid deforma-tions are more conveniently described in a *Eulerian* reference frame, i.e., with respect to their final position. In this Eulerian reference frame, the deforma-tions of the fluid registration are characterized by the Navier-Stokes partial differential equation,

$$\mu \nabla^2 \mathbf{v}(x, y, z) + (\lambda + \mu) \nabla (\nabla \cdot \mathbf{v}(x, y, z)) + \mathbf{f}(x, y, z) = 0 \quad (13.11)$$

similar to Equation (13.9) except that differentiation is carried out on the velocity field $\mathbf{v}$ rather than on the displacement field $\mathbf{u}$ and is solved for each time step. The relationship between the Eulerian velocity and displacement field is given by:

$$\mathbf{v}(x, y, z, t) = \frac{\partial \mathbf{u}(x, y, z, t)}{\partial t} + \mathbf{v}(x, y, z, t) \cdot \nabla \mathbf{u}(x, y, z, t) \quad (13.12)$$

Christensen et al.[34] suggested to solve Equation (13.11) using successive over relaxation (SOR).[31] However, the resulting algorithm is rather slow and requires significant computing time. A faster implementation has been proposed by Bro-Nielsen et al.[35] Here, Equation (13.11) is solved by deriving a convolution filter from the eigenfunctions of the linear elasticity operator. Bro-Nielsen et al.[35] also pointed out that this is similar to a regularization by convolution with a Gaussian as proposed in a nonrigid matching technique by Thirion[36] in which the deformation process is modeled as a diffusion process. However, the solu-tion of Equation (13.11) by convolution is only possible if the viscosity is assumed constant, which is not always the case. For example, Lester[37] has pro-posed a model in which the viscosity of the fluid is allowed to vary spatially, and therefore allows for different degrees of deformability for different parts of the image. In this case Equation (13.11) must be solved using conventional numerical schemes such as SOR.[31]

13.2.5 Registration Using FEM and Mechanical Models

As mentioned previously, the PDE for elastic deformations can be solved by finite element methods (FEM) which also form the topic of Chapter 15. A sim-plified version of an FEM model has been proposed by Edwards et al.[38] to model tissue deformations in image-guided surgery. They propose a three-component model to simulate the properties of rigid, elastic, and fluid structures. For this purpose the image is divided into a triangular mesh with n connected nodes ϕ_i. Each node is labeled according to the physical properties of the underlying anatomical structures: for example, bone is labeled as rigid, soft tissues as elastic, and CSF as fluid. While nodes labeled as rigid are kept fixed, nodes labeled as elastic or fluid are deformed by minimizing an energy function. Edwards et al.[38] proposed a number of different energy terms to constrain deformations: for example, nodes labeled as elastic can be constrained by a tension energy

$$E_{\text{tension}}(\phi_i, \phi_j) = \left|\phi_j - \phi_i - \phi_{i,j}^0\right|^2$$

where $\phi_{i,j}^0$ corresponds to the relaxed distance between two nodes. An alternative choice for nodes labeled as elastic is a stiffness energy term:

$$E_{\text{stiffness}}(\phi_i, \phi_j, \phi_k) = \left|\phi_j - \phi_k - 2\phi_i\right|^2$$

Nodes labeled as fluid do not have any associated tension or stiffness energy. Instead they have an associated folding energy

$$E_{\text{fold}}(\phi_i, \phi_j, \phi_k) = \begin{cases} \dfrac{A^2}{\gamma^2 A_0^2} + \dfrac{\gamma^2 A_0^2}{A^2} & \text{if } \dfrac{A}{A_0} \leq \gamma \\ 2 & \text{otherwise} \end{cases}$$

where A_0 is the area of the undeformed triangle, A is the area of the deformed triangle, and γ is a threshold for the triangular area above which the energy contribution is constant. This energy term prevents the development of singularities in the transformation, i.e., the collapsing or folding over of triangles. In the implementation proposed by Edwards et al.[38] the registration is driven by a similarity measure which minimizes the distance between corresponding landmarks, but other similarity measures can be easily integrated into the energy function.

13.2.6 Registration Using Optical Flow

A well known registration technique which is equivalent to the equation of motion for incompressible flow in physics is the so-called optical flow.[39] The concept of optical flow was originally introduced in computer vision in order to recover the relative motion of an object and the viewer in between two successive frames of a temporal image sequence. Its fundamental assumption is that the image brightness of a particular point stays constant, i.e.,

$$I(x, y, z, t) = I(x + \delta x, y + \delta y, z + \delta z, t + \delta t). \tag{13.13}$$

Using a Taylor expansion of the right side and ignoring higher-order terms, the optical flow equation (13.13) can be rewritten as

$$\frac{\partial I}{\partial x}\frac{dx}{dt} + \frac{\partial I}{\partial y}\frac{dy}{dt} + \frac{\partial I}{\partial z}\frac{dz}{dt} + \frac{\partial I}{\partial t} = 0 \qquad (13.14)$$

Alternatively this can be written as

$$\Delta I + \nabla I \cdot \mathbf{u} = 0 \qquad (13.15)$$

where ΔI is the temporal difference between the images, ∇I is the spatial gradient of the image, and $\mathbf{u}$ describes the motion between the two images. In general, additional smoothness constraints are imposed on the motion field $\mathbf{u}$ in order to obtain a reliable estimate of the optical flow. These smoothness constraints are discussed in more detail in the following section.

13.2.7   Registration as an Optimization Problem

Like many other problems in computer vision and image analysis, registration can be formulated as an optimization problem whose goal is to minimize an associated energy or cost function. The most general form of such a cost function is

$$C = -C_{\text{similarity}} + C_{\text{deformation}} \qquad (13.16)$$

where the first term characterizes the similarity between the source and target image and the second term characterizes the cost associated with particular deformations. Most of the nonrigid registration techniques discussed so far can be formulated in this framework. From a probabilistic point of view, the cost function in Equation (13.16) can be explained in a Bayesian framework.[40] In this context, the similarity measure can be viewed as a likelihood term which expresses the probability of a match between source and target image. The second term can be interpreted as a prior which represents *a priori* knowledge about the expected deformations.

The first term is the driving force behind the registration process, and aims to maximize the similarity between both images. The different similarity measures can be divided into two main categories: point based and voxel based similarity measures (a detailed discussion of those can be found in Chapter 3). Point-based similarity measures minimize the distance between features such as points, curves, or surfaces of corresponding anatomical structures and requires prior feature extraction. In recent years, voxel-based similarity measures such as sums of squared differences, cross correlation, or mutual information described in Chapter 3 have become increasingly popular. These voxel-based similarity measures have the advantage that they do not require any feature extraction process.

The second term is often referred to as the regularization or penalty function which can be used to constrain the transformation relating the source and target images. In the case of rigid or affine registration this term is normally ignored and only plays a role in nonrigid registration. For example, in elastic or fluid registration the regularization term (linear elasticity model) forms an integral part of the registration. Other regularization models are the Laplacian or membrane model:[7,41]

$$\int_{-\infty}^{\infty}\int_{-\infty}^{\infty}\int_{-\infty}^{\infty}\left[\left(\frac{\partial \mathbf{T}}{\partial x}\right)^2 + \left(\frac{\partial \mathbf{T}}{\partial y}\right)^2 + \left(\frac{\partial \mathbf{T}}{\partial z}\right)^2\right] dx\, dy\, dz$$

and the biharmonic or thin-plate model:[16,42]

$$\int_{-\infty}^{\infty}\int_{-\infty}^{\infty}\int_{-\infty}^{\infty}\left[\left(\frac{\partial^2 \mathbf{T}}{\partial x^2}\right)^2 + \left(\frac{\partial^2 \mathbf{T}}{\partial y^2}\right)^2 + \left(\frac{\partial^2 \mathbf{T}}{\partial z^2}\right)^2\right.$$
$$\left. + 2\left[\left(\frac{\partial^2 \mathbf{T}}{\partial xy}\right)^2 + \left(\frac{\partial^2 \mathbf{T}}{\partial xz}\right)^2 + \left(\frac{\partial^2 \mathbf{T}}{\partial yz}\right)^2\right]\right] dx\, dy\, dz$$

Both models have an intuitive physical interpretation. While the Laplacian model approximates the energy of a membrane (such as a rubber sheet) which is subjected to elastic deformations, the biharmonic term approximates the energy of a thin plate of metal which is subjected to bending deformations.[43] For example, Rueckert et al.[22] combine a similarity function based on mutual information with thin-plate regularization.

13.3 Applications

There are a large number of applications for nonrigid registration. Areas of considerable interest for nonrigid registration are the applications discussed in more detail in Chapter 5, in which the geometry during image acquisition is unknown or distorted, and include correction for scaling,[2] gantry tilt,[3] and magnetic field inhomogeneity.[44] Other areas of nonrigid registration can be classified into either the registration of deformable structures of the same individual (intrasubject registration) or the registration across individuals (intersubject registration). Due to the different nature of these registration tasks, the algorithms developed to solve them have quite different characteristics.

13.3.1   Intrasubject Registration

The goal of intrasubject registration is the matching and fusion of images of the same subject acquired at different times and/or with different imaging modalities. The need for nonrigid registration arises from the fact that most tissues are far from rigid and can deform considerably. This tissue deformation may be caused by patient motion, cardiac motion, or respiratory motion. For example, nonrigid registration plays an important role for contrast enhanced MR imaging of the breast. Here, the difference between the rate of uptake of contrast agent in healthy and cancerous tissue can be used to identify cancerous lesions. The rate of uptake of contrast agent is estimated as the difference between pre- and postcontrast images, and any motion between both images complicates its estimation. Due to the highly deformable nature of the breast tissue, Rueckert et al.[22] have developed a nonrigid registration technique to correct for this motion. An example of this is shown in Figures 13.3 and 13.4. A clinical evaluation in comparison

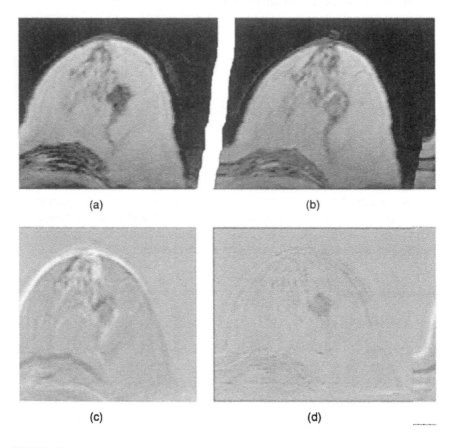

(a)   (b)

(c)   (d)

FIGURE 13.3
A contrast-enhanced MR mammography: (a) precontrast, (b) postcontrast and after subtraction (c) without registration, and (d) with nonrigid registration.[22]

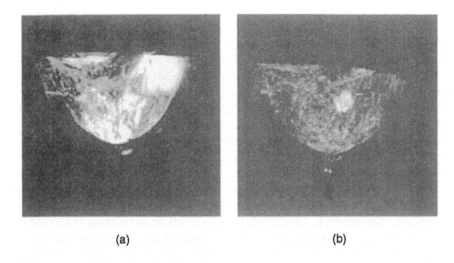

(a)   (b)

FIGURE 13.4

A maximum intensity projection (MIP) of a contrast-enhanced MR mammography: (a) without registration and (b) with nonrigid registration.[22]

with rigid and affine registration techniques has demonstrated the superior performance of the nonrigid registration technique for contrast-enhanced MR mammography.[45]

For a number of other registration tasks it is necessary to model rigid as well as nonrigid deformations. For example, in the registration of images of the spine, the vertebrae of the spine are rigid and do not deform, while the surrounding tissue can deform in a nonrigid fashion. Little et al.[18] have recently shown how the constraints of rigid bodies can be incorporated into a spline based transformation using radial basis functions. This results in an interpolating solution that is a summation of a linear term corresponding to the rigid bodies, and a basis function which smoothly tends to zero at the surface of the rigid bodies. The resulting transformation is exact at rigid bodies, given the rigid body transformation, and provides smooth interpolation elsewhere.

Other reasons for tissue deformation may be changes over time such as tumor growth or tissue deformation due to external forces. For example, in many image-guided surgery applications it is necessary to align preoperatively acquired images with intra- or postoperative images. To model soft tissue deformation in a physically more plausible way, Edwards et al.[38] developed a three-component model, described in Section 13.2.5. This model incorporates the different deformation characteristics of rigid, elastic, and fluid structures, and has been tested on CT and MR slices of the brain acquired before and after surgery for placement of electrode mats on the brain surface prior to excision of areas of focal activity in the treatment of epilepsy.

Other applications of nonrigid registration for intrasubject registration include the monitoring of temporal changes in serial MR images[46,47] and the analysis of rest and stress cardiac SPECT images.[23]

13.3.2   Intersubjection Registration

In contrast to intrasubject registration where nonrigid registration is largely used to account for the deformation of anatomical structures, the motivation for the use of nonrigid matching techniques in intersubject registration is quite different. Here, the aim of nonrigid registration is not to account for the physical deformation of the underlying anatomical structures but rather to account for the variability of these structures across different individuals. As a result, the transformations used for intersubject registration usually have a larger number of degrees of freedom and are less tightly constrained than those used for intrasubject registration.

An important application for intersubject registration is the construction and matching of computerized atlantes (also called atlases), which also forms the topic of Chapter 14. Traditional medical atlantes contain information about anatomy and function from a single individual, focusing primarily on the human brain.[48,49] Such an atlas can be made subject-specific by transforming its coordinate system to match that of another individual. This transformation removes any subject specific shape variations and allows subsequent comparison of structure and function between individuals. Consequently, a number of different elastic[26,40] and fluid[35,50,51] warping techniques have been developed for this purpose. Even though the individuals selected for these atlantes may be considered normal, they may represent an extreme of a normal distribution. To address this problem, researchers have developed probabilistic atlantes which include information from a set of subjects making them more representative of a population. These atlantes have been successfully used to investigate structural and functional differences in the human brain as part of the International Consortium for Brain Mapping (ICBM).[52] A prominent example of such a probabilistic atlantes of the human brain is the atlas developed at the Montreal Neurological Institute (MNI).[4] In this example MR images from 305 subjects were mapped into stereotactic space, intensity normalized, and averaged on a voxel-by-voxel basis.

Mapping data sets into normalized space not only accounts for anatomic and functional variations and idiosyncrasies of each individual subject, but also offers a powerful framework which facilitates comparison of anatomy and function over time, between subjects, between groups of subjects, and across sites. Another aspect of deformable atlantes is that the characteristics of the displacements required to warp the atlas onto the subject provide a method for assessing local and global shape differences and can produce valuable information about abnormalities[53] or determine gross morphometric variability.[54] An example of an MR atlas of the brain of seven normal subjects is shown in Figure 13.5. This atlas has been computed by using one subject to define a reference space and registering all other subjects to this reference space. The atlas was then constructed by averaging all MR images after they had been mapped into the reference space. This is illustrated in Figure 13.5: The top row shows the resulting atlas if a rigid transformation is used to align the images. The middle row shows the resulting atlas if an affine transformation is used to

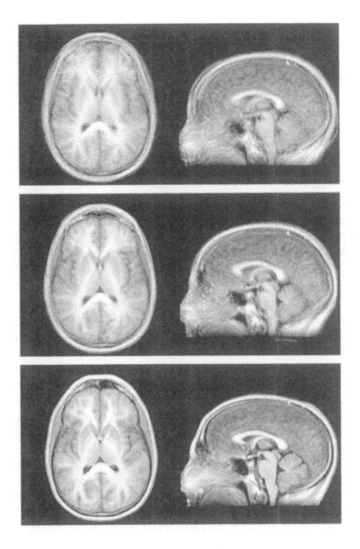

FIGURE 13.5
An example of intersubject registration: an atlas of the brain is constructed by averaging the MR images of seven normal subjects (top row) after rigid registration, (middle row) after affine registration, and (bottom row) after nonrigid registration using free form deformations.[22]

align the images. The bottom row shows the atlas obtained by using a non-rigid transformation based on freeform deformations.

Another important area of application which requires the matching of computerized atlantes is the automated segmentation and labeling of complex structures of the brain.[55,56] Many of these approaches are based on the understanding that only the use of statistical models of shape and intensity enables automatic identification of complex structures such as the human brain.

A fundamental advantage of probabilistic atlantes is that they allow for the calculation of statistical probability anatomy maps which can be used to derive statistical knowledge about the spatial position and variability of anatomical structures.

13.3.3 Analysis of Motion and Deformation Using Nonrigid Registration

In the case of rigid registration the recovered transformation itself has no clinical significance. It merely expresses the difference between the position and orientation in two images. However, in the case of nonrigid registration the recovered transformation may have clinical significance. In particular, the transformation may be used for the quantification of changes between images. In these cases the primary goal is not only the transformation which maps points in one image into their corresponding counterparts in the second image, but also the motion and deformation characteristics exhibited by this transformation.

One such example is the work of Maurer et al.,[57,58] who have used a nonrigid registration algorithm to detect and quantify intraoperative brain deformation. In this application, pre- and postoperative MR images from patients undergoing neurosurgery have been acquired using an interventional MR scanner. After rigid registration of the pre- and postoperative MR images, the images have been aligned by a nonrigid registration algorithm which maximizes the normalized mutual information between the pre- and postoperative images. The resulting deformation field can be used to calculate the volume change throughout the brain on a voxel-by-voxel basis. An example of this is shown in Figure 13.6.

In a similar effort, Thirion et al.[59] and Rey et al.[47] used a nonrigid registration algorithm to identify multiple sclerosis lesions and characterize their change over time. Finally, Thompson et al.[60] have shown that growth patterns in the developing brain can be studied and analyzed using the deformation fields obtained by nonrigid registration. From these deformation fields local rates of tissue dilation, contraction, and shear are calculated.

13.4 Conclusions

Rigid registration techniques have become widely accepted in a variety of clinical applications. In contrast, nonrigid registration is very much an area of ongoing research, and most algorithms are still in the stage of development and evaluation. One of the main reasons for the successful impact of rigid registration techniques is the fact that these techniques can be assessed and validated against a gold standard (see Chapter 6). The lack of a gold standard for assessing and evaluating the success of nonrigid registration algorithms is one of their most significant drawbacks. Currently, the only accepted method for assessing nonrigid registration is based on manually

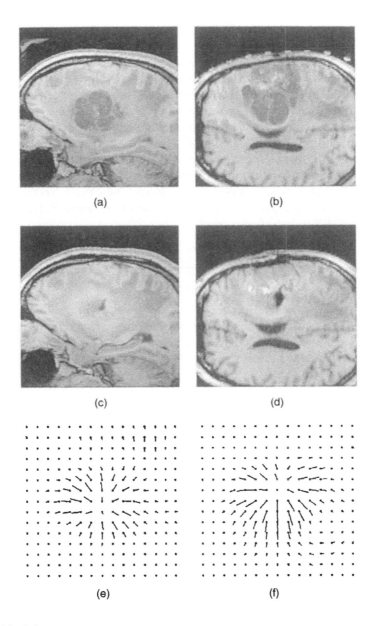

FIGURE 13.6
An example of motion and deformation analysis from intraoperative MR images using nonrigid registration:[22] (a, b) preoperative MR images, (c, d) postoperative MR images, and (e, f) the deformation field calculated by the algorithm (for better clarity the deformation vectors have been scaled by a factor of two).

identifying the position of anatomical or artificial landmarks in the source and target image and comparing those to the position predicted by the nonrigid registration algorithm.[5] In carrying out validation, it is important to consider the correspondence issues introduced in Chapter 2. An algorithm could appear to match perfectly the source image to the target image, such that all features overlap, but the transformation calculated may be completely wrong. For example, in intrasubject registration, a transformation might stretch some parts of the image and compress others to make structures appear to line up even if the underlying tissue is incompressible. In intersubject registration, an algorithm might warp structures in one image so they appear to line up with corresponding structures in a second image of a different subject, but the calculated transformation might be inappropriate for comparing functional regions identified from the two subjects. At its current stage of maturity, nonrigid registration algorithms should be used with care, especially where it is desirable to use the calculated transformation for secondary purposes such as understanding tissue deformation or studying variability between subjects.

Acknowledgments

Daniel Rueckert was a research fellow at the Computational Imaging Science Group, Department of Radiological Sciences at King's College London when most of this work was performed. He was supported by EPSRC project grant GR/L08519.

References

1. H. Lester and S.R. Arridge. A survey of hierarchical non-linear medical image registration. *Pattern Recogn.*, 32(1):129–149, 1999.
2. D.L.G. Hill, C.R. Maurer, Jr., C. Studholme, J.M. Fitzpatrick, and D.J. Hawkes. Correcting scaling errors in tomographic images using a nine degree of freedom registration algorithm. *J. Comp. Assist. Tomogr.*, 22(2):317–323, 1998.
3. C. Studholme, J.A. Little, G.P. Penney, D.L.G. Hill, and D.J. Hawkes. Automated multimodality registration using the full affine transformation: application to MR and CT guided skull base surgery. In *Proc. 4th International Conference Visualization in Biomedical Computing (VBC'96)*, pages 601–606, 1996.
4. D.L. Collins, P. Neelin, T.M. Peters, and A.C. Evans. Automatic 3D intersubject registration of MR volumetric data in standardized Talairach space. *J. Comp. Assist. Tomogr.*, 18(2):192–205, 1994.
5. R.P. Woods, S.T. Grafton, J.D.G. Watson, N.L. Sicotte, and J.C. Mazziotta. Automated image registration: II. Intersubject validation of linear and nonlinear models. *J. Comp. Assist. Tomogr.*, 22(1):153–165, 1998.
6. R. Szeliski and S. Lavallée. Matching 3-D anatomical surfaces with non-rigid deformations using octree-splines. In *IEEE Workshop on Biomedical Image Analysis*, pages 144–153, 1994.
7. Y. Amit, U. Grenander, and M. Piccioni. Structural image restoration through deformable templates. *J. Am. Statis. Ass.*, 86(414):376–387, 1991.

8. J. Ashburner and K.J. Friston. Nonlinear spatial normalization using basis functions. *Human Brain Mapping*, 7:254–266, 1999.
9. Y. Amit. A nonlinear variational problem for image matching. *SIAM J. Scien. Comp.*, 15(1):207–224, 1994.
10. F.L. Bookstein. Thin-plate splines and the atlas problem for biomedical images. In *Information Processing in Medical Imaging: Proc. 12th International Conference (IPMI'91)*, pages 326–342, 1991.
11. C.R. Meyer, J.L. Boes, B. Kim, P.H. Bland, K.R. Zasadny, P.V. Kison, K. Koral, K.A. Frey, and R.L. Wahl. Demonstration of accuracy and clinical versatility of mutual information for automatic multimodality image fusion using affine and thin-plate spline warped geometric deformations. *Med. Image Anal.*, 1(3):195–207, 1997.
12. M.H. Davis, A. Khotanzad, D.P. Flaming, and S.E. Harms. A physics-based coordinate transformation for 3-D image matching. *IEEE Trans. Med. Imaging*, 16(3):317–328, 1997.
13. J. Duchon. Interpolation des functions de deux variables suivant les principes de la flexion des plaques minces. *RAIRO Analyse Numérique*, 10:5–12, 1976.
14. J. Meinguet. Multivariate interpolation at arbitrary points made simple. *Zeitschrift für angewandte Mathematik und Physik*, 30:292–304, 1979.
15. A. Goshtasby. Registration of images with geoemtric distortions. *IEEE Trans. Geoscien. and Remote Sensing*, 26(1):60–64, 1988.
16. F.L. Bookstein. Principal warps: thin-plate splines and the decomposition of deformations. *IEEE Trans. on Pattern Anal. and Machine Intell.*, 11(6):567–585, 1989.
17. N. Arad, N. Dyn, D. Reisfeld, and Y. Yeshurun. Image warping by radial basis functions: application to facial expression. *Comp. Vision, Graphics, and Image Process. Graphical Models and Image Process.*, 56(2):161–172, 1994.
18. J.A. Little, D.L.G. Hill, and D.J. Hawkes. Deformations incorporating rigid structures. *Comp. Vision and Image Understand.*, 66(2):223–232, 1997.
19. F.L. Bookstein and W.D.K. Green. A feature space for edgels in images with landmarks. *J. Math. Imaging and Vision*, 3:231–261, 1993.
20. K. Rohr, H.S. Stiehl, R. Sprengel, T.M. Buzug, J. Weese, and M.H. Kuhn. Point-based elastic registration of medical image data using approximating thin-plate splines. In *Proc. 4th International Conference Visualization in Biomedical Computing (VBC'96)*, pages 297–307, 1996.
21. T.W. Sederberg and S.R. Parry. Free-form deformation of solid geometric models. In *Proceedings of SIGGRAPH'86, Computer Graphics*, pages 151–160, 1992.
22. D. Rueckert, L.I. Sonoda, C. Hayes, D.L.G. Hill, M.O. Leach, and D.J. Hawkes. Non-rigid registration using free-form deformations: Application to breast MR images. *IEEE Trans. Med. Imaging*, 18(8):712–721, 1999.
23. J. Declerck, J. Feldmar, M.L. Goris, and F. Betting. Automatic registration and alignment on a template of cardiac stress and rest reoriented SPECT images. *IEEE Trans. Med. Imaging*, 6(727–737), 1997.
24. J. Feldmar, J. Declarck, G. Malandain, and N. Ayache. Extension of the ICP algorithm to non-rigid intensity-based registration of 3D volumes. *Comp. Vision Image Understand.*, 66(2):193–206, 1997.
25. J. Foley, A. van Dam, S. Feiner, and J. Hughes. Computer Graphics. *ASME J. Biomech. Eng.*, 122(4):354–363, 2000.
26. R. Bajcsy and S. Kovačič. Multiresolution elastic matching. *Comp. Vision, Graphics and Image Process.*, 46:1–21, 1989.

27. G.E. Christensen. Deformable Shape Models for Anatomy. Ph.D. thesis, Washington University, 1994.
28. J.C. Gee, C. Barillot, L. Le Briquer, D.R. Haynor, and R. Bajcsy. Matching structural images of the humanbrain using statistical and geometrical features. In *Proc. 3rd International Conference Visualization in Biomedical Computing (VBC'94)*, pages 191–204, Rochester, MN, 1994.
29. C.A. Davatzikos, J.L. Prince, and R.N. Bryan. Image registration based on boundary mapping. *IEEE Trans. Med. Imaging*, 15(1):112–115, 1995.
30. P. Thompson and A.W. Toga. A surface-based technique for warping three-dimensional images of the brain. *IEEE Trans. Med. Imaging*, 15(4):402–417, 1996.
31. W.H. Press, B.P. Flannery, S.A. Teukolsky, and W. T. Vetterling. *Numerical Recipes in C*. Cambridge University Press, 2nd ed., 1989.
32. J.C. Gee, D.R. Haynor, M. Reikvich, and R. Bajcsy. Finite element approach to warping of brain images. In *Proc. SPIE Medical Imaging 1994: Image Processing*, volume 2167, pages 18–27, Newport Beach, USA, February 1994. SPIE.
33. C. Davatzikos. Spatial transformation and registration of brain images using elastically deformable models. *Comp. Vision and Image Understand.*, 66(2):207–222, 1997.
34. G.E. Christensen, R.D. Rabbitt, and M.I. Miller. Deformable templates using large deformation kinematics. *IEEE Trans. Image Process.*, 5(10):1435–1447, 1996.
35. M. Bro-Nielsen and C. Gramkow. Fast fluid registration of medical images. *Comp. Methods Biotech. Biomed. Eng.*, 3:129–146, 2000.
36. J.-P. Thirion. Image matching as a diffusion process: an analogy with Maxwell's demons. *Med. Image Anal.*, 2(3):243–260, 1998.
37. H. Lester, S.R. Arridge, K.M. Jansons, L. Lemieux, J.V. Hajnal, and A. Oatridge. Non-linear registration with the variable viscosity fluid algorithm. In *Information Processing in Medical Imaging: Proc. 16th International Conference (IPMI'99)*, pages 238–251, 1999.
38. P.J. Edwards, D.L.G. Hill, J.A. Little, and D.J. Hawkes. A three-component deformation model for image-guided surgery. *Med. Image Anal.*, 2(4):355–367, 1998.
39. B.K.P. Horn and B.G. Schnuck. Determining optical flow. *Artif. Intell.*, 17:185–203, 1981.
40. J. Gee, M. Reivich, and R. Bajcsy. Elastically deforming 3D atlas to match anatomical brain images. *J. Comp. Assist. Tomogr.*, 17(2):225–236, 1993.
41. D. Terzopoulos. Regularization of inverse visual problems involving discontinuities. *IEEE Trans. on Pattern Anal. Machine Intell.*, 8(4):413–424, 1986.
42. G. Wahba. *Spline Models for Observational Data*. Society for Industrial and Applied Mathematics, 1990.
43. R. Courant and D. Hilbert. *Methods of Mathematical Physics*, Vol. 1. Interscience, London, 1953.
44. C. Studholme, R.T. Constable, and J.S. Duncan. Incorporating an image distortion model in nonrigid alignment of EPI with conventional MRI. In *Information Processing in Medical Imaging: Proc. 16th International Conference (IPMI'99)*, pages 454–459, 1999.
45. E.R.E. Denton, L.I. Sonoda, D. Rueckert, S.C. Rankin, C. Hayes, M. Leach, D.L.G. Hill, and D.J. Hawkes. Comparison and evaluation of rigid and non-rigid registration of breast MR images. *J. Comp. Assist. Tomogr.*, 23:800–805, 1999.
46. P.A. Freeborough and N.C. Fox. Modeling brain deformations in Alzheimer disease by fluid registration of serial 3D MR images. *J. Comp. Assist. Tomogr.*, 22(5):838–843, 1998.

47. D. Rey, G. Subsol, H. Delingette, and N. Ayache. Automatic detection and segmentation of evolving processes in 3D medical images: application to multiple sclerosis. In *Information Processing in Medical Imaging: Proc. 16th International Conference (IPMI'99)*, pages 154–167, 1999.

48. G. Schaltenbrand and P. Bailey. *Introduction to Stereotaxis with an Atlas for the Human Brain*. Georg Thieme Verlag, Stuttgart, Germany, 1959.

49. J. Talairach and P. Thournoux. *Co-Planar Stereotactic Atlas of the Human Brain: 3-Dimensional Proportional System: An Approach to Cerebral Imaging*. Georg Thieme Verlag, Stuttgart, Germany, 1988.

50. G.E. Christensen, M.I. Miller, J.L. Mars, and M.W. Vannier. Automatic analysis of medical images using a deformable textbook. In *Computer Assisted Radiology*, Lemke, H., Vannier, M., Inamura, K., and Farman, A., Eds., Springer-Verlag, Berlin, Germany, June 1995, pages 146–151.

51. G.E. Christensen, S.C. Joshi, and M.I. Miller. Individualizing anatomical atlases of the head. In *Proc. 4th International Conference Visualization in Biomedical Computing (VBC'96)*, pages 434–348, 1996.

52. J. Mazziotta, A. Toga, A. Evans P. Fox, and J. Lancaster. A probabilistic atlas of the human brain: theory and rationale for its development. the international consortium for brain mapping. *NeuroImage*, 2(2):89–101, 1995.

53. P. Thompson and A.W. Toga. Detection, visualization and animation of abnormal anatomic structure with a deformable probabilistic atlas based on random vector field transformations. *Med. Image Anal.*, 1(4):271–294, 1997.

54. D.L. Collins, T.M. Peters, and A.C. Evans. An automated 3D non-linear deformation procedure for determination of gross morphometric variability in human brain. In *Proc. 3rd International Conference Visualization in Biomedical Computing (VBC'94)*, pages 180–190, Rochester, MN, 1994.

55. D.L. Collins, A.C. Evans, C. Holmes, and T.M. Peters. Automatic 3D segmentation of neuroanatomical structures from MRI. In *Information Processing in Medical Imaging: Proc. 14th International Conference (IPMI'95)*, pages 139–152, 1995.

56. T.F. Cootes, C. Beeston, G.J. Edwards, and C.J. Taylor. A unified framework for atlas matching using active appearance models. In *Information Processing in Medical Imaging: Proc. 16th International Conference (IPMI'99)*, pages 322–333, 1999.

57. C.R. Maurer, Jr., D.L.G. Hill, A.J. Martin, H. Liu, M. McCue, D. Rueckert, D. Lloret, W.A. Hall, R.E. Maxwell, D.J. Hawkes, and C.L. Truwit. Investigation of intraoperative brain deformation using a 1.5T interventional MR system: preliminary results. *IEEE Trans. Med. Imaging*, 17(5):817–825, 1998.

58. D.L.G. Hill, C.R. Maurer, Jr., A.J. Martin, S. Sabanathan, W.A. Hall, D.J. Hawkes, D. Rueckert, and C.L. Truwit. Assessment of intraoperative brain deformation using interventional MR imaging. In *Second Int. Conf. on Medical Image Computing and Computer-Assisted Intervention (MICCAI'99)*, pages 910–919, Cambridge, UK, 1999.

59. J.-P. Thirion and G. Calmon. Deformation analysis to detect and quantify active lesions in three-dimensional medical image sequences. *IEEE Trans. Med. Imaging*, 18(5):429–441.

60. P.M. Thompson, J.N. Giedd, R.P. Woods, D. MacDonald, A.C. Evans, and A.W. Toga. Growth patterns in the developing brain detected by continuum mechanical tensor maps. *Nature*, 404:190–193, March 2000.

14

Use of Registration for Cohort Studies

D. Louis Collins, Alex P. Zijdenbos, Tomáš Paus, and Alan C. Evans

CONTENTS

14.1 Introduction

The past ten years, known as the *decade of the brain,* have been marked by advances in medical tomographic imaging technology that have made it possible to acquire highly detailed volumes of human anatomy in three dimensions (3D) with magnetic resonance imaging (MRI). Such technology has facilitated the explosion of human brain mapping research, where anatomical MRI is combined with positron emission tomography

(PET) or functional magnetic resonance imaging (fMRI) to correlate structure and function in normal and diseased subjects. The combination of *in vivo* imaging data with interactive computerized visualization tools has significantly improved the understanding of gross anatomy in the living brain. Even with these new tools, traditional technical and practical difficulties have conditioned many neuroscientific studies to extrapolate findings from a relatively small sample of the population. In this chapter, our research program at the Brain Imaging Centre (BIC) of the Montreal Neurological Institute (MNI) will be used as an exemplar of the work in this field and will illustrate our perspective on this fast moving area of research.

A significant part of our research program has concentrated on the development of computerized algorithms for automated analysis of large ensembles of anatomical and functional data. These data arise from cohort studies where the number of subjects is counted in the hundreds, if not thousands. These tools are the result of our participation in the International Consortium for Brain Mapping (ICBM[1]) where the goal has been to address certain weaknesses associated with classical brain atlases (or atlantes). Such atlases are derived from a single brain, or brains from a small number of subjects.[2-6] Even though the brains selected for use in this atlas may be considered normal, they may still represent an extreme of the normal distribution. Comparison of a given subject's brain is achieved by aligning the brain with the atlas, and then using simple scaling factors in an attempt to account for variability in brain size. Unfortunately, the limited number of examples used to create the atlas prohibits quantification or representation of normal anatomical morphometric or functional variability. Thus, it is difficult to judge the degree of normalcy of a brain under study by comparison with one of these atlases.

In keeping with the goals of the Human Brain Project,[7] the thrust of the ICBM project is to characterize normal anatomy and function by building normative databases and the tools required for interaction with these databases. The primary aim of the first phase of the ICBM project was to quantify the normal range of morphometric variability and to build a probabilistic atlas of structural anatomy. In the second phase, similar tools are now being developed to capture and characterize variability of functional regions.

The methods developed in the context of the ICBM project are directly applicable to cohort studies where the goal may be to characterize the brain anatomy of a specific group of subjects or to quantify differences between two groups. For example, one might be interested in using subtle anatomical differences, such as differential rates of cerebral atrophy, to discriminate between groups of patients treated with different medications. For many of these studies, data such as blood volume, blood flow, glucose utilization, or tracer uptake must be estimated for a particular region of interest from the data set corresponding to each subject. Traditional manual definition of such regions is difficult, time consuming, and potentially unsuitable if inter- and intraobserver variability is large when compared to the size of a subtle signal difference that is to be detected.

Two basic paradigms have been proposed in the literature to replace manual segmentation methods and automate the analysis process, making it as objective as possible. The first is based on segmentation and the second is based on registration.

There have been a number of attempts at developing semiautomated[8-15] segmentation procedures that are able to identify the borders of structures of interest, with differing levels of success for different tasks. These methods require some level of manual intervention to align predefined atlas structures onto the volumetric image data. A hierarchical system is normally used, where the entire atlas is fitted with a global transformation, followed by customization of individual atlas structures. Fully automated techniques attempt to match atlas structures to the image data directly, thus obviating the need for user input, with different levels of success.[16-23]

Registration-based comparison techniques examine the data on a voxel-by-voxel basis, and thus require data to be placed into correspondence spatially to replace the aforementioned structure-by-structure comparison techniques.[24-29] These techniques have the advantage of permitting exploratory analysis of the whole brain volume without specifically identifying particular regions in each volume. The first half of this chapter will concentrate on the technical aspects of anatomical registration. The second half will summarize a number of example cohort studies that have been carried out in the BIC at the MNI.

14.2 Technical Issues

Registration-based comparison methods are based on spatial normalization where a spatial transformation is found to map similar structures (or homologous points) from different data sets to same spatial position. While the general case must concern itself with the mapping of data from different imaging modalities (intermodality registration), we deal here only with the specific case of intramodality registration of MRI data.

Four aspects of the normalization procedure must be identified and well defined before continuing:

- **Reference space:** *Which data set and coordinate system defines the reference frame used for comparisons?*
- **Spatial mapping function:** *How will brain data from a given subject be mapped or transformed from the native (original scan) representation to the reference frame?*
- **Similarity measure:** *How will a brain volume be compared to the target data set to determine value (goodness) of a given mapping function?*

- **Optimization procedure:** *What algorithm will be used to search the space of possible spatial mapping functions to determine which one yields the maximum similarity?*

These aspects will be discussed in the following sections.

14.2.1   The Reference Space

The ideal *reference space* should minimize the positional variability of homologous anatomical (or functional) features after mapping data from different subjects into the space. This frame of reference should arise directly from a simple statistical analysis of the features. However, determination of this space is dependent on the features selected in addition to the four aforementioned aspects of the spatial normalization procedure. This said, we will describe a well known, practical reference space used for neuroscientific research. Other reference spaces will be discussed in Section 14.2.5.

14.2.1.1   Talairach Stereotaxic Space

Within the brain mapping community, the *de facto* standard reference frame is based on the brain-based coordinate system first described by the French neurosurgeon Talairach.[2,30] This reference system provides a method for identifying the location of a structure so that regions of interest can be compared between brains using standard coordinates. Although originally developed to target deep brain structures for stereotaxic neurosurgical procedures using pneumoencephalography, the Talairach stereotaxic system has become an international standard for reporting the coordinates of brain locations obtained in functional activation studies. This system has facilitated the development of BrainMap, a database of spatially indexed functional brain data.[31]

The *stereotaxic space* defined by Talairach is based on the identification of a midplane line passing through the superior aspect of the anterior commissure (AC) and the inferior aspect of the posterior commissure (PC), thus defining the so-called AC-PC line. The origin of the space is defined by the intersection of a vertical perpendicular line with the AC-PC line, passing through the posterior aspect of the AC. This perpendicular is in the midplane and is known as the VAC line. The coordinate system follows the convention that the x-axis is in the left-right (LR) direction (positive towards the right), the y-axis is in the posterior-anterior (PA) direction (positive anteriorly), and the z-axis is in the caudo-cranial (CC) direction (positive superiorly).

Individual data sets can be compared with the Talairach atlas by identifying the AC-PC and VAC lines within the given volume so that they can be aligned with the atlas (thus defining the *Talairach spatial mapping function*). In order to account for different brain sizes, proportional scaling is used to partition the brain into three piecewise linear components in the PA direction (pre-AC, AC-PC, post-PC), two in the CC direction (above/below AC-PC), and two in the LR direction (one for each hemisphere).

When image volumes are transformed into this space and resampled on the same voxel grid such that all brains have the same orientation and size, voxel-by-voxel comparisons across data volumes from different populations are possible, since each voxel (i, j, k) corresponds to the same (x, y, z) points in the brain-based coordinate system. The transformation to this coordinate system also provides a means for enhancement of functional signals by averaging images in this space.[32] This paradigm allows information (anatomical, metabolic, electrophysiological, chemical, cytoarchitectonic) from different brains to be spatially organized and cataloged by mapping all brains into the same coordinate system.[31] Finally, in the original Talairach spirit, the coordinate corresponding to a particular structure, as defined by an atlas in this coordinate system, can be used to *predict* its location in a subject's brain volume when mapped into the same space. The accuracy of prediction depends greatly on the residual anatomical variability remaining after mapping a brain into this coordinate system. For thalamus and basal ganglia structures, this mapping and the corresponding prediction are quite accurate because anatomical variability of these structures in this frame of reference is low. The predictive accuracy is lower for cortical structures, mainly due to the significantly higher anatomical variability in this space.

When used for interpretation of cortical regions, there are a number of difficulties associated with the Talairach atlas. (Note the distinction between the stereotaxic *atlas* and the stereotaxic *space*.) The atlas is derived from a single cadaver brain of a right-handed, 60-year-old European female, and thus may suffer from postmortem artifacts. The atlas is defined on one hemisphere and reflected to the other hemisphere, making it completely symmetric and ignoring well known left-right hemispheric differences. With the exception of the upper midbrain, the atlas excludes the brainstem and cerebellum. It has variable slice separation, up to 4 mm. While it contains transverse, coronal, and sagittal slices, it is not contiguous in 3D nor is it entirely consistent among the three representations.[33] Finally, and perhaps most importantly, it is derived from a single subject, and thus it cannot represent statistical models of anatomical variability.

Despite the difficulties associated with the Talairach atlas, there are a number of significant advantages to using stereotaxic space for brain imaging studies, the most important of which is that this space provides a conceptual framework for the completely automated 3D analysis across subjects in cohort studies. In particular, registration of brain image volumes to this space:

- Facilitates comparisons 1) across time points for an individual subject, 2) between subjects, 3) between different groups of subjects, and 4) across acquisition sites
- Permits voxel-to-voxel averaging between subjects to detect subtle signals by increasing the signal-to-noise ratio[32]
- Allows the use of spatial masks for postprocessing[34]
- Allows the use of spatial priors (e.g., for classification)
- Allows the use of anatomical models (e.g., for segmentation)

- Provides a framework for statistical analysis with well-established random field models[35]
- Allows the rapid reanalysis of ensembles of data using different processing criteria

The uncertainties associated with the atlas, the advantages of stereotaxic space, and the availability at the MNI of a large database of MRI volumes obtained from young, normal subjects have lead our group to construct a 3D probabilistic atlas of gross neuroanatomy. This atlas is described in the next section.

14.2.1.2 MNI Stereotaxic Space

Significant morphometric variability exists between individuals.[36,37] Rather than using a single brain, we have established a model from more than 300 MRI data sets from young normals.[38,39] Our model was defined in a coordinate system similar to that proposed by Talairach;[2] however, we use a single linear transformation instead of 12 piecewise linear transformations to map a brain into stereotaxic space.

In order to build the stereotaxic space model, we proceeded with a two-stage procedure. In the first stage, each MRI volume was manually registered with the stereotaxic coordinate system using the method described by Evans et al.[36] The line defined by the AC-PC line was manually estimated by identifying the following points defined on the midsagittal plane: the occipital pole, the superior aspect of the cerebellum, the inferior aspect of the splenium of the corpus callosum, the posterior commissure, the inferior aspect of the thalamus, the anterior commissure, and the inferior aspect of the genu of the corpus callosum. A line was fitted through these points and the most anterior and most posterior aspects of the brain identified. A vertical perpendicular bisector of the AC-PC line was drawn to identify the most superior aspect of the cortex. Lateral perpendicular bisectors were drawn to identify the most lateral points of the cerebral volume. These points were used to define a **single** linear transformation required to bring each data set into stereotaxic space. Note that this is a significant difference from the method originally described by Talairach. Each volume was resampled onto a 1 mm voxel grid according to this transformation and was subsequently normalized for mean image intensity. The entire ensemble of MRI data sets was averaged to create the first-pass mean MRI brain, which was then available as a target for registration.

This first-pass mean MRI brain was degraded by random errors introduced in the alignment of each subject's AC-PC line by manual identification. A second stage was then initiated, using the first-pass mean average as the target for an automated 3D image-matching algorithm.[28] Each individual brain was again transformed from its native space to the stereotaxic space by mapping it, again with a single linear transformation (rigid body plus three scaling parameters), to the target volume. This process reduced the effect of random alignment errors and increased the contrast of the averaged result. The entire ensemble of 305 MRI data sets was averaged to create the second-pass mean MRI brain known as MNI305,[36,38,39] which has been made publicly available as a standard stereotaxic registration target within the MNI_Autoreg package* and within the statistical parametric mapping (SPM**) package developed at the Wellcome Department of Cognitive Neurology.

14.2.2 The Spatial Mapping Function

The *spatial mapping function* is used to transform coordinates from the native image volume into the reference space. There are a number of desirable characteristics for such a function. It should be continuous, unique, invertible, simple to compute, and straightforward to apply. Generally, mapping functions are divided into linear and nonlinear models.

The simplest case of linear spatial normalization involves a rigid-body transformation (translations and rotations only, no change in size or shape) and is normally applicable only for within-subject alignment. In order to account for differing head sizes, a nonrigid component of scaling can be included while maintaining shape invariance. A single scaling factor is used in the classical Procrustes mapping[40] (other Procrustes mappings are described in Chapter 3), whereas the more general use of three scaling factors yields a total of nine parameters (three translations, three rotations, and three scaling factors). These linear models are continuous, unique, invertible, simple to compute, and easy to apply when resampling data for comparisons. A variety of methods exist to compute the linear spatial mapping based on landmark matching,[36,41,42] surface matching,[43-45] or volume density matching.[28,46,47] See Chapters 2 and 3 for more detailed information on registration algorithms, in addition to the excellent reviews of van den Elsen,[48] Maintz,[49] or Hawkes.[50]

The strict piecewise linear mapping of Talairach has been implemented by Lemoine[51] using manual identification of the AC and PC landmark and by Verard[52] with automated landmark localization. This mapping method is relatively straightforward to compute, and it is easy to apply. However, it is not continuous and is only piecewise invertible. Most groups have moved to a nonlinear spatial mapping function to account for anatomical variability by allowing more degrees of freedom in the mapping function. Many of the nonrigid registration algorithms that are appropriate for intersubject registration (or spatial normalization) are described in Chapter 13.

Among the different nonlinear mapping methods, that developed by Friston et al.[53,54] is constrained to consist of a weighted linear combination of smooth basis warps that are defined by discrete cosine transforms. A similar mapping technique has been developed by Woods[55,56] except that polynomial basis functions are used. In these two methods a limited number of parameters (say, $n < 10^3$) is used to define the mapping. Bookstein has promoted a method to interpolate the 3D mapping between sparse landmarks (such as

---

* *http://www.bic.mni.mcgill.ca/software/mni_autoreg*
** *http://www.fil.ion.ucl.ac.uk/spm*

homologous points or surfaces) based on the mechanical properties of a thin metal plate with minimum bending energy.[57] Nonlinear mappings can also be constrained with elastic material properties[18,19,58,59] or the dynamics of a viscous fluid.[60] It is important to note that the underlying physical model is used only to constrain the spatial mapping function in order to yield the desired properties mentioned above. These mappings are not meant to model the true physical properties of brain tissue deformation since we are not actually physically deforming one brain into the shape of another.

14.2.3   The Similarity Measure

Ideally, the spatial mapping function will align all features of interest between a given brain volume with the corresponding features of the target in the reference space. We term the mapping that puts homologous features into correspondence *homology function*. The *similarity measure* is the practical implementation of the homology function and is used to measure the goodness of alignment between two brain volumes (for more information, see the similarity measure concept introduced in Chapter 3).

The actual definition of the homology function is highly task dependent since it relies completely on the features of interest, and many different features can be selected. For example, one might be interested only in the alignment of gross anatomical structures such as the cerebral lobes, or in the detail of particular gyri. Anatomists may be interested in the alignment of cytoarchitectonic regions across subjects. Some neuropsychologists are interested in alignment of functional regions. Even when the features have been selected, the homology function may be impossible to define in certain situations, e.g., when a certain brain region (like Heschl's gyrus) may be represented by one gyrus in one subject and by two gyri in another subject.

It is important to note that the similarity measure is only an approximation to the homology function. For example, in brain mapping, the goal is to align both anatomical and functional regions. In practice, cross-correlation,[28] a correlation ratio,[61] or mutual information[62] may be used to measure similarity between brain volumes. Since it is only an approximation, a successful registration (i.e., one that maximizes the similarity measure) may not represent the best mapping for the homology function.

14.2.4   The Optimization Procedure

The goal of the optimization procedure is to find the global maximum of the similarity measure given the domain of possible mapping functions. While not as important as the reference space, mapping function, or similarity measure, the optimization procedure must be nonetheless practical and robust—especially when one takes into account the complex shape of the similarity measure. The different procedures trade off speed, robustness, and reliability. We have found that hierarchical methods that function with data at different scales are the most robust. These methods start by blurring the data volumes, both in the given brain and the target data set, to remove detail before estimating an initial registration. This first result is used as a starting point for a second registration procedure using slightly less blurred data to refine the initial fit. When this procedure is repeated a number of times, reducing the data blur and refining the spatial mapping function, the result is both reliable and robust. This strategy has the added benefit of reducing the computational time required to compute a registration at high resolution, since the initial stages can be computed quickly on highly blurred data and the initial fits target the result and reduce the effective search space.

14.2.5 Other Brain-Based Reference Spaces

It is important to note that while versions of the Talairach coordinate system have become the *de facto* standard in much of the brain mapping field, other reference spaces exist that are applied for specific types of analysis.

In some studies, a single brain is selected as the target for registration and standardization. This method suffers from the problems associated with using a single brain (mentioned in Section 14.2.1.1) without the advantages of an atlas-based coordinate space (see Roland and Zilles for an overview of the uses of brain atlases as a research tool[63]). In neurosurgical planning of stereotactic interventions, the reference space most often used is that of the Schaltenbrand and Wahren atlas,[4] used to derive the coordinates of deep brain targets.

In contrast to 3D registration, 2D methods concentrate on registering pairs of surfaces by finding a mapping between the surfaces. Structures on the surface are used to constrain the mapping. The surface most commonly used is the outer cortical surface, i.e., the gray-matter/CSF interface. However, one could equally well use the white-matter/gray-matter boundary or a medial surface inside the gray matter. Sandor,[64] Thompson,[65] and Davatzikos[66] each developed methods that begin by automatically extracting the cortical surface followed by manual identification of a small number of sulci that are used to constrain the registration. While these techniques usually maintain the 3D geometry of the 2D surface, the methods developed by Van Essen and Drury at Washington University can be used to extract and *flatten* the cortex onto a 2D surface where one can apply surface-based coordinate systems to analyze structure and function.[15] The main difficulty with this type of technique is the spatial distortion incurred by flattening a 3D surface. The Washington University group has minimized distance and area errors by inserting *cuts* into the surface. They have applied the technique mostly to the visual system. The group at Harvard has also developed a 2D coordinate system to identify regions of interest based on automated surface extraction and flattening methods.[67,68] The extracted surface has a sphere topology, so a spherical coordinate system can be used. This method has been used to generate an average cortical folding pattern of normal anatomy.[69] Thompson and Toga have created an atlas of subjects with Alzheimer's Disease based on the surface registration of manually identified curves on the cortex.[70] Work is currently ongoing to determine which space (2D surface in 3D, flattened 2D surface, or original 3D space) is best for mapping regions of interest.

14.3 Applications

The demand for the automatic quantitative analysis in cohort studies (i.e., analysis of large medical-image data sets with hundreds or thousands of scans) has been growing over the past few years, particularly in the brain mapping community. Typical examples are the construction of probabilistic atlases of the adult and pediatric brain,[71,72] the analysis of pathology in the context of clinical research and clinical trials,[73] and the statistical analysis of functional imaging studies.[35] To address the complexities of large computer processing requirements, we have developed a production control system (PCS) that allows the rapid implementation and parallel execution of an analysis *pipeline*, a term used here to describe a sequence of processing stages applied to a collection of input data. A pipeline consists of a sequence of elementary operations that together make up a complex image analysis task. The PCS ships individual processing steps (a program with its associated data) to a free CPU on the network, monitors its progress, and reports results. This is completed for all steps in the pipeline and for all data sets in the cohort.

At the BIC, we have developed a number of pipelines to analyze large ensembles of data. Our typical pipeline for 3D brain image analysis includes a number of preprocessing steps including image intensity nonuniformity correction,[74] volume-to-target intensity normalization,[75] and noise reduction.[76] Once preprocessing is completed, the pipeline combines linear registration[28] and resampling into stereotaxic space, cortical surface extraction,[77,78] tissue classification,[79] automatic sulcal extraction,[80] and atlas matching using nonlinear registration.[19] Linear registration is achieved by maximization of the cross correlation ratio between an individual volume to be registered and average MNI305 target volume already registered to stereotaxic space.[28,36,38,39] The nonlinear registration is estimated by computing a 3D nonlinear deformation field in a piecewise linear fashion, fitting cubical neighborhoods in sequence.[19] Each data cube in one volume is translated to achieve an optimal match within the other volume. Cubes are arranged in a 3D grid to fill the volume, and each cube moves within a range defined by a grid spacing. The algorithm is applied in a multiscale hierarchy. At each step, the image volumes are preconvolved with a 3D Gaussian kernel where blurring and cube size are reduced after each stage. Initial fits are obtained rapidly since, at lower scales only gross distortions are considered, but later iterations at finer scales accomodate local differences at the price of increasing computational burden.

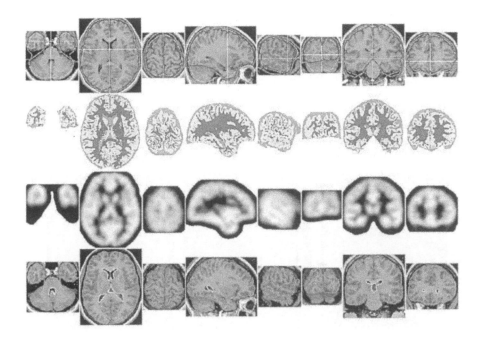

FIGURE 14.1
Example of a single-subject pipeline verification image, obtained from analysis of the brain of a healthy child. Each column shows a different slice through stereotaxic (Talairach) space, while each row shows different intermediate and final products of the automatic analysis. Top row: T1-weighted volume with several contours, showing the axes of Talairach space, the outline of the MNI 305 average brain, and a low- and high-resolution cerebral surface.[78] Second row: 3-class INSECT classification.[73] Third row: smoothed (FWHM − 10) gray matter classification.[81] Fourth row: T1-weighted image, nonlinearly deformed at low resolution to match a model brain, shown with its cerebral and ventricular contours.

After running through this basic pipeline, a subject's MRI volume can be visualized in stereotaxic space with its corresponding tissue labels, anatomical structure labels, cortical surface, and sulcal ribbons—all in 3D. As a standard procedure, a number of composite verification images are produced during processing to allow the rapid visual inspection of the results for a large number of data sets (see Figure 14.1).

The following sections describe the application of pipeline processing in cohort studies for the analysis of brain data from (1) a collection of normal young adults within the ICBM project, (2) an ensemble of children five to eighteen years of age, and (3) a group of patients suffering from multiple sclerosis.

14.3.1 Registration-Based Analysis of Normal Brain Anatomy

Figure 14.2 shows the pipeline designed for the automatic analysis of normal human brain, which has so far been applied to brain MRIs (T1-weighted 3D spoiled gradient echo acquisition with sagittal volume excitation, TR = 18, TE = 10, flip angle = 30°, 140–180 sagittal slices) obtained from 152 healthy adults (86 male, 66 female, age 24.6 ± 4.8)[1,82] and 111 healthy children and adolescents.[83]

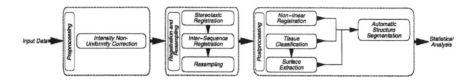

FIGURE 14.2
Flow diagram of the ICBM[1] pipeline. All MRI data is processed through the pipeline shown above. After preprocessing and stereotaxic registration, the cortical surface is extracted and the MRI data is classified into gray matter, white matter, and cerebrospinal (CSF) components.

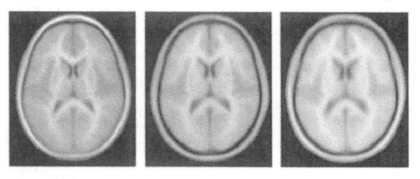

FIGURE 14.3
Average T1-weighted MRIs of, from left to right, a pediatric population ($n = 130$), healthy adults ($n = 151$), and MS patients ($n = 460$).

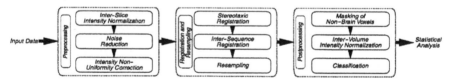

FIGURE 14.4
Flow diagram of the INSECT[73] pipeline.

After the data have been registered and resampled into stereotaxic space, they are available for processing. As a first step, voxel-by-voxel intensity averages can be computed for each group studied. Figure 14.3 shows a transverse slice through three different group averages. While useful as a qualitative indicator of local anatomical variability for the different groups, the composite MRI intensity averages are insufficient as a quantitative tool. For this purpose, the MRI intensity for each voxel must be identified with a tissue label or structure label. The former requires automated classification, while the latter requires segmentation. Figure 14.4 shows an incarnation of INSECT (intensity normalized stereotaxic environment for classification of tissues[73]), a pipeline designed for the classification of tissues in MRI. This pipeline was applied to the 152 brain volumes in the ICBM data base, classifying each voxel into gray matter, white matter, and cerebrospinal fluid. Figure 14.5 shows statistical probability anatomy maps (SPAMs) that were

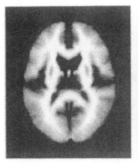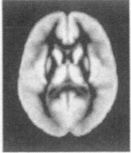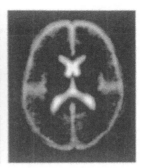

FIGURE 14.5
SPAMs of white matter, gray matter, and CSF automatically derived from 151 healthy adults.

created by voxelwise averaging of the 152 classified volumes. In these images, the voxel intensity is directly proportional to the probability of the given tissue type at that voxel location. These tissue SPAMs can therefore be used as priors for automated (Bayesian, among others) classification methods.

The classified data have been used to study structural asymmetries in the human brain[84] where the binary mask for each tissue class was smoothed with a 10 mm full width at half maximum (FWHM) Gaussian filter to produce a *tissue density map*. These maps were then flipped about the $x = 0$ axis (i.e., the longitudinal fissure) and the mirror images were subtracted from the original map. After correcting for multiple comparisons, a voxelwise t-test analysis of the difference images confirmed known existing asymmetries for the planum temporale and for frontal and occipital petalias. The technique has also demonstrated interesting differences for other regions such as the head of the caudate nucleus ($r > l$).

To study brain development we have used voxelwise regression analysis to investigate relationships between structural features and a combination of independent variables. Three examples are described here. In the first, we were interested in characterizing age-related changes in local white matter signal throughout the brain using an MRI data base of children and adolescents aged 4 to 17 years (66 boys, age 10.7 ± 3.8 years; 45 girls, age 11.5 ± 3.7 years).[85] The significance of the relation between age and white matter density was assessed for each voxel in the volume by means of simple linear regression. T-values were computed by dividing the voxel slope estimate by its standard deviation. The presence of regions that were significantly correlated with age was determined using the 3D Gaussian random field theory developed by Worsley.[35] This analysis showed significant regions in the internal capsule (see Figure 14.6) and the posterior portion of the left arcuate fasciculus.

In the second example of regression analysis, we were interested in the anatomy of the hippocampus. Eighty subjects were selected from the ICBM data base (41 females, 39 males, 25 ± 4.9 years old). Their hippocampi were manually segmented and averaged to create hippocampal SPAMs.[86] Even though it is generally believed that the age-related decline in hippocampal volume occurs in late adulthood and is independent of gender, we found

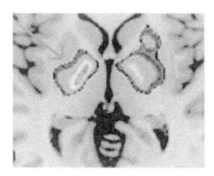

FIGURE 14.6
Voxelwise regression analysis: The maps of t-statistic values are superimposed on an axial MR section from a single subject. The image depicts the exact locations in the internal capsule (indicated by the arrow) that showed statistically significant correlations between white matter density and the subject's age.

a significant negative correlation with age for both left and right hippocampal volume in men ($r = -.46$ and $r = -.43$, respectively) but not in women ($r = .01$ and $r = .02$, respectively) in this group of young adults. Voxel-based regression analysis was used to determine which part of the hippocampus is correlated with age. Here, the subject's age acts as independent variable and the MR image signal intensity of each voxel as dependent variable in the regression. After statistical analysis (as described above), the regression analysis revealed that the volume loss occurred mostly in the head and tail of the hippocampus (see Color Figure 14.7*).

The last example does not use image data in the regression analysis. Instead, age is correlated with deformation vectors (a byproduct of a nonlinear registration procedure). Previous work has suggested that the size of the brain changes little after the age of five years.[72] We sought to address the possibility that after this age the human brain continues to grow, albeit in a region-specific fashion.[82] Each of the brains in the children/adolescent MRI data base described above was registered with a nonlinear transformation to match a single "template" volume resident in stereotaxic space. The deformation fields represent the local difference at each voxel between the subject and template, and as such are indicators of individual anatomical variability. These fields were used in voxelwise linear regression analysis to identify regions in which age correlated with a local change in X, Y, and/or Z vectors. Hotelling's F statistic was employed to evaluate statistical significance of such correlations; $F > 9$ was deemed significant after correcting for multiple comparisons. Significant correlations ($30 < F < 60$) between age and the local vectors around both the temporal lobes and the ventral aspects of the frontal lobes were found. Analysis of the X, Y, and Z vectors indicates a possible overall growth of the temporal lobes and/or their downward and lateral "movement." In contrast, no significant correlations were observed around

---

* Color Figures follow page 22.

the corpus callosum, basal ganglia, thalamus, or lateral ventricles. These findings suggest that in the range between 5 and 18 years, the brain continues to change its shape locally. It remains to be determined what underlies such changes in the brain's gross anatomy.

14.3.2 Segmentation-Based Analysis of Normal Brain Anatomy

The previously described procedures do not rely on *a priori* regional identification in each volume. Therefore, localization of the results must be interpreted with respect to the blurred anatomy visible in the average MRI volumes in conjunction with brain atlases registered within the same space. Region of interest (ROI) analysis, respecting specific anatomical boundaries in each subject's brain, requires segmentation of regions (or volumes) of interest within each MR image volume.

Segmentation can be accomplished using manual tools that allow the user to identify the voxels of a given structure by voxel painting using *Display*, a computer program developed in our laboratory[87] that shows four 2D orthogonal slices (transverse, coronal, sagittal, and user defined oblique) through the volume with arbitrary pan, zoom, and intensity mapping on each slice. Display also includes a 3D graphics window capable of displaying 3D geometric objects such as the cortical surface. The cursor can be placed in any of the 2D or 3D windows, and its position is simultaneously updated in the other views. Voxel labels are painted on any of three orthogonal views with simultaneous update in all other views. Within our group at the MNI, this painting technique has been used to characterize the normal anatomy of the cingulate and paracingulate sulci in 105 subjects,[88] the corpus callosum in 100 subjects,[89] the planum temporale in 50 subjects,[90] the hippocampus and amygdala in 80 subjects,[86] the lobes and fissures of the cerebellum in 12 subjects,[91] as well as the distribution of frontal and lateral gyri,[92] orbitofrontal gyri,[93] and the region of the parieto-temporo-occipital cortex.[94] The manual method has also been used to identify and then compare the frontal lobe anatomy of patients with schizophrenia with age-matched control subjects.[95]

Since manual labeling is prohibitively time consuming and error prone, we have designed an automated procedure called ANIMAL (automatic nonlinear image matching and anatomical labeling) to segment objectively gross anatomical structures from 3D MRIs of normal brains.[19,96] Automatic segmentation is achieved by estimating the nonlinear spatial transformation required to register all voxels from a subject's MRI volume with an average MRI brain that is coregistered with a SPAM atlas in a Talairach-like stereotaxic space.[71] The atlas' 90 average gross anatomical structures are mapped through the inverse transform to effectively define customized masks on the subject's MRI for the *most-likely* region for each structure. Tissue classes such as gray matter, white matter, and CSF, identified by a minimum distance classifier, are masked by these regions to complete the segmentation. This methodology was applied to the collection of 152 MRI brains in the ICBM data base.[82]

Since each structure has been segmented, it is possible to compute its native volume (reported in cm^3 in Figure 14.8 and Table 14.1). Table 14.1

TABLE 14.1

Structure Volumes: in cm³ (mean ± sd) for
Structures Not Visible in Figure 14.8

Structure	Left Mean(sd)	Right Mean(sd)
Insula	8.8(1.1)	8.8(1.1)
Caudate	5.4(0.7)	5.1(0.6)
Putamen	5.4(0.7)	5.5(0.7)
Globus pallidus	0.9(0.2)	1.4(0.2)
Thalamus	8.3(0.9)	9.0(1.0)
Nucleus accumbens	0.3(0.1)	0.4(0.1)
Subthalamic nucleus	0.1(0.0)	0.1(0.0)
Anterior internal capsule	3.3(0.5)	3.0(0.6)
Posterior internal capsule	1.6(0.3)	1.6(0.3)
Lateral ventricle	8.9(3.6)	8.0(3.4)
Corpus collosum	10.9(1.5)	
Fornix	0.3(0.1)	

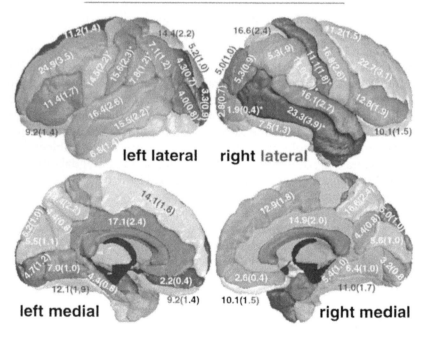

FIGURE 14.8
Structure volumes: These images show different views of the SPAM atlas with the volumes in cm³ (mean ± sd) for each structure. Structures with a significant ($p < 0.01$) left-right difference are indicated with a '*'. The isosurface of each SPAM was extracted at the 50% probability level.

shows volumes for structures not visible in the surface renderings of Figure 14.8. Significant hemispheric left-right differences ($p < 0.01$, two-tailed student's t-test with Bonferoni correction) were found for the precentral gyrus (left smaller than right), postcentral gyrus (left larger than right), middle temporal gyrus (left smaller than right), angular gyrus (left smaller than right),

TABLE 14.2

Lobe Volumes: in cc^3 (mean ± sd). Only Temporal (Left Larger Than Right) and Parietal (Left Smaller Than Right) Lobe Volume Differences are Significant ($p < 0.05$)

Lobe	Left Mean(sd)	Right Mean(sd)
Frontal	175.0(25.3)	174.0(25.0)
Temporal	119.3(18.1)	109.8(16.4)
Parietal	95.0(13.7)	99.3(14.3)
Occipital	44.8(7.9)	45.9(8.2)

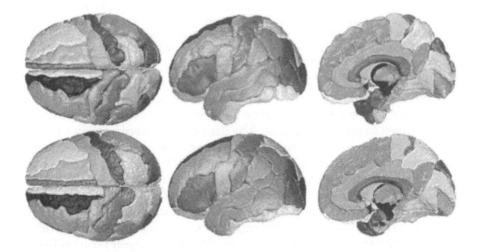

FIGURE 14.9
3D renderings of structure SPAMs, automatically generated from (top) 152 healthy adults (age 24.6 ± 4.8) and (bottom) 110 children and adolescents (age 11.2 ± 3.6). From left to right: top view, lateral view of left hemisphere, medial view of right hemisphere.

and inferior occipital gyrus (left larger than right). The left-right volume difference for temporal (left larger than right) and parietal (left smaller than right) lobes are significant at the $p = 0.05$ level (see Table 14.2). The method presented here is completely automatic, fully objective, and has been applied to a large ensemble of brain volumes. The resulting volume statistics will prove useful as a normative data base for comparisons in future studies of normal or pathological brains. Figure 14.9 compares the average segmentations of the ICBM young adult brains with the child/adolescent MRI data base.

14.3.3 Analysis of Normal Anatomical Variability

Besides segmentation, ANIMAL has been applied to nonrigid registration and to the analysis of morphometric variability. To quantify anatomical variability, it is necessary to identify homologous features between the source and target volumes and to measure the difference in position between them, within the

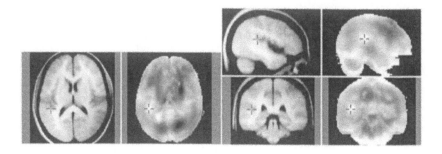

FIGURE 14.10
Variability Map
The images show the average intensity volume of 17 ICBM subjects mapped into stereotaxic space nonlinearly along with the corresponding slices through the average variability map. The cross marker ($x = -44$ mm, $y = -37$ mm, $z = 14$ mm) is near the planum temporale on the left side, a region known to be variable, measured here to be 6.3 mm 3-D FWHM, and appearing more variable than the right.

stereotaxic space. This identification can be achieved automatically by ANIMAL, since the recovered deformation field essentially establishes correspondence between homologous points. The field can be interpreted as a map of "positional differences" between individual source (after affine transformation) and target volumes. In other words, for every 3D coordinate in the target space, the registration procedure yields a vector-valued estimate of the difference in position between the two data sets.

This information derived from the deformation fields, and when averaged over a large number of individual/target pairs, can yield estimates of normal anatomical variability. The standard deviation at each voxel position (for 17 subjects from the ICBM data base) is computed separately for each of the x, y, and z components. These values are combined to yield a single number for each voxel measuring intersubject variability (ISV), equivalent to a 3D FWHM measure. For a Gaussian distribution:

$$fwhm = 2.35\sqrt{(\sigma_x^2 + \sigma_y^2 + \sigma_z^2)/3}$$

The 17 deformation fields were used to compute the anatomical variability map shown in Figure 14.10. The regions of largest neuroanatomical variability were posterior poles of the lateral ventricles, the region near the fourth ventricle, the cingulate sulcus (slightly more on the left than the right), the inferior frontal lobe, and the area just above the splenium of the corpus callosum. The anatomical variability map is not symmetric on left and right sides. The left frontal lobe and right parieto-occipital lobe appear to be more variable than their counterparts. These data have been partially validated with manual estimates of intersubject anatomical variability (regression coefficient of 0.867) demonstrating good correlation between both automatic and manual methods at the 1% significance level.[97]

14.3.4   Analysis of Brain Anatomy in Multiple Sclerosis

Besides applications which are primarily research-oriented, automatic analysis of medical image data is becoming increasingly important in the evaluation of drug therapies. Especially in phase II/III clinical trials, accurate and reproducible quantification of disease-specific features in MRI data is key to the acceptance of new treatments.

For example, the quantification of total lesion load (TLL), sometimes referred to as "burden of illness," in T2-weighted MRI scans of patients with multiple sclerosis (MS) has become a standard surrogate endpoint in clinical trials. To date, a modified version of the INSECT pipeline has been used to quantify TLL in two large-scale, multicenter clinical trials in MS: (i) phase III, 600 patients, scanned 3 times on a yearly basis using T1-, T2-, and PD-weighted MRI; and (ii) phase II, 150 patients, scanned 6 times on a monthly basis using T1-, T2-, PD-weighted, and FLAIR MRI. The MRI acquisiton protocol used in these studies was uniform accross centers and the resulting image data were carefully controlled for quality.

The version of INSECT used for the quantification of MS lesion volume differs somewhat from the one used for the study of normal brain. First, a standard stereotaxic brain mask is used to eliminate false positive lesions possibly detected outside the brain area, and stereotaxic SPAMs of WM, GM, and CSF are included as extra features in the classification process to suppress false positive lesions inside the brain based on their (stereotaxic) location. Second, the MRI data volumes are all intensity-normalized to a standard brain model in stereotaxic space, allowing for the use of a once-trained, fixed classifier across all acquisitions in the study. The classifier used is an artificial neural network, trained to separate MS lesion from other tissues on a limited number of hand-labeled volumes. The resulting output is a binary map of MS lesions for each patient scan. The accuracy of INSECT-obtained MS lesion measurements has been validated against those obtained manually by experts.[98] Figure 14.11 shows the MS lesion SPAM generated from a total of 460 automatically segmented patient data sets.

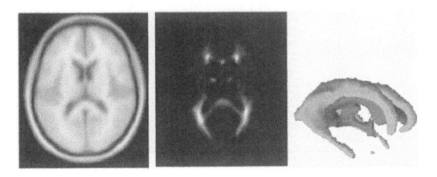

FIGURE 14.11
Average MS T1-weighted data and lesion SPAM ($n = 460$), shown in transverse cross-section and rendered with the CSF SPAM shown in Figure 14.5.

14.3.5   Analysis of Brain Metabolism in Multiple Sclerosis

Metabolite images generated from magnetic resonance spectroscopy imaging (MRSI) are often difficult to interpret because of low signal-to-noise ratio (SNR) and imaging artifacts. SNR is increased with spatial standardization and image averaging as is done with PET data,[24] and may thus reveal subtle consistent changes when comparing images from two groups. Our strategy has been to define the transformation that best maps a subject's MRI into the standardized stereotaxic brain space, and then apply the same transformation to the inherently registered MRSI. Once in stereotaxic space, MRSIs from different subjects can be directly compared on a voxel-to-voxel basis.

Proton MRSIs (90° - 180° - 180° sequence, TR 2 sec, TE 272 msec, 32 $\times$ 32 voxels, 25 cm field of view, 2 cm slice thickness) were acquired of a 10 $\times$ 10 $\times$ 2 cm volume of interest that was roughly parallel to the AC-PC line and centered on the corpus callosum. Post processing was applied to correct for residual field inhomogeneity, phase roll, and eddy currents.[99] Metabolite concentration images for N-acetylaspartase (NAA), choline (Cho), and creatine (Cr) were reconstructed by integration between automatically chosen frequency limits surrounding each peak. To correct for remaining B_0 and radio frequency inhomogeneities, ratio images were also created. After registration, resampling, and averaging in stereotaxic space, the average metabolite images for normal subjects show a decrease in NAA signal intensity corresponding to the partial volume effect due to the lateral ventricles. Although not apparent on individual MRSIs, comparison of average metabolite images in stereotaxic space enables us to determine that Cho and Cr are not uniformally distributed in periventricular region. This nonuniformity is due not only to the presence of the ventricles, but also to metabolic specific differences in distribution in periventricular tissues. Figure 14.12 shows an average ratio image of Naa/(Cho + Cr).

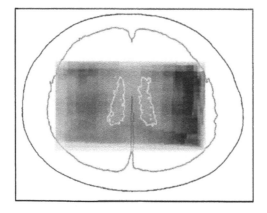

FIGURE 14.12
Stereotanic average MRSI of NAA/(Cho + Cr) for seven normals; contours of scalp, cortex, and ventricles from matched MRI.

14.4 Conclusion

The production control system that we have developed allows the rapid implementation and efficient parallel execution of processing pipelines on large amounts of data. PCS has shown its usefulness in a number of application areas as shown by the examples, and it is currently in routine use at the BIC for the automatic analysis of MRI data in a multicenter, mass production setting. The use of stereotaxic space combined with automated image processing tools yields a powerful qualitative and quantitative data analysis paradigm that facilitates comparisons over time for an individual, between subjects, between different groups of subjects, and between acquisition sites. Furthermore, the brain-based coordinate system permits anatomically-based processing and hypothesis testing, such as using spatial masks to limit processing to a specific region or using anatomical information as spatial priors. The combination of stereotaxic space with the collection of automated image processing tools makes it possible to embark on a myriad of studies that were previously impractical.

References

1. J. Mazziotta, A. Toga, A. Evans, P. Fox, and J. Lancaster, A probabilistic atlas of the human brain: theory and rationale for its development. The international consortium for brain mapping, *NeuroImage*, vol. 2, no. 2, pp. 89–101, 1995.
2. J. Talairach and P. Tournoux, *Co-planar Stereotactic Atlas of the Human Brain: 3-Dimensional Proportional System: an Approach to Cerebral Imaging.* Stuttgart: Georg Thieme Verlag, 1988.
3. G. Schaltenbrand and P. Bailey, *Introduction to Stereotaxis with an Atlas of the Human Brain.* Stuttgart: Georg Thieme Verlag, 1959.
4. G. Schaltenbrand and W. Wahren, *Atlas for Stereotaxy of the Human Brain.* Stuttgart: Yearbook Med, 1959.
5. K. Brodmann, *Vergleichende Lokalisationlehre der Grosshirnrinde in ihren Prinzipien dargestellt auf Grund des Zellenbaues.* Leipzig: J.A. Barth, 1909.
6. T. Matsui and A. Hirano, *An Atlas of the Human Brain for Computerized Tomography.* Tokyo: Igaku-Shoin, 1978.
7. M. Huerta, S. Koslow, and A. Leshner, The Human Brain Project: an international resource, *Trends Neurosci.*, vol. 16, pp. 436–438, 1993.
8. A.C. Evans, C. Beil, S. Marrett, C.J. Thompson, and A. Hakim, Anatomical functional correlation using an adjustable MRI based atlas with PET, *J. Cereb. Blood Flow Metab.*, vol. 8, no. 4, pp. 813–830, 1988.
9. A.C. Evans, S. Marrett, J. Torrescorzo, S. Ku, and L. Collins, MRI-PET correlation in three dimensions using a volume-of-interest (VOI) atlas, *J. Cereb. Blood Flow Metab.*, vol. 11, pp. A69–78, Mar. 1991.
10. C. Bohm, T. Greitz, R. Seitz, and L. Eriksson, Specification and selection of regions of interest (rois) in a computerized brain atlas, *J. Cereb. Blood Flow Metab.*, vol. 11, pp. A64–8, Mar. 1991. Review.

11. F. Bookstein, Thin-plate splines and the atlas problem for biomedical images, in *12th International Conference, Information Processing in Medical Imaging* (A. Colchester and D. Hawkes, eds.), vol. 511 of *Lecture Notes in Computer Science*, (Wye, UK), pp. 326–342, IPMI, Springer-Verlag, July 1991.
12. S.U. Berlangieri, T. Schifter, J.M. Hoffman, T.C. Hawk, S.M. Hamblen, and R.E. Coleman, An interactive, computer-based atlas of neurologic positron emission tomographic studies for use in teaching, *AJR Am. J. Roentgenol.* vol. 160, pp. 1295–8, Jun. 1993.
13. M.I. Kazarnovskaya, S.M. Borodkin, V.A. Shabalov, V.Y. Krivosheina, and A.V. Golanov, 3-D computer model of subcortical structures of human brain, *Comput. Biol. Med.*, vol. 21, no. 6, pp. 451–7, 1991.
14. E.D. Lehmann, D.J. Hawkes, D.L. Hill, C.F. Bird, G.P. Robinson, A.C. Colchester, and M.N. Maisey, Computer-aided interpretation of SPECT images of the brain using an MRI-derived 3D neuro-anatomical atlas, *Med. Inf. (Lond)*, vol. 16, pp. 151–66, Apr.–Jun. 1991.
15. D.C. Van Essen and H.A. Drury, Structural and functional analyses of human cerebral cortex using a surface-based atlas, *J. Neurosci.* vol. 17, pp. 7079–102, Sep. 15 1997.
16. A.P. Dhawan and L. Arata, Knowledge-based multi-modality three-dimensional image analysis of the brain, *Am. J. of Physiol. Imaging*, vol. 7, pp. 210–9, Jul.–Dec. 1992.
17. R. Bajcsy, R. Lieberson, and M. Reivich, A computerised system for the elastic matching of deformed radiographic images to idealized atlas images, *J. of Comp. Assist. Tomogr.*, vol. 7, no. 4, pp. 618–625, 1983.
18. J.C. Gee, M. Reivich, and R. Bajcsy, Elastically deforming 3D atlas to match anatomical brain images, *J Comput Assist Tomogr*, vol. 17, pp. 225–36, Mar.–Apr. 1993.
19. D.L. Collins, C.J. Holmes, T.M. Peters, and A.C. Evans, Automatic 3D model-based neuroanatomical segmentation, *Human Brain Mapping*, vol. 3, no. 3, pp. 190–208, 1995.
20. G. Christensen, S. Joshi, and M. Miller, Volumetric transformation of brain anatomy, *IEEE Trans. on Med. Imaging*, vol. 16, no. 6, pp. 864–77, 1996.
21. S. Sandor and R. Leahy, Surface-based labeling of cortical anatomy using a deformable atlas, *IEEE Trans. Med. Imaging*, vol. 16, pp. 41–54, Feb. 1997.
22. P.M. Thompson, D. MacDonald, M.S. Mega, C.J. Holmes, A.C. Evans, and A.W. Toga, Detection and mapping of abnormal brain structure with a probabilistic atlas of cortical surfaces, *J. Comput. Assist. Tomogr.*, vol. 21, pp. 567–81, Jul.–Aug. 1997.
23. C. Bohm, T. Greitz, D. Kingsley, B.M. Berggren, and L. Olsson, Adjustable computerized stereotaxic brain atlas for transmisison and emission tomography, *Am. J. of Neuroradiology*, vol. 4, pp. 731–733, May/June 1983.
24. P.T. Fox, J.S. Perlmutter, and M.E. Raichle, A stereotactic method of anatomical localization for positron emission tomography, *J. of Comp. Assist. Tomogr.*, vol. 9, no. 1, pp. 141–153, 1985.
25. H. Steinmetz, G. Furst, and H. Freund, Cerebral cortical localization: application and validation of the proportional grid system in MR imaging, *J. Comp. Assist. Tomogr.*, vol. 13, pp. 10–19, Jan.–Feb. 1989.
26. K. Friston, C. Frith, P. Liddle, and R. Frackowiak, Plastic transformation of PET images, *J. Comp. Assist. Tomogr.*, vol. 15, no. 1, pp. 634–639, 1991.
27. D. Lemoine, C. Barillot, B. Gibaud, and E. Pasqualini, A 3D C^1 stereotactic deformation model to merge multimodality images and atlas data, in *Proceed. of Comp. Assist. Radiol.*, pp. 665–668, 1991.

28. D.L. Collins, P. Neelin, T.M. Peters, and A.C. Evans, Automatic 3D inter-subject registration of MR volumetric data in standardized Talairach space, *J. of Comp. Assist. Tomogr.*, vol. 18, pp. 192–205, March/April 1994.

29. P. van den Elsen, Multi-modality Matching of Brain Images. Ph.D. thesis, Utrecht University, Netherlands, 1993.

30. J. Talairach, G. Szikla, and P. Tournoux, *Atlas d'Anatomie Stereotaxique du Telencephale*. Paris: Masson, 1967.

31. P.T. Fox, S. Mikiten, G. Davis, and J.L. Lancaster, BrainMap: A database of functional brain mapping, in *Functional Neuroimaging, Technical Foundations* (R.W. Thatcher, M. Hallett, T. Zeffiro, E.R. John, and M. Heurta, Eds.), pp. 95–105, San Diego, CA.: Academic Press, 1994.

32. P.T. Fox, M.A. Mintun, E.M. Reiman, and M.E. Raichle, Enhanced detection of focal brain responses using intersubject averaging and change-distribution analysis of subtracted PET images, *J. of Cerebral Blood Flow and Metabolism*, vol. 8, pp. 642–653, 1988.

33. W. Nowinski, A. Fang, B. Nguyen, J. Raphael, L. Jagannathan, R. Raghavan, R. Bryan, and G. Miller, Multiple brain atlas database and atlas-based neuroimaging system, *Comp. Aided Surg.*, vol. 2, pp. 42–66, 1997.

34. F. Riahi, A. Zijdenbos, S. Narayanan, D. Arnold, G. Francis, J. Antel, and A.C. Evans, Improved correlation between scores on the expanded disability status scale and cerebral lesion load in relapsing remitting multiple sclerosis. Results of the application of new imaging methods, *Brain*, vol. 121, pp. 1305–12, July 1998.

35. K. Worsley, S. Marrett, P. Neelin, A. Vandal, K. Friston, and A. Evans, A unified statistical approach for determining significant signals in images of cerebral activation, *Human Brain Mapping*, vol. 4, pp. 58–73, 1996.

36. A.C. Evans, S. Marrett, P. Neelin, D.L. Collins, K. Worsley, W. Dai, S. Milot, E. Meyer, and D. Bub, Anatomical mapping of functional activation in stereotactic coordinate space, *NeuroImage*, vol. 1, no. 1, pp. 43–53, 1992.

37. H. Steinmetz and R. Seitz, Functional anatomy of language processing: neuroimaging and the problem of individual variability, *Neuropsychologia*, vol. 29, no. 12, pp. 1149–1161, 1991.

38. A.C. Evans, D.L. Collins, and B. Milner, An MRI-based stereotactic atlas from 250 young normal subjects, *Soc. Neurosci. Abstr.*, vol. 18, p. 408, 1992.

39. A. Evans, M. Kamber, D. Collins, and M.D, An MRI-based probabilistic atlas of neuroanatomy, in *Magnetic Resonance Scanning and Epilepsy* (S. Shorvon, D. Fish, F. Andermann, G. Bydder, and H. Stefan, Eds.), vol. 264 of *NATO ASI Series A, Life Sciences*, pp. 263–274, Boston, Plenum Press, 1994.

40. R. Sibson, Studies in the robustness of multidimensional scaling: perturbation analysis of classical scaling, *J.R. Statist. Soc.*, vol. 41, no. 2, pp. 217–229, 1979.

41. P. Neelin, J. Crossman, D.J. Hawkes, Y. Ma, and A.C. Evans, Validation of an MRI/ PET landmark registration method using 3D simulated PET images and point simulations, *Comp. Med. Imaging and Graphics*, vol. 17, pp. 351–6, Jul.–Oct. 1993.

42. Y. Ge, J. Fitzpatrick, R. Kessler, and R. Margolin, Intersubject brain image registration using both cortical and subcortical landmarks, in *Proceed. of SPIE Med. Imaging*, vol. 2434, pp. 81–95, SPIE, 1995.

43. C.A. Pelizzari, G.T.Y. Chen, D.R. Spelbring, R.R. Weichselbaum, and C.T. Chen, Accurate three-dimensional registration of CT, PET and MRI images of the brain, *J. Comp. Assist. Tomogr.*, vol. 13, no. 1, pp. 20–26, 1989.

44. B. Payne and A. Toga, Surface mapping brain function on 3D models, *IEEE Comp. Graphics and Appl.*, vol. 10, pp. 33–41, 1990.
45. C. Mauer Jr., R. Maciunas, and J. Fitzpatrick, Registration of head CT images to physical space using a weighted combination of points and surfaces, *IEEE Trans. on Med. Imaging*, vol. 17, pp. 753–61, Oct. 1998.
46. R. Woods, J. Mazziotta, and S. Cherry, MRI-PET registration with automated algorithm, *J. Comp. Assist. Tomogr.*, vol. 17, pp. 536–546, 1993.
47. A. Collingnon, F. Maes, D. Delaere, D. Vandermeulen, P. Suetens, and G. Marchal, Automated multi-modality image registration based on information theory, in *Proceed. of Inf. Process. in Med. Imaging*, (Brest, France), pp. 263–274, June 1995.
48. P. van den Elsen, E. Pol, and M. Viergever, Medical image matching—a review with classification, *IEEE Eng. Med. and Biol.*, vol. 12, pp. 26–39, Mar. 1993.
49. J.B.A. Maintz and M.A. Viergever, A. survey of medical image registration, *Med. Image Anal.*, vol. 2, no. 1, pp. 1–36, 1998.
50. D. Hawkes, Algorithms for radiological image registration and their clinical application, *J. Anat.*, vol. 193, no. Pt 3, pp. 347–61, 1998.
51. D. Lemoine, C. Barillot, B. Gibaud, and E. Pasqualini, An anatomically-based 3D registration of multimodality and atlas data in surgery, in *12th International Conference, Information Processing in Medical Imaging* (A. Colchester and D. Hawkes, Eds.), (Wye, UK), p. 188, IPMI, Springer-Verlag, July 1991.
52. L. Verard, P. Allain, J. Travere, J. Baron, and D. Bloyet, Fully automatic identification of AC and PC landmarks on brain MRI using scene analysis, *IEEE Trans. on Med. Imaging*, vol. 16, no. 5, pp. 610–616, 1998.
53. K. Friston, J. Ashburner, C. Frith, J.-B Poline, J. Heather, and R. Frackowiak, Spatial registration and normalization of images, *Human Brain Mapping*, vol. 1, no. 2, pp. 1–25, 1995.
54. J. Ashburner and K. Friston, Fully three-dimensional nonlinear spatial normalisation: a new approach, in *2nd International Conference on Functional Mapping of the Human Brain* (J. Belliveau, D. Kennedy, and B. Rosen, eds.), (Boston), p. 169, Organization for Human Brain Mapping, June 1996.
55. R. Woods, S. Grafton, C. Holmes, S. Cherry, and J. Mazziotta, Automated image registration: I. General methods and intrasubject, intramodality validation., *J. Comp. Assist. Tomogr.*, vol. 22, pp. 139–152, Jan.–Feb. 1998.
56. R. Woods, S. Grafton, J. Watson, N. Sicotte, and J. Mazziotta, Automated image registration: II. Intersubject validation of linear and nonlinear models., *J. Comp. Assist. Tomogr.*, vol. 22, pp. 153–165, Jan.–Feb. 1998.
57. F.L. Bookstein, Principal warps: thin-plate splines and the decomposition of deformations, *IEEE Trans. Pattern Anal. and Machine Intell.*, vol. PAMI-11, no. 6, pp. 567–585, 1989.
58. R. Bajcsy and S. Kovacic, Multiresolution elastic matching, *Comp. Vision, Graphics, and Image Process.*, vol. 46, pp. 1–21, 1989.
59. G. Christensen, R. Rabbitt, and M. Miller, 3D brain mapping using a deformable neuroanatomy, *Physics in Med and Biol*, vol. 39, pp. 609–618, 1994.
60. G. Christensen, R. Rabbitt, and M. Miller, Deformable templates using large deformation kinematics, *IEEE Trans. on Image Process.*, vol. 5, no. 10, pp. 1435–1447, 1996.
61. A. Guimond, A. Roche, N. Ayache, and J. Meunier, Multimodal brain warping using the demons algorithm and adaptative intensity corrections, Tech. Rep. 3796, INRIA Research Report, 1999.
62. F. Maes, A. Collignon, D. Vandermeulen, G. Marchal, and P. Suetens, Multimodality image registration by maximization of mutual information, *IEEE Trans. on Med. Imaging*, vol. 16, no. 2, pp. 187–198, 1997.

63. P.E. Roland and K. Zilles, Brain atlases—a new research tool, *Trends Neurosci.*, vol. 17, no. 11, pp. 458–467, 1994.

64. S. Sandor and R. Leahy, Towards automated labelling of the cerebral cortex using a deformable atlas, in *14th International Conference, Information Processing in Medical Imaging* Y. Bizais, C. Barillot, and R. DiPaola, Eds., (Brest, France), pp. 127–138, IPMI, Kluwer, Aug 1995.

65. P. Thompson and A. Toga, A surface-based technique for warping 3-dimensional images of the brain, *IEEE Trans. Med. Imaging*, vol. 15, no. 4, pp. 383–392, 1996.

66. C. Davatzikos, Spatial normalization of 3D brain images using deformable models, *J. Comput. Assist. Tomogr.*, vol. 20, pp. 656–65, Jul–Aug 1996.

67. B. Fischl, M. Sereno, and A. Dale, Cortical surface-based analysis. II: inflation, flattening, and a surface-based coordinate system, *Neuroimage*, vol. 9, no. 2, pp. 195–207, 1999.

68. A. Dale, B. Fischl, and M. Sereno, Cortical surface-based analysis. I. Segmentation and surface reconstruction, *Neuroimage*, vol. 9, pp. 179–194, 1999.

69. B. Fischl, M. Sereno, R. Tootell, and A. Dale, High-resolution intersubject averaging and a coordinate system for the cortical surface, *Human Brain Mapping*, vol. 8, no. 4, pp. 272–84, 1999.

70. P.M. Thompson, R.P. Woods, M.S. Mega, and A.W. Toga, Mathematical/computational challenges in creating deformable and probabilistic atlases of the human brain, *Human Brain Mapping*, vol. 9, pp. 81–92, 2000.

71. A. Evans, D. Collins, and C. Holmes, Computational approaches to quantifying human neuroanatomical variability, in *Brain Mapping: The Methods* (J. Mazziotta and A. Toga, Eds.), pp. 343–361, Academic Press, San Diego, 1996.

72. J. Giedd, J. Snell, N. Lange, J. Rajapakse, B. Casey, P. Kozuch, A. Vaituzis, Y. Vauss, S. Hamburger, D. Kaysen, and J. Rapoport, Quantitative magnetic resonance imaging of human brain development: ages 4–18, *Cereb. Cortex*, vol. 6, no. 4, pp. 551–60, 1996.

73. A.P. Zijdenbos and A.C. Evans, Stereotaxic mapping in automatic quantification of neuropathology: application to multiple sclerosis, in *Proceed. of the Third Int. Conf. on Functional Mapping of the Human Brain*, Copenhagen, p. 396, May 1997.

74. J.G. Sled, A.P. Zijdenbos, and A.C. Evans, A non-parametric method for automatic correction of intensity non-uniformity in MRI data, *IEEE Trans. on Med. Imaging*, vol. 17, no. 1, pp. 87–97, Feb. 1998.

75. A.P. Zijdenbos, B.M. Dawant, and R.A. Margolin, Inter- and intra-slice intensity correction in MRI, in *Proceed. the 14th Int. Conf. Inf. Process. in Med. Imaging (IPMI)*, (France), pp. 349–350, June 1995.

76. G. Gerig, O. Kübler, R. Kikinis, and F.A. Jolesz, Nonlinear anisotropic filtering of MRI data, *IEEE Trans. on Med. Imaging*, vol. 11, pp. 221–232, June 1992.

77. D. MacDonald, D. Avis, and A.C. Evans, Multiple surface identification and matching in magnetic resonance images, in *Proceed. of the 3rd Int. Conf. Visualization in Biomed. Computing*, SPIE, vol. 2359, pp. 160–169, 1994.

78. D. MacDonald, Identifying Geometrically Simple Surfaces from Three Dimensional Data. PhD thesis, McGill University, Montreal, Canada, December 1994.

79. A.P. Zijdenbos, A.C. Evans, F. Riahi, J. Sled, J. Chui, and V. Kollokian, Automatic quantification of multiple sclerosis lesion volume using stereotaxic space, in *Proceed. 4th Int. Conf. Visualization in Biomed. Computing*, vol. 1131 of *Lecture Notes in Computer Science*, pp. 439–448, Springer-Verlag, Heidelberg, Sept. 1996.

80. G.L. Goualher, C. Barillot, and Y. Bizais, Three-dimensional segmentation and representation of cortical sulci using active ribbons, in *Int. J. Pattern Recogn. Artif. Intell.*, vol. 11, no. 8, pp. 1295–1315, 1997.

81. I.C. Wright, P.K. McGuire, J.-B. Poline, J.M. Travere, R.M. Murray, C.D. Frith, R.S.J. Frackowiak, and K.J. Friston, A voxel-based method for the statistical analysis of gray and white matter density applied to schizophrenia, *Neuroimage*, vol. 2, pp. 244–252, 1995.

82. D.L. Collins, N.J. Kabani, and A.C. Evans, Automatic volume estimation of gross cerebral structures, in *4th International Conference on Functional Mapping of the Human Brain* (A. Evans, Ed.), (Montreal), Organization for Human Brain Mapping, June 1998. abstract no. 702.

83. A. Zijdenbos, A. Jimenez and A. Evans, Pipelines: large scale automatic analysis of 3D brain data sets, in *4th International Conference on Functional Mapping of the Human Brain* (A. Evans, Ed.), (Montreal), Organization for Human Brain Mapping, June 1998. abstract no. 783.

84. K. Watkins, T. Paus, A. Zijdenbos, D. Collins, J. Lerch, P. Neelin, K. Worsley, and A. Evans, Detecting structural brain asymmetries using voxel-based morphometry, in *Proceed. of the Int. Conf. on Human Brain Mapping, Neuroimage*, vol. 11, No. 5, May 2000, Part 2 of 2, p. 548, 2000.

85. T. Paus, A. Zijdenbos, K. Worsley, D.L. Collins, J. Blumenthal, J.N. Giedd, J.L. Rapoport, and A.C. Evans, Structural maturation of neural pathways in children and adolescents: *in vivo* study, *Science*, vol. 283, pp. 1908–1911, Mar 19 1999.

86. J.C. Pruessner, L.M. Li, W. Serles, M. Pruessner, D.L. Collins, N. Kabani, S. Lupien, and A.C. Evans, Volumetry of hippocampus and amygdala with high-resolution MRI and three-dimensional analysis software: minimizing the discrepancies between laboratories, *Cerebral Cortex*, 10(4):p. 433–442, 2000.

87. D. MacDonald, *Display: A User's Manual*, tech. rep., McConnell Brain Imaging Centre, Montreal Neurological Institute, McGill University, Montreal, Sept 1996.

88. T. Paus, N. Otaky, Z. Caramanos, D. MacDonald, A. Zijdenbos, D.D.'Avirro, D. Gutmans, C. Holmes, F. Tomaiuolo, A.C. Evans. *In-vivo* morphometry of the intrasulcal gray-matter in the human cingulate, paracingulate and superior-rostal sulci: hemispheric asymmetries and gender differences. *J. Compar. Neurology* vol. 376, pp. 664–673, 1996.

89. P. Bermudez, R. Zatorre, and A. Evans, Human corpus callosum measures from 3-D MRI: morphometry, sex differences, and probability maps, *Soc. Neurosci. Abstr.*, vol. 23, Part 1, p. 212, 1997.

90. C. Westbury, R. Zatorre, and E. A.C., Quantifying variability in the planum temporale: a probability map, *Cereb. Cortex*, vol. 9, no. 4, pp. 392–405, 1999.

91. J. Schmahmann, J. Doyon, D. McDonald, C. Holmes, K. Lavoie, A. Hurwitz, N. Kabani, A. Toga, A. Evans, and M. Petrides, Three-dimensional MRI atlas of the human cerebellum in proportional stereotaxic space, *Neuroimage*, vol. 10, no. 3 Part 1, pp. 233–260, 1999.

92. Z. Caramanos, R. Venugopal, D. Collins, D. MacDonald, A. Evans, and M. Petrides, Human brain sulcal anatomy: an MRI-based study, in *Third International Conference on Functional Mapping of the Human Brain*, vol. 5, no. 4, (Copenhagen), p. S350, Human Brain Map, May 1997.

93. M. Chiavaras, G. Le Goualher, A.C. Evans, and M. Petrides, The human orbitofrontal cortex: sulcal patterns and probabilistic analysis, in *Human Brain Mapping, HBM'98*, vol. 7, no. 4, p. S731, 1998.

94. S. Dumoulin, R. Bittar, N. Kabani, C.J. Baker, G. Le Goualher, G. Pike, and A. Evans, Quantification of the variability of human area V5/MT in relation in to the sulcal pattern in the parieto-temporo-occipital cortex: a new anatomical landmark, *Cerebral Cortex*, vol. 10, no. 5, pp. 454–463, 2000.

95. R. Mandl, H.H. Pol, D. Collins, N. Ramsey, A. Evans, W. Barré, W. Staal, and R. Kahn, A comparison of linear and non-linear automatic frontal lobe volume measurement in schizophenia, *NeuroReport*, submitted.

96. D.L. Collins, A.P. Zijdenbos, W.F.C. Baaré, and A.C. Evans, Animal+insect: improved cortical structure segmentation, in *16th International Conference, Information Processing in Medical Imaging* (A. Kuba, Ed.), vol. 1613, pp. 210–223, IPMI, Springer, Hungary LLCS, Aug 1999.

97. C. Sorlié, D.L. Collins, K.J. Worsley, and A.C. Evans, An anatomical variability study based on landmarks, McConnell Brain Imaging Centre Technical Report, Mc Gill University, Montreal, Sept. 1994.

98. A. Zijdenbos, R. Forghani, and A. Evans, Automatic quantification of MS lesions in 3D MRI brain data sets: validation of INSECT, in *First International Conference on Medical Image Computing and Computer-Assisted Intervention* (W.M. Wells, A. Colchester, and S. Delp, eds.), Lecture notes in computer science, pp. 439–448, Berlin, Springer, 1998.

99. J. den Hollander, B. Oosterwaal, H. van Vroonhoven, and P. Luyten, Elimination of magnetic field distortions in 1h NMR spectroscopic imaging, *Proc. Soc. Magn. Reson. Med*, vol. 1, pp. 472–472, 1991.

15

Biomechanical Modeling for Image Registration: Applications in Image Guided Neurosurgery

Keith D. Paulsen and Michael I. Miga

CONTENTS

15.1 Introduction

The majority of the chapters of this book discuss methods for rigid-body registration and applications (especially of the brain in the closed skull) where these methods can be used for intermodality, intramodality, or image to physical space registration. There is increasing interest now in nonrigid registration, which is more generally applicable. Chapter 13 reviewed the main approaches to nonrigid registration. These methods are almost invariably used for intramodality registration of images from the same or different subjects. Chapter 14 discusses the intersubject registration of brain images in detail. For image-to-physical registration, as used for image-guided surgery and also for intermodality applications, nonrigid registration is a harder problem because of the difference in the information available in the spaces being aligned. In these cases, biomechanical models of the sort described in this chapter have the potential to provide model-based registration techniques that can align an image collected on one occasion with a very different image or the coordinates of a surgical instrument at a later time. These models can take into account the mechanical properties of the tissue, the operative conditions, and the presence of surgical instruments such as retractors. Furthermore, sparse intraoperative information, such as photographs of the site of resection or ultrasound images, can be used as constraints on the models to improve accuracy.

Modeling activities associated with surgical simulation have been explored for a number of years, and important progress continues to be reported.[1,2] The goal of these virtual reality experiences is to produce a video-like visualization of a deforming tissue that appears to be real. For these simulations, there is a fundamental shift from the traditional emphasis on predictive modeling with secondary interest in computational speed to a situation where these priorities are exactly reversed—the primary interest is speed of computation to enable real-time interaction, and physical accuracy is of less concern. In contrast, the modeling efforts described in this chapter are intended to impact intraoperative clinical decision making within the image-guided framework; hence, there is an emphasis not only on modeling accuracy and speed (although not at the real-time or video refresh rate) but also on the use of both preoperative and intraoperative data to define/confine model parameters and outcomes.

The motivation for the deployment of such physically defined deformation models of brain tissue has been the recognition and recent characterization and quantification of brain motion during surgery. A number of studies have tracked both surface and subsurface points in the brain and reported that movements on the order of a centimeter or more can occur intraoperatively.[3,4] During image-guided procedures this motion manifests as a dynamic registration error which erodes the effectiveness of image guidance when the operating room (OR) is registered with the statistically defined preoperative image space. While it is clear that intraoperative brain motion is significant and can severely compromise the added advantage of image-based surgical navigation, strategies to address this source of error intraoperatively are in early stages of development. One intriguing approach is to employ computational methods based on physical models of tissue deformation to compensate for intraoperative brain motion.

A conceptually powerful paradigm would be to:

- Update preoperative images intraoperatively by generating a patient-specific computational model based on segmentation of high resolution preoperative scans
- Collect readily accessible but incomplete intraoperative information relevant to brain motion with low cost tracking technology

- Modify the model based on this data coupled to a mathematical description of tissue deformation
- Update (i.e., deform) the preoperatively obtained high resolution images according to the computed three-dimensional deformation field

This approach exploits the wealth of high resolution preoperative data which is routinely available on a case-by-case basis, while taking advantage of incomplete intraoperative information and low-cost, high-performance computing to reduce registration errors which develop concurrent with surgery. If this form of preoperative image compensation can be developed, it may be possible to address the problem of tissue motion during image-guided procedures in many instances without involving volumetric intraoperative imaging, which, while intuitively appealing, can be both expensive and cumbersome within the traditional OR environment. Even in the setting where high resolution intraoperative MR is available,[5,6] computational estimates of volumetric tissue displacement are likely to be useful, for example, as an intermediate update path between full intraoperative image acquisitions as in the case of a twin operating theater (surgery + imaging), or when preoperative information cannot be duplicated in the OR as in the case of functional studies (e.g., fMRI). Hence, there is considerable rationale for and interest in developing computational models of tissue deformation for improving image guidance.

Interestingly, the potential of using model-based computations in the context of image registration has been recognized for a number of years. There is a significant body of literature associated with the matching of medical images when deformation is involved, which are reviewed in Chapter 13. Typically, pre- and postcondition images exist which need to be matched or a patient-specific image is conformed to a reference atlas. Approaches for elastically matching two existing images usually involve the optimization of a prescribed cost function, and a variety of techniques have been developed (e.g., see references 7 and 8, among others). In all of these efforts, the primary task has been to transform one known image into the shape of another known image without any knowledge of the physical driving forces involved. Intraoperatively, one has the luxury of being able to model the physical events which take place during surgery in order to account for tissue motion.

This chapter focuses on these later models. It provides an abbreviated historical perspective on brain tissue mechanical modeling and some of the mathematical options that are available for representing brain tissue mechanical response to surgical interventions. Of these options, consolidation theory is followed as an example framework for discussing computational implementation and validation. Discussion of the types of model parameters and sources of data input needed for model computations is highlighted. Examples of updated images from *in vivo* modeling, including in the human OR, are described. The focus here is modeling for neurosurgical image guidance, but many of the principles presented could be adapted to other applications where tissue motion may compromise the value of image-guided surgery when preoperative scans form the only basis for image-to-patient registration.

15.2   Brain Tissue Modeling: An Abbreviated Review

The literature contains a number of physical descriptions of the brain as a mechanical medium. Hakim et al. made the important observation that brain tissue acts like a sponge, providing impetus to consider the brain as a porous biphasic system.[9] While quantitative information on the brain's mechanical properties is sparse, especially *in vivo*, its mechanical behavior has been qualitatively studied and recently reviewed.[10] Typically, gray matter is regarded as stiffer and less porous than white matter. According to Doczi, gray matter can increase its water content by approximately 1.5% while white matter can increase by as much as 10%. In addition, the number of capillaries in gray matter exceeds that of white, which can influence brain osmotics causing volume changes by fluid transport through the vasculature. Typically, volume regulation is maintained by lymphatic drainage and plasma-to-tissue exchange. When compressed, brain tissue responds by displacing fluid from its veins and extracellular space which comprise 3% and 20% of the cranial tissue volume, respectively.[10] Doczi also points out that when the blood brain barrier is compromised, the driving force for fluid movement becomes hydrostatic pressure, which lends itself nicely to modeling hydrocephalus and edema.

With respect to the physics involved, several different continuum descriptions have found their way into mathematical forms which could serve as the basis for modeling tissue motion during surgery. In general these have fallen into two classes: (1) single-phase viscoelastic and (2) biphasic elastic representations. For example, Mendis et al.[11] developed a single phase nonlinear viscoelastic model for brain tissue experiencing large deformation. Their approach is based on the strain energy density function which is assigned a polynomial form with time dependent coefficients, making it particularly applicable to high strain rate loading conditions associated with traumatic injury. A related formulation has been developed by Miller and Chinzei which has been demonstrated to be an appropriate description of brain tissue deformation under compression at the much slower strain rates that would be expected to occur during surgery.[12]

Poroelastic biphasic prescriptions of soft tissue mechanics have been popular as well.[13,14] In particular, adaptations of Biot's consolidation theory[15] have found their way into the brain modeling literature. Nagashima and colleagues have demonstrated that a wide range of pathophysiologies can be simulated from this perspective, including hypdrocephalus and vasogenic edema;[16,17] this approach continues to appear as the mathematical model of choice in many cases,[18] in large part because of its linearity, which translates into computational advantages that are lost when complex constitutive relationships are modeled.

Very recently, brain deformation modeling has appeared in the context of image-guided neurosurgery as a vehicle for estimating tissue motion during surgical intervention.[19,20] The study by Edwards et al.[21] represented the brain as a three-compartment system consisting of bone, fluid, and soft tissue where rigid-body transformations were applied to bone, fluid regions were unconstrained, and smooth deformation was applied to the parenchyma. Several energy models were compared in 2D with data from an epilepsy patient where preoperative MR and postoperative CT were available for analysis. The Skrinjar et al.[20] study modeled the brain as a homogeneous linear viscoelastic medium with finite elements on relatively coarse discretizations of the tissue continuum ($\approx$250 nodes in 2D, 1000 nodes in 3D). Simulations of an artificial parietal craniotomy were reported in two and three dimensions, illustrating time sequences of the computed deformation field which showed settling effects due to gravity that cause not only posterior movements near the craniotomy but also motion in the superior and inferior directions.

The remainder of this chapter focuses on the work of Paulsen and Miga[19,22,23] as representative of the state of the art in biomechanical modeling with finite elements for intraoperative use during image guidance. These investigators have developed a 3D computational framework based on consolidation which exploits high resolution meshes derived from high definition preoperative medical images. Studies of the performance of both the computational mathematics and the computational physics have been undertaken through benchmark problem analysis and *in vivo* experiments in animal and human brains. As such, this work can be used to illustrate many of the issues associated with this type of modeling which are generic to the concept of intraoperative updating of preoperative images with deformation models driven by the physical events occurring in the OR. It is worth noting that finite element models are also being exploited in the more conventional image registration and segmentation contexts.[24,25]

15.3 Brain Tissue Model Description

In the neurosurgery setting, consolidation theory represents the brain as a linearly elastic biphasic medium consisting of a solid matrix with interstitial fluid saturating the intramatrix spaces. Tissue motion is characterized by an instantaneous displacement at the site of mechanical loading followed by additional deformation resulting from hydrodynamic changes from prescribed or strain-induced pressure gradients in the interstitial fluid. The equations of motion can be written as coupled partial differential equations (PDEs) involving a force balance and conservation statement

$$\nabla \cdot G\nabla\mathbf{u} + \nabla\frac{G}{1-2\nu}\nabla\cdot\mathbf{u} - \alpha\nabla p + (\rho_t - \rho_f)\mathbf{g} = 0 \qquad (15.1a)$$

$$\alpha\frac{\partial}{\partial t}(\nabla\cdot\mathbf{u}) - \nabla\cdot k\nabla p + \frac{1}{S}\frac{\partial p}{\partial t} = 0 \qquad (15.1b)$$

where G is the shear modulus, ν is Poisson's ratio, $\mathbf{u}$ is the displacement vector, p is the pore fluid pressure, α is the ratio of fluid volume extracted to volume change of tissue under compression, k is the hydraulic conductivity, $1/S$ is the amount of fluid which can be forced into tissue under constant volume, ρ_t and ρ_f are the densities of tissue and surrounding fluid, respectively, and $\mathbf{g}$ is the gravitational acceleration vector.

In Equation (15.1a), the first two terms are the classic PDE describing mechanical equilibrium in a linearly elastic solid, i.e., the stress of the solid matrix is linearly proportional to the strain. The third term reflects an applied body force which is a function of interstitial pressure gradients arising from hydraulic loading conditions, e.g., cerebrospinal fluid drainage, hyperosmotic drugs, capillary transport, etc. The last term in Equation (15.1a) approximates the effects of gravity on brain tissue. Here, a reduction in buoyancy forces is modeled by changes in the density of the fluid surrounding tissue which has become exposed to air (i.e., ρ_f becomes the density of air).

In Equation (15.1b), the first term reflects the time rate of dilatational changes of the solid matrix. The second term in the equation is a conservation of mass statement. It contains (within the divergence operator) Darcy's law, which linearly relates the movement of interstitial fluid to the pressure gradient acting across the tissue, i.e., $v = k\nabla p$ where v is the velocity of the interstitial fluid. These first two terms taken together state that volumetric changes correlate directly with the transport of fluid into and out of a control volume. The last term in (15.1b) represents an accumulation of pressure which allows compressibility of the interstitial fluid. This term may be used in cases where the tissue is not completely saturated with fluid, i.e., small voids of air or gas are present. Generally, the brain is considered to be a fully saturated medium which sets α to unity and eliminates the time rate of change of pressure from (15.1b).

To first order, this characterization of brain tissue would seem to be a reasonable starting point for modeling, especially under the acute loading conditions associated with surgery and given that the mechanical properties for brain tissue are not agreed to universally. As an aid to better understanding the physical behavior associated with Equations (15.1a–b), Figure 15.1 shows a fully saturated porous medium undergoing compression by a perforated piston. In this example, the material is placed under compression ΔP and drainage is allowed through the holes in the piston face. Figure 15.2 illustrates the

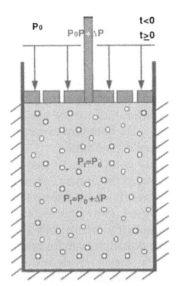

FIGURE 15.1
Illustrative example to demonstrate deformation
and hydraulic behavior of porous medium.

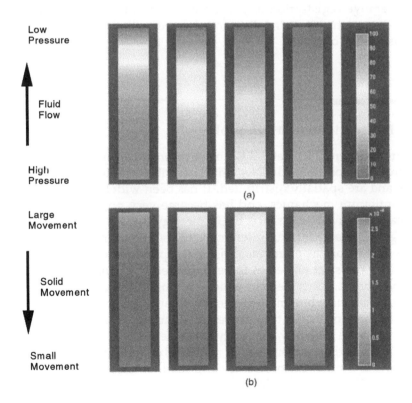

FIGURE 15.2
Consolidation of a column of porous medium under top surface compression; (a) time course
of interstitial pressure along the column, (b) time course of absolute vertical displacement
along the column.

time course of displacement and pressure experienced in the column. Initially, there is instant drainage and deformation at the surface, with the load supported by the interstitial fluid at depth. This generates a pressure gradient acting directionally opposite to the deformation source (i.e., high pressure at depth and low pressure at the surface). Over time as more fluid drains (i.e., gradual reduction in the gradient over time), the load is transferred from the interstitial fluid to the solid matrix (i.e., gradual increase in deformation at depth). The behavior exemplified here is often compared to that of deforming a saturated sponge.

There is little doubt that the microscale events occurring during surgical loading of the brain are complex. However, consolidation theory provides a framework which captures the bulk deformation and hydraulic behavior associated with surgical deformations. Although a viscoelastic response was not explicitly incorporated in the above description, alteration of the constitutive equations can be readily accomplished to include these effects. However, further investigation in the context of surgical loading is needed to better understand which modeling terms are most important for nonrigid intraoperative registration of preoperative data. In the next section, we briefly discuss the issues involved in solving equations such as (15.1a-b) on complex spatial domains.

15.4 Finite Element Methodology

The finite element (FE) method is a classical engineering analysis technique that produces solutions to PDEs which describe complex systems and processes and are spatially distributed. It has been widely used in structural and continuum mechanics, and has become very popular in biomedical applications as well. In essence, the FE strategy divides the domain of interest (e.g., the brain) into an interconnected set of subregions or elements which fill the volume of interest. Discrete approximations to the PDEs that govern the physical processes to be simulated (e.g., consolidation theory) are developed on each element which can possess its own local properties (e.g., gray versus white matter), thereby allowing complicated geometries and tissue heterogeneties to be represented through a simple building block structure. In the limit of vanishingly small elements, the FE approximation to the PDE solution converges to its analytical continuum, provided that the principles of numerical consistency and stability are satisfied (e.g., see reference 26). Thus, given sufficient resolution of the geometry of interest, FE methods produce highly accurate solutions to complex equations under realistic conditions.

Following the development by Paulsen et al.,[19] Galerkin weighed residual discretization of Equation (15.1) begins with volume integration after multiplication by a suitable, spatially continuous weighting function ϕ_i

$$\langle \phi_i \nabla \cdot G\nabla \mathbf{u} \rangle + \left\langle \phi_i \nabla \frac{G}{1-2\nu}(\nabla \cdot \mathbf{u}) \right\rangle - \langle \phi_i \nabla p \rangle = \langle (\rho_f - \rho_t)\mathbf{g}\phi_i \rangle \qquad (15.2a)$$

$$\left\langle \phi_i \frac{\partial}{\partial t}(\nabla \cdot \mathbf{u}) \right\rangle - \langle \phi_i \nabla \cdot k\nabla p \rangle = 0 \qquad (15.2b)$$

where $\langle \cdot \rangle$ indicates integration over the problem space. Here, ϕ_i is the ith member of a complete set of scalar functions of position (which is ultimately truncated as part of the discretization process), in particular, the standard C° locally defined Lagrange polynomial interpolants associated with finite elements. Applying divergence and gradient integral theorems to the second derivative terms in Equation (15.2) leads to

$$\langle G\nabla \mathbf{u} \cdot \nabla \phi_i \rangle + \left\langle \frac{G}{1-2\nu}(\nabla \cdot \mathbf{u})\nabla \phi_i \right\rangle + \langle \phi_i \nabla p \rangle = \langle (\rho_f - \rho_t)\mathbf{g}\phi_i \rangle$$

$$+ \oint G\hat{n} \cdot \nabla u \phi_i \, ds + \oint \frac{G}{1-2\nu}\hat{n}(\nabla \cdot \mathbf{u})\phi_i \, ds \qquad (15.3a)$$

$$\left\langle \phi_i \frac{\partial}{\partial t}(\nabla \cdot \mathbf{u}) \right\rangle + \langle k\nabla p \cdot \nabla \phi_i \rangle = \oint k\hat{n} \cdot \nabla p \phi_i \, ds \qquad (15.3b)$$

where $\oint$ denotes integration over the boundary which encloses the brain volume and $\hat{n}$ is the outward pointing normal direction to this boundary. Spatial discretization of Equation (15.3) is completed by expanding the unknown displacement vector, $\mathbf{u}$, and fluid pressure, p, as sums of time-varying (but spatially constant) coefficients multiplied by known (time-invariant) functions of position which produces the coupled set of ordinary differential equations.

$$\sum_j \mathbf{u}_j \langle G\nabla \phi_j \cdot \nabla \phi_i \rangle + \sum_j \mathbf{u}_j \cdot \left\langle \nabla \phi_j \frac{G}{1-2\nu}\nabla \phi_i \right\rangle \sum_j p_j \langle \nabla \phi_j \phi_i \rangle =$$

$$\langle (\rho_f - \rho_t)\mathbf{g}\phi_i \rangle + \oint G\hat{n} \cdot \nabla \mathbf{u} \phi_i \, ds + \oint \frac{G}{1-2\nu}\hat{n}(\nabla \cdot \mathbf{u})\phi_i \, ds \qquad (15.4a)$$

$$\sum_j \frac{\partial \mathbf{u}_j}{\partial t} \langle \nabla \phi_j \ \phi_i \rangle + \sum_j p_j \langle k\nabla \phi_j \cdot \nabla \phi_i \rangle = \oint k\hat{n} \cdot \nabla p \phi_i \, ds \qquad (15.4b)$$

Equation (15.4) can be integrated in time using a simple two-point weighting

$$\int_{t_n}^{t_{n+1}} f(t)dt = \Delta t[\theta f(t_{n+1}) + (1-\theta)f(t_n)] \qquad (15.5)$$

where $\Delta t = t_{n+1} - t_n$ and $0 \le \theta \le 1$. This generates a two-time-level, fully discrete system that is expressible as matrix equation

$$AU^{n+1} = BU^n + C^{n+\theta} \qquad (15.6)$$

where the entries matrices A and B and column vector C are constructed from spatial integrations of known functions as defined in references 19 and 27 for Cartesian coordinates. Provided tissue material property coefficients do not vary in time, matrices A and B are stationary and can be constructed once. Because the weighting functions, ϕ_i, and, correspondingly, the solution basis functions have local support, A and B are extremely sparse relative to their overall rank (four times the number of sample positions or nodes used to represent the brain geometry) which lends them to sparse storage methods and iterative solution schemes that become essential in 3D problems. Hence, the displacement vector and pressure field evolve by one time increment through iterative matrix solution to the sparse linear system described symbolically in Equation (15.6).

15.5   Model Validation

The process of model validation involves answering two questions: (1) does the discrete model represent the continuum mathematics as posed, and (2) does the discrete model emulate physical reality? The first question is relatively straightforward to answer, and a number of analysis tools and techniques are available. One of the keys to this form of validation is to exercise the model under a number of different conditions where known solutions exist. For example, benchmark problems of increasing complexity ranging from a relatively simple 1D column consolidation problem to a 3D concentric sphere case intended to correspond to infusion-induced brain swelling have been considered in Paulsen et al.[19] There, computational accuracies of 1 to 2% in both displacement and pressure fields have been readily achieved with moderate levels of finite element discretization.

Another aspect of examining the mathematical integrity of computed results involves investigation of the propagation of errors during time evolution of the solution, since numerical convergence on vanishingly small element sizes requires numerical stability. Miga et al. have conducted a Fourier analysis of the spectrum of modes which are sustainable by the discrete FE equations of consolidation on an infinite mesh having uniform node-to-node sample spacing.[28] This so-called Von Neumann stability analysis shows that two dimensionless groups along with the time integration weighting used in Equation (15.5) control the stability of error propagation for changes in physical property and mesh discretization parameters. The results indicate that the presence and persistence of stable spurious oscillations in the pore pressure which have been attributed to incorrect initial incompressibility constraints[29,30] are in fact controlled by the ratio of time-step size to the square of the space-step for fixed time integration weightings and physical property selections. In general, increasing the time-step or decreasing the mesh spacing has a smoothing effect on the discrete solution; however, special cases exist that violate this generality which can be readily identified through the Von Neumann approach.[28] The analysis also reveals that explicitly dominated schemes ($\theta < 0.5$ in Equation 15.5) are not stable for saturated media ($\alpha = 1, 1/S = 0$) and only become possible through a decoupling of the mechanical equilibrium (Equation 15.1a) and continuity (Equation 15.1b) equations. In the case of unsaturated media, a breakdown in the Von Neumann results has been demonstrated to occur due to boundary conditions which also influence numerical stability.[28]

In practice, meshes are not uniform and problem geometries are irregular and complex; hence, a useful approach for determining the computational integrity of numerical solutions is to perform a mesh convergence study where the finite element grid is successfully refined for the actual problem of interest. This type of study would fall into the category of demonstrating that the finite element model solutions are mathematically robust. An example of a mesh convergence study reported by Miga et al. is described later in this section.[23]

The second, more important, and difficult question of model validation is to determine the extent to which the model equations (e.g., the consolidation Equations (15.1a) and (15.1b)) represent enough of the physics involved in brain tissue deformation to be useful intraoperatively. Model validation in this context is often confounded by the fact that the rationale for using a computational model in the first place is that detailed measurements are difficult to obtain in the setting of interest. Hence, a dilemma often arises and two approaches emerge: (1) simplify the setting of interest to the point where detailed measurements become possible and assume that the findings extrapolate to the actual situation, or (2) obtain limited, often less accurate measurements in the setting of interest and assume that agreement with a sparsely sampled response is indicative of results that would be obtained throughout the volume if detailed measurement maps were possible. An example of the former approach is nicely illustrated by the recent work of Miller.[12,31] Here, *ex vivo* pig brain specimens were prepared and micromechanical manipulations performed in order to develop a multiparametered viscoelastic constitutive relationship as a means of defining and validating a computational model for robotic surgery and virtual reality surgical systems.

Fortunately, the availability of volumetric noninvasive imaging makes possible model validation studies which can be carried out *in vivo* in both animal and human brains where detailed measurement maps of tissue displacements can be obtained. As a result, there is a rich opportunity to complete model validation studies in the actual setting of interest. An interesting example of an initial phase of *in vivo* model validation has been provided in previous work.[23,32] A representative quantitative result is presented in Figure 15.3, which

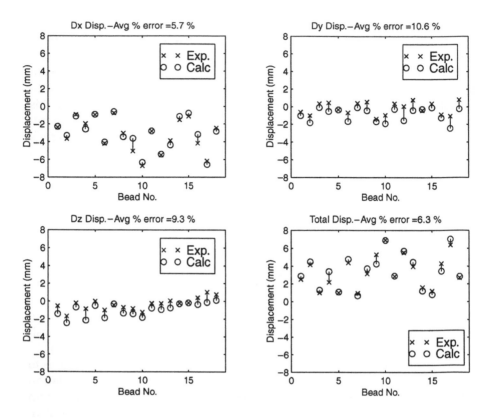

FIGURE 15.3

Trajectory and total displacement comparisons between experimental and calculated values of bead movement for the pig brain under a 12 mm piston-induced displacement in the temporal lobe (i.e., shown are Dx (top left), Dy (top right), Dz (bottom left), and total displacement (bottom right)). A good correspondence is achieved when the distance between measured displacement (X) and predicted displacement (O) is small (i.e., line connecting (X) and (O) at each point is small).

shows a set of point-by-point comparisons of the Cartesian components of computed and measured displacement vectors in the porcine brain *in vivo*. These investigators opted to develop an experimental animal system where point displacement vectors could be measured as a strategy for beginning the model validation process in the neurosurgery setting. They chose to implant templates of small (1 mm) stainless steel beads through stereotactic technique in the closed cranium and then to insert some form of displacement source to impart a mechanical load. Figure 15.4 is a fluoroscope film illustrating a completed bead implant. Preprocedure MR scans were used to define a finite element mesh of the pig brain for modeling purposes. Issues related to anatomical mesh generation from high resolution preoperative scanning are discussed in the next section. Tissue deformation and concomitant bead movement were tracked with intraoperative CT which allowed detailed 3D maps of bead motion to be deduced from a series of CT scans. Several different types of loads

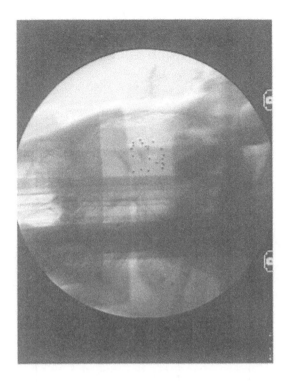

FIGURE 15.4
Examples of an experiment in progress with a fluoroscopic film illustrating a complete implant.

have been used, including a temporally mounted piston[32] and temporally and intraparenchymally located balloon catheters.[33] These deformation sources were moved incrementally in a controlled fashion with full CT image acquisitions occurring between each intervention event. Rigid-body image registration was maintained from scan to scan by the stereotactic frame which was in place and the fact that the animal's position was not changed once inside the CT scanner.

Interestingly, this group chose to use MR images to define their computational model, but CT scans to track deformation events. MR scanning for model construction is a logical choice because of its superior soft tissue contrast, allowing computational models which differentiate gray and white matter to be employed. In terms of deploying the CT for deformation tracking, they have clearly traded off the error induced by having to coregister the model (constructed from MR) with the CT images obtained during an experiment with the fast image acquisition and artifact reduction (around the small metallic tissue markers) afforded by the CT. The investigators have quantified the impact of registration error on model validation by randomly perturbing the starting location of each bead in the model (i.e., the uncertainty of bead location resulting from potential registration error) up to 5 mm, and concluded that model comparisons vary no more than 10%. Figure 15.5 shows a

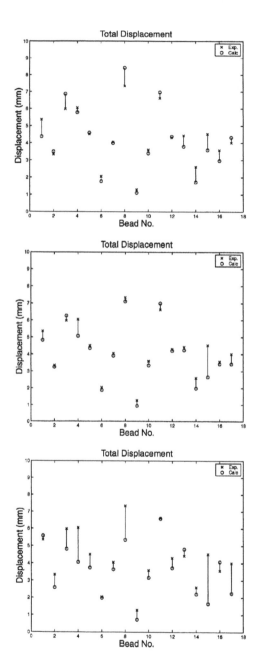

FIGURE 15.5

Total displacement variations in computed bead position from 0 mm, 2 mm, and 5 mm randomly applied displacement offsets to initial bead positions which simulate CT/MR registration errors. These induced offsets resulted in less than a 10% change in the overall data-model match. A good correspondence is achieved when the distance between measured displacement (X) and predicted displacement (O) is small (i.e., line connecting (X) and (O) at each point is small).

sample comparing total bead displacement with 0 mm, 2 mm, and 5 mm random perturbations on starting bead locations. The most striking feature of Figure 15.5 is the fact that the bead trajectories are very similar across these cases.

A mesh convergence study has also been performed on these pig brain calculations in order to ensure that numerical discretization error is sufficiently small that differences between predicted and measured bead locations can be assigned to data model mismatch associated with physical conditions. Shown in Figure 15.6 are results from a study involving computations in a pig brain model where solutions are compared under increasing levels of discretization with the goal of defining a solution-independent mesh resolution. Figure 15.6 displays changes in displacement and pressure at several distances from the deformation source under increasing mesh discretization. These surface plots are quite informative and indicate that the calculations which produced the results in Figure 15.3 can be considered well resolved. In these plots, six levels of mesh discretization are reported which illustrate a maximum solution variance of 1 mm in displacement and 2 mm Hg in pressure at the coarsest mesh scale (less than 5000 nodes) and less than 0.1 mm and 0.3 mmHg at mesh resolutions of more than 16,000 nodes. The computations reported by Miga and colleagues have typically used meshes with resolutions in the 18,000 to 20,000 range, making them highly accurate from the point of view of numerical discretization error.

Once valid model calculations have been obtained, their intraoperative value depends on whether they can be utilized in a form that is familiar to the neurosurgeon. Towards this end, the Dartmouth group has developed a strategy to deform the preoperative MR images based on the volumetric displacement field computed with their model. Figure 15.7 dramatically illustrates the point by showing a set of preoperative MR slices adjacent to their model-deformed counterparts for a pig brain experiment where significant intraoperative tissue motion has been induced. The algorithm in place is conceptualized in Figure 15.8 which shows that the displacement is computed at each image voxel using the finite element basis functions expressed in the coordinate frame of the deformed finite element mesh. These points are then undeformed to the original image space in order to define the voxel intensity value, which should be assigned to each image voxel in the deformed image space.

Within this framework, these investigators have defined a percent recapture metric in order to quantify the accuracy of the model in the image-guided setting. The percent recapture is the difference between the remaining absolute total bead displacement error (difference between measured and computed displacements) and the average total bead displacement, which can be viewed as the amount of motion recovered by the model which would have been unaccounted for if preoperative images were used as the basis for image guidance. Across the series of *in vivo* pig brain experiments reported by Miga et al.,[32] this percentage has ranged from 75 to 85% which is quite encouraging, especially given that there are many ways in which the modeling can be enhanced.

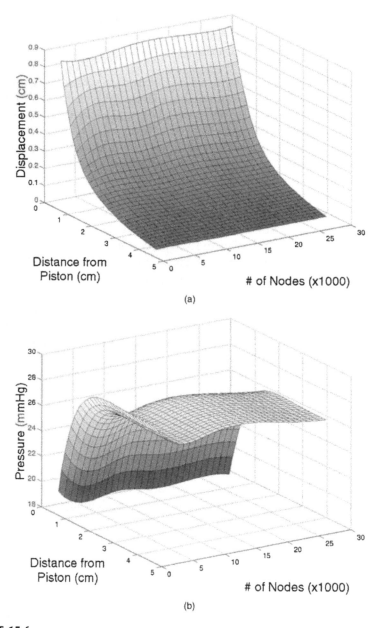

FIGURE 15.6

Mesh convergence study where the solution for displacement and pressure is compared at several distances from the deformation source at increasing mesh resolutions. The goal is to define a solution independent mesh resolution which ensures numerical fidelity.

More surgically relevant simulations of pig brain interventions are also under way. Figure 15.9 illustrates the sequence of events needed to model tissue retraction. First, the geometry of the retractor blade is predefined as a wireframe description which can be inserted into the model in an arbitrary location

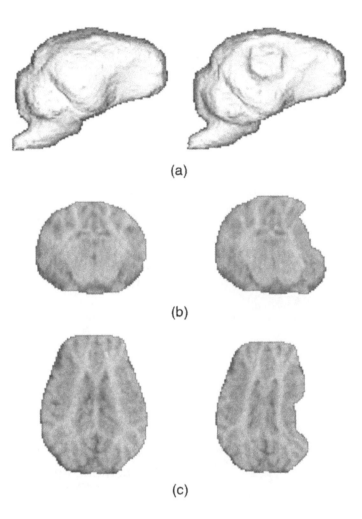

FIGURE 15.7
Model-updated images of a pig brain experiencing a 1 cm piston-induced displacement of the temporal lobe: (a) volumetric segmented brain surface, (b) coronal cross-sectional image, and (c) axial cross-sectional image. Notice the visible collapsing of ventricular space as well as the compression of white matter tracks in the deformed image volume.

(Figure 15.9a). Once inserted, brain model nodes nearest the retractor are moved onto the defining surface and duplicated to create two coincident nodal positions that will represent independent degrees of freedom once the blade begins to move (Figure 15.9b). Movement of the blade (Figure 15.9c) occurs by applying boundary conditions, either fixed displacements or normal stresses in the direction of retraction, for one set of the coincident nodes defining the blade geometry while the second set of nodes become stress free and able to move according to the equations of consolidation. Once the boundary conditions are applied and the calculations completed, the tissue deformation map

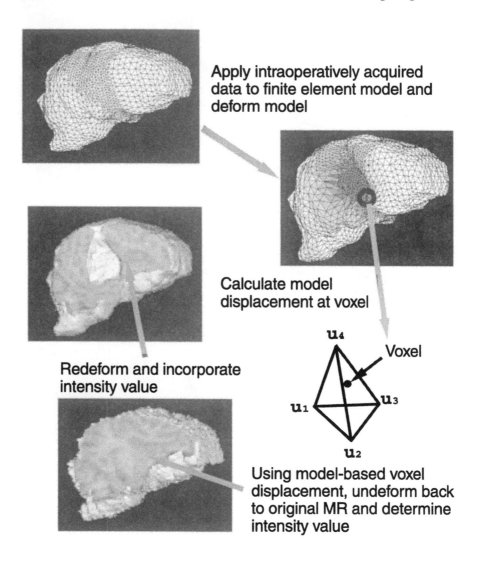

Apply intraoperatively acquired
data to finite element model and
deform model

Calculate model
displacement at voxel

Redeform and incorporate
intensity value

Using model-based voxel
displacement, undeform back
to original MR and determine
intensity value

FIGURE 15.8
Intraoperative image updating algorithm based on model calculated deformation.

can be used to update the undeformed preoperative images. Implementation in
3D is reasonably straightforward, as illustrated in Color Figure 15.10.* These
calculations show an interesting tissue bulge in the retraction direction. Figure
15.11a presents an intraoperative CT image of the *in vivo* pig brain under retraction. The motion of the blade and implanted bead markers is evident along with
a bulging of tissue in the retraction direction as suggested by the model. Note
that in this case tissue on the "back side" of the retractor appears to adhere to

_____
* Color Figures follow page 22.

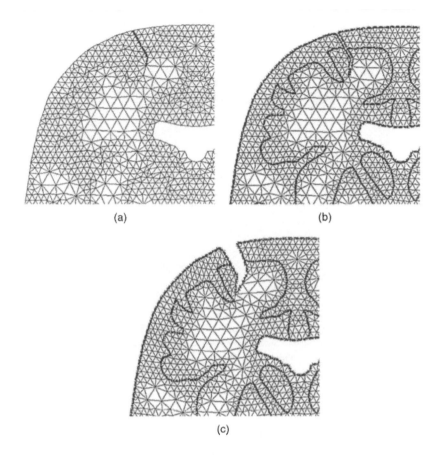

FIGURE 15.9
Computational procedure to simulate intraoperative retraction: (a) the retractor blade is described by a patch description inserted into the model, (b) the patch description guides the splitting of the finite element mesh, (c) the retraction occurs with the application of boundary conditions separating the tissue.

the blade, whereas in the simulation it separates. Clearly, boundary conditions on both sides of the blade-tissue interface require further study. Figure 15.11b contains additional data acquired by placing a small pressure sensor on the face of the retractor blade which could be helpful in this regard and easily deployed in the human OR as well. The recordings show a pressure spike immediate to the initialization of a retraction event followed by a period of transient decay until the next retraction occurs. This information could be useful for defining appropriate boundary conditions for retraction on a case-by-case basis. If both displacement and normal stresses at the retractor surface can be measured, the opportunity also exists to estimate local mechanical properties *in vivo*.

Interestingly, the pressure measurements at the retractor surface in Figure 15.11b are similar in character to interstitial pressure measurements which

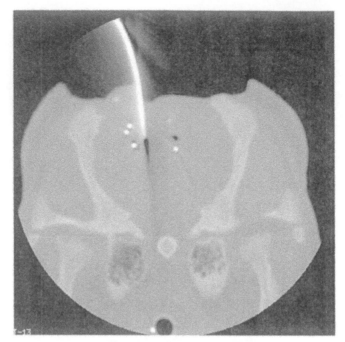

Retractor Pressure vs Time

(a)

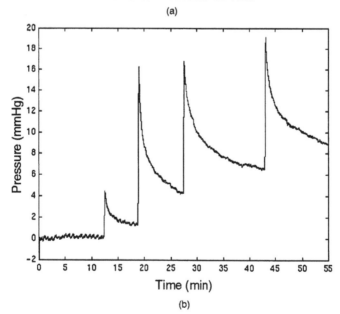

(b)

FIGURE 15.11

Experimental techniques to validate computational procedures for tissue retraction: (a) porcine system for characterizing *in vivo* retraction, and (b) sensored retractors to measure forces applied.

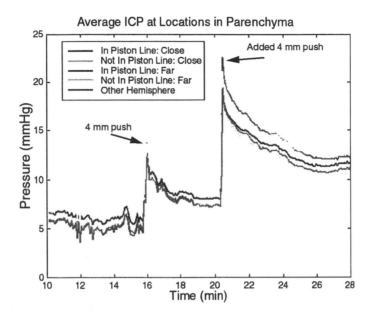

FIGURE 15.12
Interstitial pressure traces over time recorded during a deformation experiment.

are potentially important determinants of brain tissue mechanical response. Studies performed by Wolfla et al.[34,35] have shown that significant pressure gradients can occur when the brain is subjected to large displacements. Under conditions of acute mass expansion in the porcine brain, their interstitial pressure curves exhibited a characteristic spike in interstitial pressure corresponding to expansion followed by a period of exponential decay between expansions, with a gradual accumulation of strain-induced gradients across the brain. These measurements are very similar to Figure 15.11b and other data/calculations obtained in the pig brain for the types of loading conditions used by Miga et al.[23] In additional pig experiments, pressure sensors are implanted in the brain and monitored while the subject is undergoing a temporally located load. Figure 15.12 shows the pressure time traces measured in the pig brain at several locations in the cranium under two successive piston displacements of 4 mm and 8 mm, respectively, which mimic the behavior noted by Wolfla et al.[35] Comparable pressure responses have been produced with a consolidation model approach, although the computed absolute peak pressure levels have generally exceeded those measured experimentally, depending on the tissue property and cortical surface boundary condition assumptions that have been invoked.[23]

15.6   Model Inputs

One of the intriguing aspects of employing a computational model to update images during image-guided neurosurgery is the opportunity to maximize the utility of both preoperative and intraoperative data for neuronavigation. This seems important at the present time given the wealth of preoperative information and planning which accompanies most neurosurgical cases, yet there is the potential for loss of or de-emphasis on this information with adoption of intraoperative MR imaging. Preoperatively, image scans can be employed to define the patient-specific computational model to be deformed intraoperatively. The possibility of using additional MR sequences to derive patient specific brain tissue properties through the emerging techniques of diffusion tensor imaging[36,37] and elastography[38,39] also exists. Once in the OR, several forms of reduced or incomplete data (short of volumetric imaging with CT and MR) are also available for incorporation within the model. Specifically, cortical surface motion can be monitored with automated surface digitalization techniques such as laser scanning. Coregistered ultrasound provides another information source on the movement of some subsurface structures; for example, the ventricular system, which can provide internal constraints on the computed deformation field. In this section, examples of model inputs available from both preoperative and intraoperative data are briefly illustrated.

15.6.1   Preoperative Data

Prior to surgery, high resolution MR imaging is routinely acquired and is ideal for model discretization purposes. Following this image series, a 3D representation can be constructed from the MR slices by segmenting the brain from the cranium using an image manipulation platform such as **Analyze AVW** (Biomedical Imaging Resource—Version 2.5, Mayo Foundation, Rochester, MN). After the extraction, each voxel within the volume can be saturated to a constant intensity value and a marching cubes algorithm[40] used to generate a surface description characterized by triangular patches. Armed with the resulting patch description, a 3D tetrahedral mesh can be generated.[41] If internal structures are to be preserved, the process of image segmentation and boundary generation can be employed for each constituent of interest in order to define a composite wire-frame boundary to guide the mesh generation process.

An alternate strategy which is particularly helpful for incorporating complex structures such as gray/white matter boundaries is to use an image-to-grid segmentation scheme. In this case, the average voxel intensity from the MR image volume can be determined for each individual element within the finite element mesh. An intensity-to-material-property map can then be defined by the user. For example, a strict binary thresholding can be employed to discriminate gray from white matter. The beauty of this approach is that alternate intensity-to-property maps can be identified by the user, depending on problem requirements. Figure 15.13 shows an example of mesh generation at several stages of completion, including wireframe descriptions with and without internal boundaries which define model geometry, and image-to-grid segmentations based on gray/white matter intensity thresholding. The figure makes it clear that high resolution computational models which faithfully capture patient-specific geometry and tissue types can be routinely produced.

Utilizing preoperative MR data to estimate tissue elastic properties may also become a reality in the near future. Computational models of tissue deformation play an important role here as well. By imparting small amplitude (10 μm) displacement to tissue at low frequencies (100 Hz) synchronized with specialized MR pulse sequences, it is possible to measure 3D displacement fields at the MR voxel level. These displacement patterns are a complex synthesis of dilatational and shear waves that are functions not only of the local tissue properties, but also of the boundary conditions and stimulation forces that are applied. Hence, estimation algorithms are needed to infer intrinsic tissue mechanical properties from the MR-measured displacements. An example of a recently reported finite element technique is illustrated in Figure 15.14.[42] The reconstruction of an elastic property map is based on a simulation, but is none-theless quite impressive, especially given the fact that the synthetic measurements have been corrupted with 10% added noise, yet detailed discrimination of differences in modulus between gray and white matter is quite clear. If this technology can be developed, it is quite conceivable that patient-specific, spatially resolved mechanical property maps would be available for modeling purposes in the OR to improve the ability to account for intraoperative tissue motion through a model-based approach.

15.6.2 Intraoperative Data

Tracking of instruments and cortical surface movement in the OR can be accomplished with a variety of tools. Figure 15.15 illustrates one option which consists of an operating microscope attached to a ceiling-mounted robotic platform which maintains knowledge of a coordinate system in the OR. The realization in Figure 15.15 is the Surgiscope System manufactured by Elekta AB (Stockholm, Sweden). It offers a number of precision tracking functions including a continuous readout of microscope location and orientation, memorization of a particular location (and orientation) which can be returned to at any time, and laser beam positioning within the optics of the microscope convergent at its focus. Coregistered digital photographs can be acquired of the surgical field and used to capture cortical motion as illustrated in Figure 15.16, which shows two photographs recorded at different

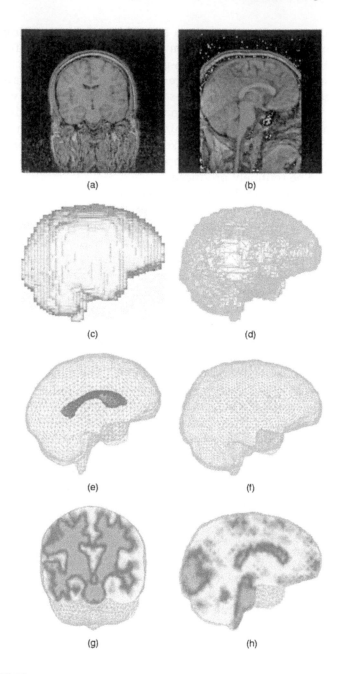

FIGURE 15.13
Steps in computational model generation: (a, b) coronal and sagittal MR cross sectional
images, (c) segmented region of interest surface, (d) marching cubes boundary patch description of region of interest, (e, f) generation of volumetric tetrahedral mesh with and
without boundary-defined internal structures, (g, h) coronal and sagittal cross sections of
material property heterogeneity pattern using image-to-grid thresholding.

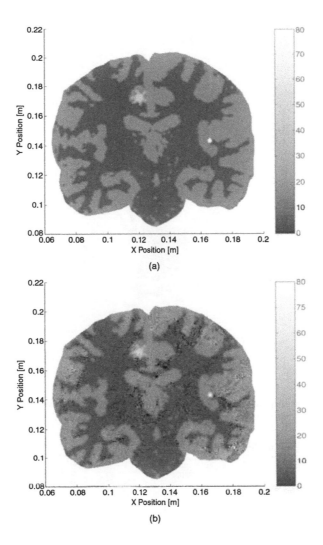

FIGURE 15.14
Simulated reconstruction of Young's Modulus in a coronal brain cross section where (a) is the original Young's Modulus distribution provided by image-to-grid segmentation as described in Figure 15.13 and (b) is the reconstructed modulus distribution from synthetic displacement measurements having 10% noise.

times from the same location that have been processed to extract feature movement within the image pair.

Intraoperative ultrasound is a low-cost imaging technology which can also be registered in the OR coordinate system and potentially provide control points as model constraints during intraoperative image updating.[43–46] Figure 15.17 illustrates how this might function. At the start of a case, ultrasound image sweeps can be recorded (Figure 15.7a), echogenic structures (e.g., ventricles,

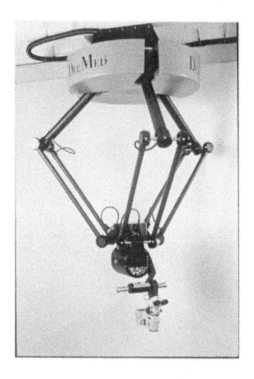

FIGURE 15.15
Surgiscope System manufactured by Elekta AB (Stockholm, Sweden) which can be used for the tracking of instruments and cortical surface movement in the OR.

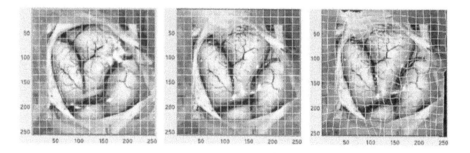

FIGURE 15.16
Using high-resolution digital photographs captured in the OR (left two images), cortical surface patterns can be manipulated with image morphing techniques (right image) to generate a spatial distribution of cortical surface movement that can subsequently be used as input for model updates.

tumor) segmented (Figure 15.17b) and overlayed (Figure 15.17d) with the pre-operative MR (Figure 15.17c), and also registered in OR coordinates in order to define baseline conditions and estimate registration errors. From this established state, subsequent movements in these boundaries can be followed with the ultrasound and supplied to the model as known data. The model is

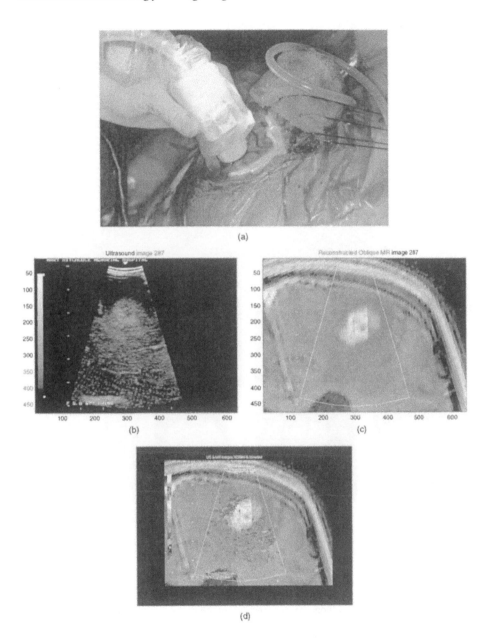

FIGURE 15.17

Low-cost imaging modalities can serve as a source of incomplete intraoperative data. For example, (a) spatially registered intraoperative ultrasound image acquisition in the OR can be employed to: (b) display an ultrasound image, (c) define the spatially equivalent preoperative MR image, and (d) generate an overlay superimposing the intraoperative ultrasound on the preoperative MR to monitor tissue motion at selected subsurface locations.

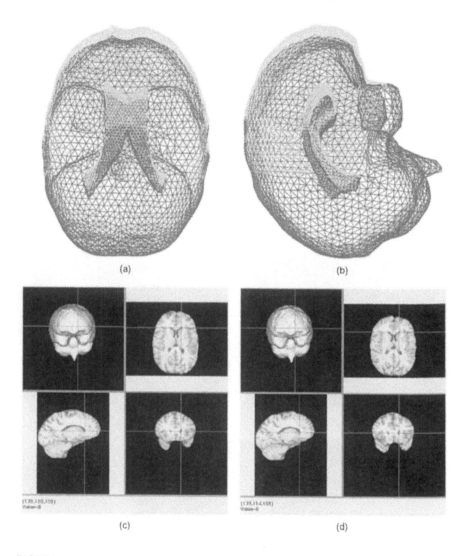

FIGURE 15.18
A finite element intraoperative update based on gravity-induced shift during a clinical case: overlay of undeformed and deformed finite element mesh boundaries for (a) axial and (b) sagittal orientations. Preoperative orthogonal cross sections of the image volume are shown in (c) with their intraoperatively updated counterpart presented in (d). Model predictions show an approximate 6 mm shift of the lateral ventricle tip highlighted by the cursor cross-hairs in these images.

deformed by this and other OR inputs (e.g., cortical surface motion) in order to create the volumetric update of the preoperative MR images as surgery progresses.

To complete this illustration, an example of a clinical update of gravity-induced deformation performed retrospectively to the actual surgery is shown in Figure 15.18. These results are discussed more fully in references 27 and 47. They are important because they indicate how the finite element models of Figure 15.13 which are unfamiliar to the neurosurgeon can provide deformation data that can be used to update image formats which are the basis of navigation for the surgeon. In addition, they show that volumetric motion of tissue structures can be many millimeters, making the static preoperative MR images of less value for navigational decisionmaking as the surgery progresses.

15.7 Conclusions

The opportunity to exploit computational models of tissue deformation in the OR as an aid to updating preoperative image information to reflect tissue motion that occurs during surgery appears to be quite promising. This is an appealing approach because it integrates the high resolution preoperative images which are routinely available in all image-guided surgeries with the acquisition of incomplete intraoperative data that can be recorded at low cost and modest inconvenience within the traditional OR environment. Many of the basic building blocks necessary to implement such a strategy already exist or have been recently developed. Undoubtedly, there is much more work to be done to advance the modeling to include more complex surgical interventions, (for example, tissue resection) and questions of the value-added by model updating and the degree to which high resolution, 3D computations can be performed directly in the OR still persist. Issues related to the most appropriate mathematical description to use and whether patient specific mechanical properties can be deduced or are even necessary are important as well. Increased research activity can be expected to occur over the coming years in order to sort out many of the remaining questions and hopefully demonstrate that a model-based methodology is one viable solution to the image registration problem which results from intraoperative brain tissue motion.

References

1. M. Bro-Nielsen, Finite element modeling in medical VR, *J. IEEE*, vol. 86, no. 3, pp. 490–503, 1998.
2. K.V. Hansen and O.V. Larsen, Using region-of-interest based finite element modelling for brain-surgery simulation, *Lecture Notes in Computer Science: Medical Image Computing and Computer-Assisted Intervention—MICCAI'98*, vol. 1496, pp. 305–316, 1998.
3. N.L. Dorward, A. Olaf, B. Velani, F.A. Gerritsen, W.F. J. Harkness, N.D. Kitchen, and D.G.T. Thomas, Postimaging brain distortion: magnitude, correlates, and impact on neuronavigation, *J. Neurosurg.*, vol. 88, pp. 656–662, 1998.

4. C.R. Maurer, D.L.G. Hill, A.J. Martin, H. Liu, M. McCue, D. Rueckert, D. Lloret, W.A. Hall, R.E. Maxwell, D.J. Hawkes, and C.L. Truwit, Investigation of intra-operative brain deformation using a 1.5-t interventional MR system: preliminary results, *IEEE Trans. Med. Imaging*, vol. 17, no. 5, pp. 817–825, 1998.
5. T.M. Moriarty, R. Kikinis, F.A. Jolesz, P.M. Black, and E. Alexander 3rd, Magnetic resonance imaging therapy. Intraoperative MR imaging, *Neurosurg. Clin. N. Am.*, vol. 7, pp. 323–331, 1996.
6. R. Steinmeier, R. Fahlbusch, O. Ganslandt, C. Nimsky, M. Buchfelder, M. Kaus, T. Heigl, R. Kuth, and W. Huk, Intraoperative magnetic resonance imaging with the Magnetom open scanner: Concepts, neurosurgical indications, and proce-dures: a preliminary report, *Neurosurgery*, vol. 43, no. 4, pp. 739–748, 1998.
7. R. Bajcsy, R. Lieberson, and R. Reivich, A computerized system for the elastic matching of deformed radiographic images to idealized atlas images, *J. Comp. Assist. Tomogr.*, vol. 7, pp. 618–625, 1983.
8. G.E. Christensen, R.D. Rabbitt, and M.J. Miller, Deformable templates using large deformation kinematics, *IEEE Trans. on Image Process.*, vol. 5, no. 10, pp. 1435–1447, 1996.
9. S. Hakim, J.G. Venegas, and J.D. Burton, The physics of the cranial cavity, hy-drocephalus and normal pressure hydrocephalus: mechanical interpretation and mathematical model, *Surg. Neurol.*, vol. 5, pp. 187–210, 1976.
10. T. Doczi, Volume regulation of the brain tissue—a survey, *Acta Neurochirurgica*, vol. 121, pp. 1–8, 1993.
11. K.K. Mendis, R.L. Stalnaker, and S.H. Advani, A constitutive relationship for large deformation finite element modeling of brain tissue, *ASME J. Biomech. Eng.*, vol. 117, pp. 279–285, 1995.
12. K. Miller and K. Chinzei, Constitutive modeling of brain tissue: experiment and theory, *J. Biomechanics*, vol. 30, no. 11/12, pp. 1115–1121, 1997.
13. B.R. Simon, J.P. Laible, D. Pflaster, Y. Yuan, and M.H. Krag, Poroelastic finite element formulation including transport and swelling in soft tissue structures, *ASME J. Biomech. Eng.*, vol. 118, pp. 1–9, 1996.
14. R.L. Spilker and J.K. Suh, Formulation and evaluation of a finite element model for the biphasic model of hydrated soft tissue, *Comp. Struct.*, vol. 35, no. 4, pp. 425–439, 1990.
15. M.A. Biot, General theory of three-dimensional consolidation, *J. App. Physics*, vol. 12, pp. 155–164, 1941.
16. T. Nagashima, T. Shirakuni, and S.I. Rapoport, A two-dimensional, finite element analysis of vasogenic brain edema, *Neurol. Med. Chir.*, vol. 30, pp. 1–9, 1990.
17. T. Nagashima, N. Tamaki, M. Takada, and Y. Tada, Formation and resolution of brain edema associated with brain tumors. A comprehensive theoretical model and clinical analysis, *Acta Neurochirurgica, Suppl.*, vol. 60, pp. 165–167, 1994.
18. A. Pena, M.D. Bolton, H. Whitehouse, and J.D. Pickard, Effects of brain ventri-cular shape on periventricular biomechanics: a finite-element analysis, *Neurosur-gery*, vol. 45, no. 1, pp. 107–118, 1999.
19. K.D. Paulsen, M.I. Miga, F.E. Kennedy, P.J. Hoopes, A. Hartov, and D.W. Roberts, A computational model for tracking subsurface tissue deformation during ster-eotactic neurosurgery, *IEEE Trans. Biomed. Eng.*, vol. 46, no. 2, pp. 213–225, 1999.
20. O. Skrinjar, D. Spencer, and J. Duncan, Brain shift modeling for use in neurosur-gery, *Lecture Notes in Computer Science: Medical Image Computing and Computer-Assisted Intervention—MICCAI'98*, vol. 1496, pp. 1067–1074, 1998.

21. P. Edwards, D. Hill, J. Little, and D. Hawkes, A three component deformation model for image-guided surgery, *Med. Image Anal.*, vol. 2, no. 4, pp. 355–367, 1998.
22. M.I. Miga, Development and Quantification of a 3D Brain Deformation Model for Model-Updated Image-Guided Stereotactic Neurosurgery, Ph.D. thesis, Dartmouth College, Thayer School of Engineering, Hanover, N.H., 1998.
23. M.I. Miga, K.D. Paulsen, P.J. Hoopes, F.E. Kennedy, A. Hartov, and D.W. Roberts, *In vivo* modeling of interstitial pressure in the brain under surgical load using finite elements, *ASME J. Biomech. Eng.*, (in press), 1999.
24. S.K. Kyriacou and C. Davatzikos, A biomechanical model of soft tissue deformation, with applications to non-rigid registration of brain images with tumor pathology, *Lecture Notes in Computer Science: Medical Image Computing and Computer-Assisted Intervention—MICCAI'98*, vol. 1496, pp. 531–538, 1998.
25. F.S. Yaacobson and D. Giovoli, An adaptive finite element procedure for image segmentation problem, *Communic. Numer. Methods Eng.*, vol. 14, no. 7, pp. 621–632, 1998.
26. L. Lapidus and G.F. Pinder, *Numerical Solution for Partial Differential Equations in Science and Engineering*, John Wiley & Sons, New York, 1982.
27. M.I. Miga, K.D. Paulsen, J.M. Lemery, S.D. Eisner, A. Hartov, F.E. Kennedy, and D.W. Roberts, Model-updated image guidance: initial clinical experiences with gravity-induced brain deformation, *IEEE Trans. Med. Imaging*, vol. 18, no. 10, pp. 866–874, 1999.
28. M.I. Miga, K.D. Paulsen, and F.E. Kennedy, Von Neumann stability analysis of Biot's general two-dimensional theory of consolidation, *Int. J. Numer. Methods Eng.*, vol. 43, pp. 955–974, 1998.
29. M. Murad and A. Loula, Improved accuracy in finite element analysis of Biot's consolidation problem, *Comput. Methods Appl. Mech. Eng.*, vol. 95, pp. 359–382, 1992.
30. M. Murad and A. Loula, On stability and convergence of finite element approximations of Biot's consolidation problem, *Int. J. Numer. Methods Eng.*, vol. 37, pp. 645–667, 1994.
31. K. Miller, Constitutive model of brain tissue suitable for finite element analysis of surgical procedures, *J. Biomechanics*, vol. 32, pp. 531–537, 1999.
32. M.I. Miga, K.D. Paulsen, P.J. Hoopes, F.E. Kennedy, A. Hartov, and D.W. Roberts, *In vivo* quantification of a homogeneous brain deformation model for updating preoperative images during surgery, *IEEE Trans. Biomed. Eng.*, vol. 47, no. 2, pp. 266–273, 2000.
33. M.I. Miga, K.D. Paulsen, P.J. Hoopes, F.E. Kennedy, A. Hartov, and D.W. Roberts, *In vivo* analysis of heterogeneous brain deformation computations for model-updated image guidance, *Comp. Methods Biomechanics Biomed. Eng.*, 2000.
34. C.E. Wolfla, T. G. Luerssen, R.M. Bowman, and T.K. Putty, Brain tissue pressure gradients created by expanding frontal epidural mass lesion, *J. Neurosurg.*, vol. 84, pp. 642–647, 1996.
35. C.E. Wolfla, T.G. Luerssen, and R.M. Bowman, Regional brain tissue pressure gradients created by expanding extradural temporal mass legion, *J. Neurosurg.*, vol. 86, pp. 505–510, 1997.
36. P.J. Basser, J. Mattiello, and D. Le Bihan, Estimation of the effective self-diffusion tensor from the NMR spin echo, *J. Magn. Reson., Series B*, vol. 103, pp. 247–254, 1994.

37. J. Mattiello, P.J. Basser, and D. Le Bihan, The b matrix in diffusion tensor echo-planar imaging, *Magn. Reson. Med.*, vol. 37, pp. 292–300, 1997.
38. R. Muthupillai, P.J. Rossman, D.J. Lomas, J.F. Greenleaf, S.J. Riederer, and R.L. Ehman, Magnetic resonance elastography by direct visualization of propagating acoustic strain waves, *Science*, vol. 269, pp. 1854–1857, 1995.
39. E.E. W. Van Houten, J.B. Weaver, M.I. Miga, F.E. Kennedy, and K.D. Paulsen, Elasticity reconstruction from experimental MR displacement data: initial experience with an overlapping subzone finite element inversion process, *Med. Physics*, vol. 27, no. 1, pp. 101–107, 2000.
40. W. Schroeder, K. Martin, and B. Lorensen, *The Visualization Toolkit: An Object-Oriented Approach to 3D Graphics*, Prentice Hall, New Jersey, 1996.
41. J.M. Jr. Sullivan, G. Charron, and K.D. Paulsen, A three dimensional mesh generator for arbitrary multiple material domains, *Finite Element Anal. Design*, vol. 25, pp. 219–241, 1997.
42. E.E.W. Van Houten, K.D. Paulsen, M.I. Miga, F.E. Kennedy, and J.B. Weaver, An overlapping subzone technique for MR-based elastic property reconstruction, *Magn. Reson. Med.*, vol. 42, no. 4, pp. 779–786, 1999.
43. J.W. Trobaugh, W.D. Richard, K.R. Smith, and R.D. Bucholz, Frameless stereotactic ultrasonography: methods and applications, *Comp. Med. Imaging Graphics*, vol. 18, no. 4, pp. 235–246, 1994.
44. H. Erbe, A. Kriete, A. Joe, W. Deinsberger, and D.K. Boker, 3D ultrasonography and image matching for detection of brain shift during intracranial surgery, *Comp. Assist. Rad.*, pp. 225–230, 1996.
45. R.M. Comeau, A. Fenster, and T.M. Peters, Intraoperative US in interactive image-guided neurosurgery, *Radiographics*, vol. 18, no. 4, pp. 1019–1027, 1998.
46. A. Hartov, S.D. Eisner, D.W. Roberts, K.D. Paulsen, L.A. Platenik, and M.I. Miga, Error analysis for a freehand 3D ultrasound system for neuronavigation, *Neurosurgical Focus*, vol. 6, no. 3, article 5, 1999.
47. D.W. Roberts, M.I. Miga, F.E. Kennedy, A. Hartov, and K.D. Paulsen, Intraoperatively updated neuroimaging using brain modeling and sparse data, *Neurosurgery*, vol. 45, no. 5, pp. 1199–1207, 1999.

16

View of the Future

Joseph V. Hajnal, Derek L.G. Hill, and David J. Hawkes

CONTENTS

16.1 Introduction

Over the past 15 years image registration has been a very successful topic in the application of computer technology to medical image processing and analysis. In terms of satisfying the technical requirements of robustness and accuracy with minimal user interaction, rigid-body registration is considered by many working in the field to be a solved problem. Despite the technical success and widespread use in medical research, image registration has had less impact on routine healthcare than many proponents expected.

This situation is beginning to change. Rigid-body registration is now used routinely in image-guided surgery systems for neurosurgery and orthopedic surgery. Well validated algorithms are beginning to appear in radiology workstations for rigid-body intermodality registration and serial MR registration. One factor holding up routine use of this technology has been that many medical images, although intrinsically digital in origin for some time, continue to be stored and reviewed in analog form, usually as "radiographic films." Fast and convenient access to digital image data is now rapidly becoming feasible with the increase in use of digital image archiving and communication. This provides the necessary infrastructure for combining images from different modalities or images taken at widely separated time intervals. Another factor is that image registration is often only one component in an image processing and analysis package directed to a specific clinical problem. Progress needs to be made in other areas, most notably image segmentation, before a wide range of image analysis protocols can enter routine clinical use.

16.2   Future Application of Image Registration

Below are a few personal observations and predictions on where this exciting technology will lead in the next few years, and where to expect significant progress.

16.2.1   Perfusion Studies

Rigid and nonrigid registration are essential enabling technologies for perfusion imaging because patients cannot be relied on to stay sufficiently still during dynamic studies lasting many minutes. (This is especially relevant in MRI.) Perfusion imaging is likely to have many clinical applications. Cardiac MR imaging is progressing fast, and interest in tumor metabolism and angiogenesis is driving advances in MR imaging for oncology.

16.2.2   Registration in Multimedia Electronic Patient Records

Multimedia electronic patient record systems will soon be widely used in hospitals. These incorporate radiological images as well as much other nontext-based information about patients. Integrating this information and relating it to atlas data could be achieved transparently with the potential for improved diagnosis and decision support. Indeed, once such systems are established, it will seem strange not to align all the images acquired from a patient.

16.2.3   The Role of Deformation Fields Generated by Nonrigid Registration

Medical image registration, and nonrigid registration in particular, have great potential beyond simply lining up images. Some of these applications have already been discussed in this book, but it is worth highlighting them again here.

As discussed in Chapter 13, the deformation field produced by nonrigid intra-subject registration algorithms can quantify normal development and contribute to an understanding of disease processes and aging. The nonrigid registration algorithms used in these applications will soon be reliable enough to enter clinical use, providing valuable tools for diagnosis and monitoring disease progression.

16.2.4 Group Differences and Postgenomic Registration

When nonrigid intersubject registration algorithms are applied to cohorts of patients and matched normals, the calculated deformation field has the potential to provide a very sensitive measure of structural differences between the groups. Much work has already been done in the study of schizophrenia, but deformation fields might reveal effects in other disorders that interfere with structure. This should contribute to a better understanding of disease and perhaps even provide a link between genes, structure, and function. Integrating imaging information obtained *in vivo* may provide direct and powerful insights into gene function and genetic control in whole functioning organisms as opposed to model systems or *ex vivo* specimens. Postgenomic registration studies are beginning to be applied to the study of gene expression in mice, and intersubject registration of human subjects correlated with sequenced genomes could be even more revealing. This is likely to be a key tool in studying gene-environment interactions.

16.2.5 Registration for and Combined with Image Segmentation

The difficult problem of image segmentation has traditionally been thought of as quite a different research topic to image registration, but several groups have now demonstrated that good segmentation can be achieved by lining up a subject's images to an atlas using a nonrigid registration algorithm (e.g., Dawant et al.[1]). Labeled structures in the atlas can then be used to split up the images into anatomical and pathological components for visualization or quantification. A related use of image registration is to fuse functional and metabolic information obtained by methods that reveal little of the structural information onto segmented anatomical images, or vice versa. For example, high resolution data segmented by tissue classification may allow much more subtle changes in metabolism or perfusion to be detected. Several applications of this general type have been discussed in this book, but further developments and widespread use are likely to allow much more effective use of the data.

16.2.6 Registration to Improve Image Acquisition

Registration is beginning to be used to improve image acquisition. For example, on-the-fly registration can be used to dynamically adjust slice position in MR scans to compensate prospectively for subject motion (e.g., Thesen et al.[2]) Registration of previously acquired images could also be used to reduce the field of view when using ionizing radiation, and hence reduce patient dose. Spectroscopic or perfusion acquisitions can be defined to interrogate specific tissues of interest, delineated in a previously acquired high resolution image, rather than a fixed region relative to the scanner. Specific tissue regions could be followed as the patient moves or is repositioned. These applications are likely to grow as algorithms become faster and scanner computing power increases.

Another set of applications relates to use of registration methods to improve image quality or reduce acquisition time by aligning new data with previously obtained calibration data or patient-specific information.

16.2.7   Registration of Intraoperative and Preoperative Images in Image-Guided Interventions

Commercially available image-guided surgery systems are currently restricted to applications in which patient anatomy can be treated as a rigid-body, yet this technology has great potential in soft tissues away from bone, where there is frequently considerable deformation. Several imaging modalities are being developed with interventional applications in mind. These include MR, CT, x-ray fluoroscopy, and ultrasound as well as optical images from endoscopes, microscopes, and arrays of free-standing cameras. Registration methods could be used to update the spatial information in accurate and detailed representations of the patient generated from preoperative images using often incomplete and much lower quality information from intraoperative images.

16.3   Remaining Research Challenges

For all these exciting potential applications of image registration to be realized, several challenges remain, including:

- Developing a validation methodology for nonrigid registration algorithms
- Devising faster and more accurate algorithms (especially nonrigid). For on-the-fly registration, run times of hundreds of milliseconds are desirable
- Inventing similarity measures that are more robust to image artifacts including intensity shading, ghosting, streaking, etc., that can be applied to more modality combinations
- Devising algorithms that can distinguish between situations where tissue volume is preserved or changing, where some structures are rigid and others are not, and change in one subject over time compared to differences between subjects

- Developing novel display techniques that make it easy to relate information in different images with very different resolutions, and for nonrigid registration, to provide intuitive visualization of the deformation field which may have scalar, vector, or tensor values, depending on the application
- Developing and validating complete applications. Registration is but one component in what may be a sophisticated chain of processing tasks. Solving the whole image processing and analysis task for specific clinical applications will be an important focus

In thinking about future image registration development, it is important to return to the topic of correspondence introduced in Chapter 2. Image registration is about establishing point-by-point correspondence between two images (or an image and physical space). While the basic definition of correspondence is clear, its meaning in particular applications may not be. For example, when tracking change in one subject over a short time interval, correspondence refers to a specific element of tissue within the patient. This is less clear when comparing one subject with another where correspondence could be related to shape, histological characteristics, or metabolic function. Correspondence between images of a patient who has changed position (where no tissue is gained or lost) is different from studying images of a patient over time, where tissue may grow, shrink, or be surgically removed. It is not yet clear whether these different registration problems will be solved by quite different algorithms, or whether an underlying unified approach will be successful. The next few years will be very interesting in the field of image registration as greater clinical use is made of techniques that have become established in research literature, and as new techniques are devised, in particular for different applications of nonrigid registration.

References

1. Dawant, B.M., Hartmann, S.L., Thirion, J.P., Maes, F., Vandermeulen, D., and Demaerel, P., Automatic 3-D segmentation of internal structures of the head in MR images using a combination of similarity and free-form transformations: Part I, methodology and validation on normal subjects. *IEEE Trans. Med. Imaging* 18: 909–916, 1999.
2. Thesen, S., Heid, O., Mueller, E., and Schad, L.R., Prospective acquisition correction for head motion with image-based tracking for real-time fMRI. *Mag. Reson. Med.* 44: 457–463, 2000.

Index

A

Abdomen
  protocols for registering images from, 212
  surgery of, 272
Absolute total bead displacement error, 345
Acoustic position sensors, 108, 257
Acquisition geometry, distortions intrinsic to, 98
Activation
  image, 195
  maps, 197
Active/passive optical tracker, 107, 258
Adult
  infarction, 173
  neurosurgery, 227, 271, 332
Affine transformation, 19, 46, 282, 320
AIR algorithm (*see* ratio image uniformity)
Algorithm(s)
  AIR (*see* ratio image uniformity)
  automated 3D image-matching, 308
  head and hat, 23, 50
  intensity remapping, 53, 225
  iterative closest point, 25, 51
  nonrigid registration, 30
  partitioned intensity uniformity, 28, 56
  point registration, 47
  ratio image uniformity, 26, 56
  SPM, 54
  variance of intensity ratios, 26
Alignment errors, 49, 119, 124
Alzheimer's disease, 178, 312
Anatomically guided reconstruction, 243
Angiography, dynamic contrast-enhanced, 180
ANIMAL, see Automatic nonlinear image matching and anatomical labeling
Artifact(s)
  failed registration and, 164
  generation mechanisms, 89, 93
  ghost, 223
  misregistration, 150
  motion, 206
  susceptibility, 165
Astrocytoma, 148, 176, 177

Attenuation effects, 100
Auditory activation clusters, 190
Automatic nonlinear image matching and anatomical labeling (ANIMAL), 317, 319
Axial resolution, 104

B

Background noise, 145
Baseline images, interpretation of, 148
Basis functions, registration using, 283
BIC, see Brain Imaging Centre
Biharmonic model, 291
Biomechanical modeling, for image registration, 331–362
  brain tissue modeling, 334–335
  brain tissue model description, 335–338
  finite element methodology, 338–340
  model inputs, 352–359
    intraoperative data, 353–359
    preoperative data, 352–353
  model validation, 340–351
Biopsy(ies)
  application of stereotactic frames to, 259
  functionally guided, 248
Blade-tissue interface, 349
Blood
  flow, distribution of, 201
  oxygenation level dependent (BOLD) effect, 184
  vessels, 163
Blurring
  /distortion, depth-dependent, 106
  due to limited spatial resolution, 242
  interpolation related, 188
BMP, see Microsoft window bitmap
BOLD effect, see Blood oxygenation level dependent effect
Bone marrow transplantation, 179
Bonferoni correction, 318
Bootstrapping, 123
Border zone shifts, 152, 167
Bow-tie effect, 93

369

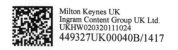

9 780367 397203